Symposium in Immunology VIII

Springer

*Berlin
Heidelberg
New York
Barcelona
Hong Kong
London
Milan
Paris
Singapore
Tokyo*

M. M. Eibl   C. Huber
H. H. Peter   U. Wahn (Eds.)

Symposium in Immunology VIII

Inflammation

With 44 Figures and 11 Tables

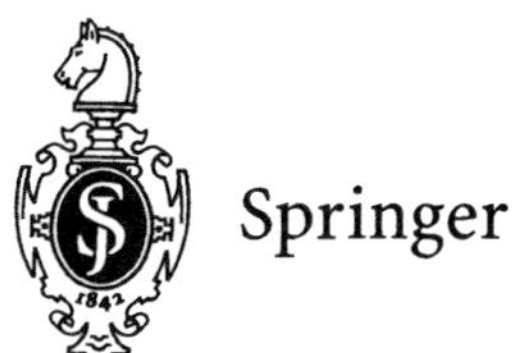

Springer

Prof. Dr. MARTHA M. EIBL
Institut für Immunologie der Universität Wien
Borschkegasse 8 a
1090 Wien
Austria

Prof. Dr. CHRISTOPH HUBER
Department of Hematology
Johannes Gutenberg Universität
Langenbeckstr. 1
55101 Mainz
Germany

Prof. Dr. HANS H. PETER
Abteilung für Rheumatologie und
Klinische Immunologie
Medizinische Universitätsklinik
Hugstetter Str. 55
79106 Freiburg
Germany

Prof. Dr. ULRICH WAHN
Pädiatrische Pneumologie und Immunologie
Universitäts-Klinikum Rudolf-Virchow
Standort Charlottenburg
Heubnerweg 6
14059 Berlin
Germany

ISBN-13: 978-3-540-64722-5   e-ISBN-13: 978-3-642-59947-7
DOI: 10.1007/978-3-642-59947-7

Library of Congress Cataloging-in-Publication Data
Symposium in Immunology (8th : 1998 : Budapest, Hungary) Symposium in Immunology VIII : Inflammation / M. M. Eibl ... [et al.]. p. cm. Symposium held in Budapest in April, 1998. Includes bibliographical references and index. ISBN-13: 978-3-540-64722-5 (softcover : alk. paper) 1. Inflammation – Immunological aspects – Congresses. 2. Inflammation – Mediators – Congresses. I. Eibl, Martha M. II. Title. III. Title: Symposium in Immunology 8. IV. Title: Symposium in Immunology eight. V. Title: Inflammation. [DNLM: 1. Inflammation – immunology congresses. 2. Inflammation – therapy congresses. QW 700 S9885s 1998] RB 131.S92 1998 616.07'9 – dc21 DNLM/DLC for Library of Congress

Production: PRO EDIT GmbH, D-69126 Heidelberg
Typesetting: Zechnersche Buchdruckerei, D-67346 Speyer
Cover design: design & production GmbH, D-69121 Heidelberg
SPIN: 10686206   27/3136/ – 5 4 3 2 1 0

Contents

Basic Mechanisms 1

Complement and Inflammation
H. R. COLTEN 3

Role of Phospholipases A2 in Inflammation
J. PFEILSCHIFTER 15

Acivation of NF-κB by Inflammatory Cytokines
M. ROTHE 31

Interaction of the Parasite *Echinococcus granulosus*
with Host Innate Immunity
A. J. DIAZ, A. M. FERREIRA, F. IRIGOIN, M. BREIJO, and R. B. SIM . . . 43

Endo- and Exotoxins and Soluble Receptors 61

Nitric Oxide, Systemic Inflammatory Response Syndrome
and Circulatory Shock
C. THIEMERMANN 63

Intracellular Protein Modification and Signal Transduction
in Response to Lipopolysaccharide
S. Hauschildt and H. Heine 79

Bacterial Lipopolysaccharides: Chemical Constitution,
Endotoxic Activity, and Biological Neutralization
W. BRABATZ, U. MAMAT, C. ALEXANDER, and E. TH. RIETSCHEL 89

Membrane-Damaging Toxins and Inflammation
S. BHAKDI 123

Treatment Perspectives 133

The Interleukin-6 Family: Biological Function
of the Soluble Receptors
S. ROSE-JOHN, P. VOLLMER, M. PETERS, P. MÄRZ, and J. MÜLLBERG . . 135

IgE-Mediated Allergen Presentation via FcεRIαγ Complexes
on Dendritic Antigen-Presenting Cells
D. MAURER and G. STINGL 159

Anti-Inflammatory Effects of Intravenous Immunoglobulin (IVIg)
Y. BAR-DAYAN, S. V. KAVERI, Y. BAR-DAYAN, A. PASHOV, Y. SHOENFELD,
and M. D. KAZATCHKINE 171

Gene Therapeutic Strategies in Inflammatory Bowel Diseases
M. F. NEURATH, S. WIRTZ, C. BECKER, K. BARBULESCU,
and S. FINOTTO 185

Pathology of Rheumatoid Arthritis:
Molecular and Inflammatory Aspects
S. GAY and R. E. GAY 199

Subject Index 205

Contributors

ALEXANDER, C.
Research Center Borstel, Center for Medicine and Biosciences,
Department of Immunochemistry and Biochemical Microbiology,
Parkallee 22, 23845 Borstel, Germany

BARBULESCU, K.
Laboratory of Immunology, I. Medical Clinic, University of Mainz,
Langenbeckstr. 1, 55101 Mainz, Germany

BAR-DAYAN, YARON
INSERM U430, and Université Pierre et Marie Curie, Hôpital Broussais,
96 Rue Didot, 75014 Paris, France
and
Department of Medicine "B" and Research Unit of Autoimmune Diseases,
Sheba Medical Center, Tel Aviv, Israel

BAR-DAYAN, YOSEFA
INSERM U430, and Université Pierre et Marie Curie, Hôpital Broussais,
96 Rue Didot, 75014 Paris, France

BECKER, C.
Laboratory of Immunology, I. Medical Clinic, University of Mainz,
Langenbeckstr. 1, 55101 Mainz, Germany

BHAKDI, S.
Institute of Medical Microbiology and Hygiene,
Johannes Gutenberg-Universität Mainz, Hochhaus am Augustusplatz,
55101 Mainz, Germany

BRABETZ, W.
Research Center Borstel, Center for Medicine and Biosciences,
Department of Immunochemistry and Biochemical Microbiology,
Parkallee 22, 23845 Borstel, Germany

BREIJO, M.
Cátedra de Immunología, Facultad de Veterinaria,
Universidad de la República, Montevideo, Uruguay

Colten, H. R.
Northwestern University Medical School, Morton Building 4-656,
303 East Chicago Avenue, Chicago, Illinois 60611-3008, USA

Diaz, A. J.
MRC Immunochemistry Unit, Department of Biochemistry,
Oxford University, South Parks Road, Oxford OX1 3QU, UK
and
Cátedra de Immunología, Facultad de Química/Facultad de Ciencias,
Universidad de la República, Montevideo, Uruguay

Ferreira, A. M.
Cátedra de Immunología, Facultad de Química/Facultad de Ciencias,
Universidad de la República, Montevideo, Uruguay
and
MRC Immunochemistry Unit, Department of Biochemistry,
Oxford University, South Parks Road, Oxford OX1 3QU, UK

Finotto, S.
Laboratory of Immunology, I. Medical Clinic, University of Mainz,
Johannes Gutenberg Universität Mainz, Langenbeckstr. 1,
55101 Mainz, Germany

Gay, R. E.
WHO Collaborating Center for Molecular Biology
and Novel Therapeutic Strategies for Rheumatic Diseases,
Department of Rheumatology, University Hospital,
8091 Zurich, Switzerland

Gay, S.
WHO Collaborating Center for Molecular Biology
and Novel Therapeutic Strategies for Rheumatic Diseases,
Department of Rheumatology, University Hospital,
8091 Zurich, Switzerland

Hauschildt, S.
Institute of Zoology, Department of Immunobiology, University of Leipzig,
Talstr. 33, 04103 Leipzig, Germany

Heine, H.
Maxwell Finland Laboratory for Infectious Diseases,
774 Albany Street, Boston, MA 02118, USA
and
Research Center Borstel, Center for Medicine and Biosciences,
Parkallee 22, 23845 Borstel, Germany

IRIGOIN, F.
Cátedra de Immunología, Facultad de Química/Facultad de Ciencias,
Universidad de la República, Montevideo, Uruguay
and
MRC Immunochemistry Unit, Department of Biochemistry,
Oxford University, South Parks Road, Oxford OX1 3QU, UK

KAVERI, S. V.
INSERM U430, and Université Pierre et Marie Curie, Hôpital Broussais,
96 Rue Didot, 75014 Paris, France

KAZATCHKINE, M. D.
INSERM U430, and Université Pierre et Marie Curie, Hôpital Broussais,
96 Rue Didot, 75014 Paris, France

MÄRZ, P.
I. Medical Clinic, Department of Pathophysiology,
Johannes Gutenberg-Universität Mainz,
Obere Zahlbacher Str. 63, 55101 Mainz, Germany

MAMAT, U.
Research Center Borstel, Center for Medicine and Biosciences,
Department of Immunochemistry and Biochemical Microbiology,
Parkallee 22, 23845 Borstel, Germany

MAURER, D.
Division of Immunology, Allergy, and Infectious Diseases (DIAID),
Department of Dermatology, University of Vienna Medical School,
Währinger Gürtel 18-20, 1090 Vienna, Austria

MÜLLBERG, J.
I. Medical Clinic, Department of Pathophysiology,
Johannes Gutenberg-Universität Mainz,
Obere Zahlbacher Str. 63, 55101 Mainz, Germany

NEURATH, M. F.
Laboratory of Immunology, I. Medical Clinic, University of Mainz,
Langenbeckstr. 1, 55101 Mainz, Germany

PASHOV, A.
INSERM U430, and Université Pierre et Marie Curie, Hôpital Broussais,
96 Rue Didot, 75014 Paris, France

PETERS, M.
I. Medical Clinic, Department of Pathophysiology,
Johannes Gutenberg-Universität Mainz,
Obere Zahlbacher Str. 63, 55101 Mainz, Germany

PFEILSCHIFTER, J.
Zentrum der Pharmakologie,
Klinikum der Johann Wolfgang Goethe-Universität,
Theodor Stern-Kai 7, 60590 Frankfurt, Germany

RIETSCHEL, E. Th.
Research Center Borstel, Center for Medicine and Biosciences,
Department of Immunochemistry and Biochemical Microbiology,
Parkallee 22, 23845 Borstel, Germany

ROSE-JOHN, S.
I. Medical Clinic, Department of Pathophysiology,
Johannes Gutenberg-Universität Mainz,
Obere Zahlbacher Str. 63, 55101 Mainz, Germany

ROTHE, M.
Tularik, Inc., Two Corporate Drive, South San Francisco, CA 94080, USA

SHOENFELD, Y.
Department of Medicine "B" and Research Unit of Autoimmune Diseases,
Sheba Medical Center, Tel Aviv, Israel

SIM, R. B.
MRC Immunochemistry Unit, Department of Biochemistry,
Oxford University, South Parks Road, Oxford OX1 3QU, UK

STINGL, G.
Division of Immunology, Allergy, and Infectious Diseases (DIAID),
Department of Dermatology, University of Vienna Medical School,
Währinger Gürtel 18–20, 1090 Vienna, Austria

THIEMERMANN, C.
The William Harvey Research Institute, St. Bartholomew's
and the Royal London School of Medicine and Dentistry,
Charterhouse Square, London EC1M 6BQ, UK

VOLLMER, P.
I. Medical Clinic, Department of Pathophysiology,
Johannes Gutenberg-Universität Mainz, Obere Zahlbacher Str. 63,
55101 Mainz, Germany

WIRTZ, S.
Laboratory of Immunology, I. Medical Clinic, University of Mainz,
Langenbeckstr. 1, 55101 Mainz, Germany

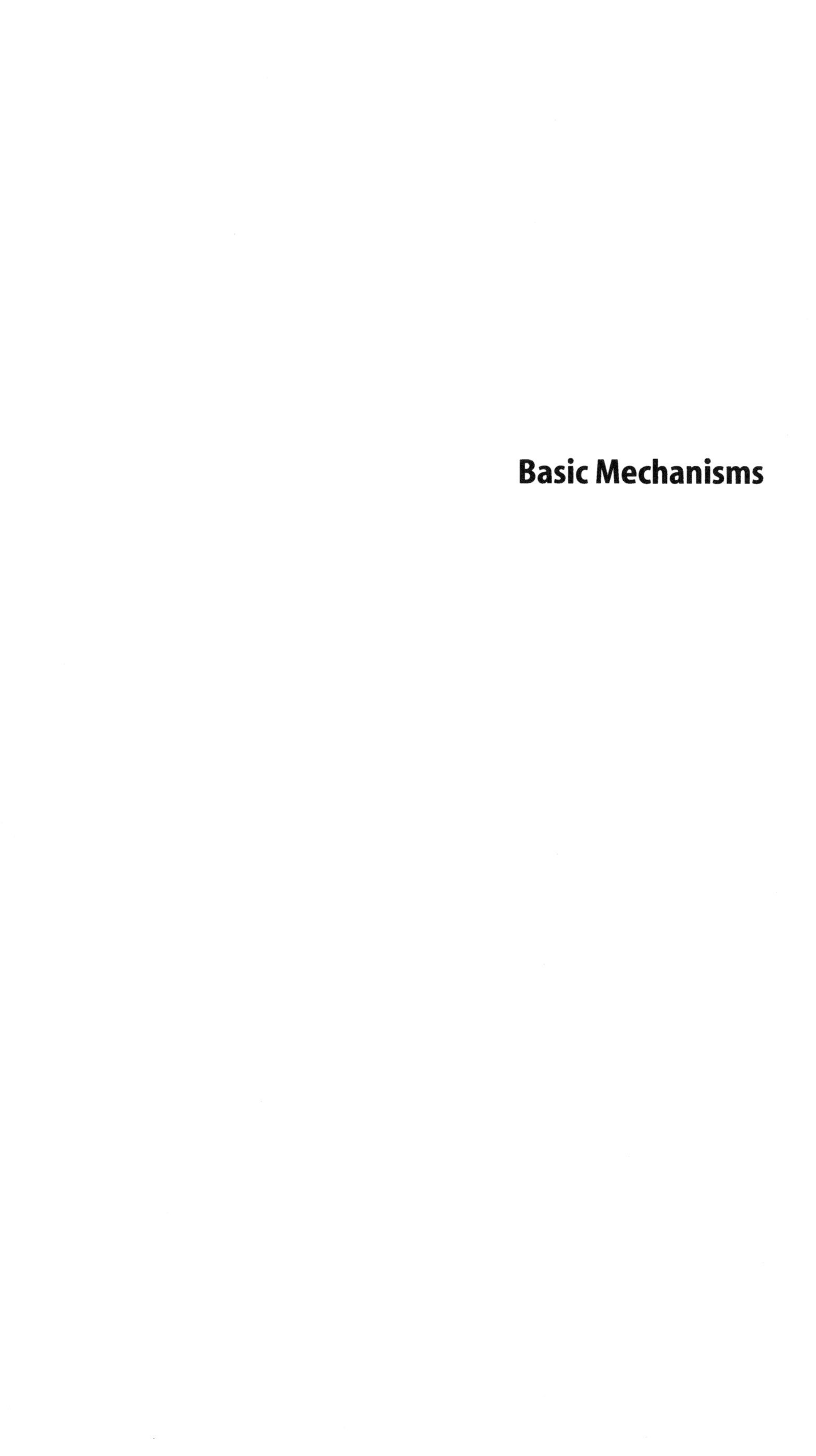

Basic Mechanisms

Complement and Inflammation

H. R. COLTEN

Inflammation is a programmed response to tissue injury and microbial agents. In primitive multicellular organisms, humoral and cellular constituents of host defenses are focused by the presence of a foreign body or at a site of tissue injury. The evolution in higher organisms of a discrete circulatory system introduced complexity that imposed a need for mechanisms regulating changes in permeability of the circulatory system and for margination/ directed migration of circulating cellular elements. For instance, an array of regulated genes expressed in endothelium, blood leukocytes, and in extravascular cells direct the accumulation of white cells to sites of inflammation. Proteins within the selectin family (McEver 1991) displayed on the majority of lymphocytes, neutrophils, monocytes, and the corresponding cytokine-regulated proteins on endothelium, are critical for the recruitment of white cells to an inflammatory site. Similar general functions are served by adhesion molecules of the integrin and immunoglobulin (Ig) families (Springer 1990; Kishimoto et al. 1989). Small molecular species such as nitric oxide (Kubes et al. 1991), arachadonic acid metabolites (Smith et al. 1980), and reactive oxygen radicals (Patel 1991) generated at inflammatory sites, play modulating and direct roles in leukocyte adherence, migration, and activation. This process involves elaborate control mechanisms and is highly redundant even when considering only the intravascular elements. In addition, separate vascular and peripheral tissue sources of the critical constituents evolved. This has resulted in separate regulatory mechanisms that govern availability of the intravascular and extravascular components of the inflammatory response.

Interest in the specificity of host responses to microbes was the basis for the development of immunology as a distinct discipline in the late nineteenth century. Elucidation of the mechanisms generating diversity of specific antibody and the cellular responses to antigen has been a central goal of immunologists. It was clear, however, even from early studies, that an effective inflammatory response can dispose of toxins, microbes, and tissue debris even in the absence of specific immunity.

The complement system is an important effector mechanism of humoral immunity. It consists of 30 plasma and cell-membrane proteins that work in defense against bacterial and viral infections, as a mediator of immunopath-

Symposium in Immunology VIII
Eibl/Huber/Peter/Wahn (Eds.)
© Springer Verlag Berlin Heidelberg 1999

ological inflammation, and that amplify immune responsiveness. The complement system is activated by two distinct pathways, the classical and the alternative pathways, which share the terminal sequence of the cascade (Fig. 1). The classical pathway is an effector system that is triggered by antibody in complex with antigen. The activation of the classical pathway is initiated primarily by binding of subcomponent C1q to the Fc region of IgG or IgM antibody in immune complexes. This activates the C1 enzymes, subcomponents C1r and C1s. The latter cleaves C4 and C2 complement proteins. The surface-bound C4 fragment, C4b, and the C2 fragment, C2a, together form a complex C4bC2a, a C3 cleaving enzyme (C3 convertase of the classical pathway) (Muller-Eberhard 1975, 1988). Viruses, DNA, C-reactive protein and mitochondrial membranes can induce antibody-independent activation of the classical pathway (Welsh et al. 1975; Cooper et al. 1976; Bartholomew et al. 1980; Kaplan et al. 1974; Richards et al. 1977; Storrs et al. 1981).

The alternative pathway is activated by a wide range of nonimmunoglobulin activators such as yeast and other fungi, lipopolysaccharide, many viru-

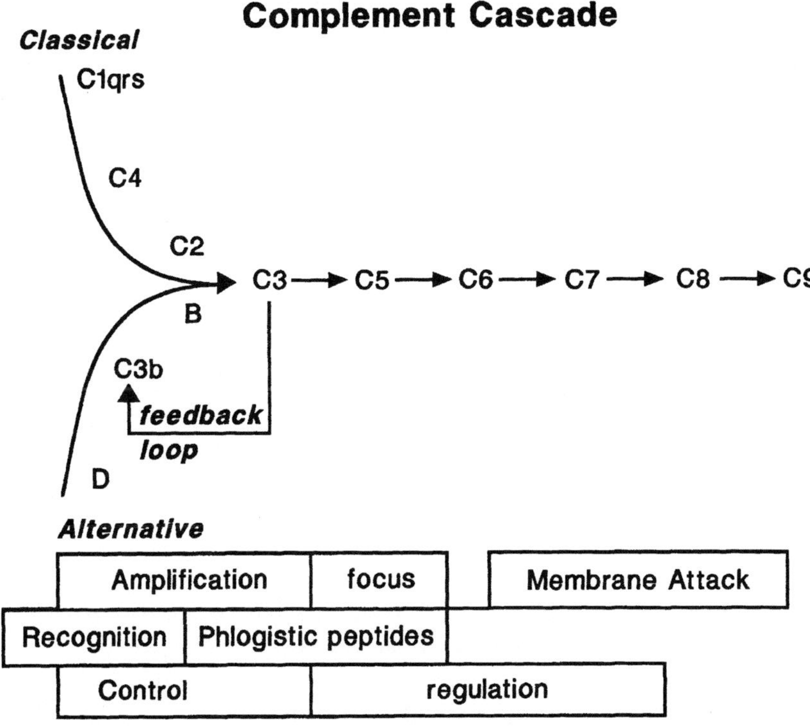

Fig. 1. The two complement activation pathways with biochemical/ biological effects identified in the *boxes* at the approximate steps in the sequence where they are manifested. (Reprinted with permission from Blackwell Science)

ses, and virus-infected cells (as well as by complexes of IgG, IgA, and IgE) (Pangburn et al. 1984; Cooper and Nemerow 1983). In the initiation of complement activation through the alternative pathway, a C3 fragment (C3b) reacts with factor B. The factor B is cleaved by the serine protease factor D to form the C3 convertase (C3bBb). If C3b binds to the surface of host cells, efficient soluble and cellular regulatory molecules prevent further activation. If it binds to substances that limit regulatory control, C3bBb cleaves C3 to generate C3a and C3b. Thus, C3b generates an amplification loop resulting in further C3b production (Vogt et al. 1997; Fearon et al. 1973). Activation of either the classical or alternative pathways of the complement cascade produce C3a and C3b. The C3a fragment is a potent anaphylatoxin causing smooth muscle contraction, increased vascular permeability, basophil/mast cell degranulation, and lysosomal enzyme release. The C3b fragment reacts covalently with cell surface molecules of bacteria, viral pathogens, and immune complexes. Bound C3b via the cell membrane receptors CR1 (CD35) and CR3 (CD11b/CD18) enhances adherence and phagocytosis by leukocytes and the solubilization and clearance of immune complexes (Hugli 1986; Frank and Fries 1991). Surface-bound C3b in complex with the C3 convertase forms trimolecular complexes (C4bC2aC3b or C3bBbC3b), which serve as the C5 convertases, cleaving C5 protein to C5a and C5b fragments. C5a is a potent chemotactic agent for neutrophils acting through the C5a receptor (C5aR), a G protein-coupled receptor bearing seven transmembrane domains. It also increases neutrophil adherence and release of intracellular enzymes, reactive oxygen, and arachidonate metabolites. C5b is the nidus for the assembly of the terminal cytolytic C5b–9 membrane attack complex (MAC) (Schifferli et al. 1982).

The complement cascade has several natural regulators. Protein factor I has specificity for C3b and C4b. Factor H and C4-binding protein (C4bp) facilitate and enhance the cleavage by factor I of C3b to C3c and C3d (Muller-Eberhard 1986; Zipfel and Skerka 1994). Vitronectin, or S-protein, functions as an inhibitor of the membrane attack complex and C1-inhibitor (C1-INH) is the major inhibitor of the C1r and C1s enzymes (Hourcade et al. 1989; Podack and Muller-Eberhard 1985). The membrane bound complement regulators include: (a) membrane cofactor protein (MCP, CD46), a protein that facilitates factor I cleavage of C3b/C4b (Salvesen et al. 1985); (b) decay-accelerating factor (DAF, CD55) that facilitates decay and dissociation of the C3 and C5 convertases (Atkinson and Farries 1987; Liszewski et al. 1994); and (c) homologous restriction factor (HRF) and CD59 that inhibit complement-mediated cytotoxicity by restricting the activity of the MAC complex (Kinoshita et al. 1985). The receptor for C3b binding (complement receptor type 1, CR1, CD35) also serves as a membrane-bound regulator, mediating the decay and dissociation of the C3 convertases and as a cofactor for factor I cleavage of C3b on leukocytes (Lublin and Atkinson 1989).

The discovery of C-reactive protein (CRP) by Tillett and Francis (1930) prompted the concept of acute-phase responses summarized in Kushner (1982). Changes in plasma protein concentrations (100–1000-fold for CRP and serum amyloid A) occur within hours after tissue injury or infection. In addition, fever, leukocytosis, changes in nitrogen balance, fat, carbohydrate, and heavy metal metabolism are features of the acute-phase response. None is dependent on specific immune mechanisms. The acute-phase reaction, therefore, provides a rapid response to noxious stimuli, and also facilitates the acquisition of specific immunity. Proteins of the complement system are among the acute-phase proteins that are important in both nonspecific and specific host defenses. The increase in complement proteins is neither quantitatively nor kinetically the most impressive among the acute-phase plasma proteins. For example, serum concentrations of C3 protein rise only about twofold over baseline within 1 week following an acute-phase stimulus (tissue injury or infection), but the elevation is sustained for several days.

The serum complement proteins are primarily of hepatic origin (Alper et al. 1980). Nevertheless, a substantial amount of plasma complement is derived from extrahepatic sites of synthesis. For instance, about 3% of complement protein C3 is produced in marrow and an additional 5% in nonmarrow extrahepatic tissues (Naughton et al. 1996). For complement protein C7, about 20% and 30% are from marrow and nonmarrow extrahepatic sources, respectively (Naughton et al. 1996). These studies underestimate the complement proteins produced in extrahepatic sites, i.e., the complement produced in extrahepatic tissue that remains in the extravascular space. The kinetics of extrahepatic induction of complement genes in vivo is not known, but data from Katz et al. (1988) show that acute-phase-induced changes in extrahepatic complement gene expression is quantitatively much greater than in hepatocytes. Several studies suggest that this is also true in vivo. For example, the increase in extrahepatic complement expression exceeds severalfold the increase in liver-derived complement in animal models of systemic lupus erythematosus (SLE) and in human disorders (Passwell et al. 1988, 1990; Ahrenstedt et al. 1990; Welch et al. 1991).

The complement system is a complex network of soluble and cell-associated proteins which functions not only in host defense against pathogens, but also in the pathophysiology of immune-mediated tissue injury. As noted above, alterations in plasma complement levels occur during inflammation. Plasma levels of the third component of complement and the alternative pathway protein factor B rise as a result of new synthesis following acute-phase stimuli (Perlmutter and Colten 1992). Immune complex-mediated disorders, such as active SLE membranoproliferative glomerulonephritis (MPGN), and acute poststreptococcal glomerulonephritis, lead to depressed plasma C3 complement levels as a result of decreased hepatic synthesis, increased catabolism, or both (Alper and Rosen 1967; Peters, Martin et al. 1972).

Complement protein (C3) is found along the tubular basement membrane in human MPGN type I, in lupus nephritis (Striker et al. 1990), and in experimental interstitial nephritis in guinea pigs (Rudofsky and Pollara 1981). Linear deposits of C3 and factor B are also present along the tubular basement membrane in allograft rejection (Mathew and Bolten 1988). Some of this C3 is produced locally. For example, Welch et al. found C3 mRNA in tubular epithelial cells in several types of immune complex-mediated renal disease, but not in normal kidneys, nor in several types of nonimmune renal disease (Welch et al. 1991). Brooimans et al. (1991) demonstrated synthesis of C3 protein in vitro by cultured human proximal tubular epithelial cells (Brooimans, Stegman et al. 1991). C3-specific mRNA is detected at low levels in normal mouse kidney and is markedly up-regulated by intraperitoneal endotoxin (lipopolysaccharide; LPS) injection (Falus, Beuscher, et al. 1987). Some of this C3 is produced locally and increased C3 expression has been observed in two models of murine lupus nephritis at a time when plasma C3 levels are actually depressed (Passwell, Schreiner et al. 1988; Passwell, Schreiner et al. 1990). The cell type expressing C3 in these two models of renal inflammation differ; that is, LPS induces increased C3 expression in tubular epithelium and in murine SLE the C3 is produced primarily in perivascular inflammatory cells (Ault and Colten 1994).

Activation of C3 and the generation of the lytic membrane attack complex can proceed even when a protein of one of the two activation pathways is deficient. Complete deficiency of one of the proteins of the shared terminal sequence will block the assembly of MAC. Deficiencies of the regulatory proteins generally result in spontaneous and sustained activation of the corresponding pathway, leading to a secondary deficiency of complement effector protein(s) or injury to host cells. The naturally occurring complement deficiencies and targeted deletion of complement genes in experimental animals has provided important insight into the role of complement in inflammatory and host defenses. Several examples will suffice to illustrate the importance of this approach to the study of the physiological functions of complement in vivo.

Deficiencies of nearly all of the complement effector and control proteins have been recognized in humans with medical problems and in population surveys among different ethnic groups. The clinical manifestations vary among individuals with genetically determined complement deficiencies. Some are asymptomatic, but most display symptoms of increased susceptibility to infection, rheumatological diseases, or angioedema (Winkelstein, Colten 1993). Increased susceptibility to infection is the predominant feature in patients with deficiencies of: (a) complement protein C3, (b) control proteins such as factor I and H, the absence of which leads to wasteful consumption of C3, (c) the receptor for a C3 cleavage product (CD11b/18, leukocyte adhesion deficiency), and (d) C5, C6, C7, and C8 (members of the membrane-attack complex). Encapsulated pyogenic bacteria are the predominant organisms affecting patients with C3 deficiency or CD11b/18 deficiencies, reflecting the importance of C3 as an opsonin and its receptors as mediators of opsonization. Recurrent neisserial infections are characteristic of patients with deficiences of C5–C8, indicating that bacterolysis is an important host defense against this bacterial species.

Rheumatological disorders are the major clinical manifestations of classical pathway complement deficiencies, C3 deficiency, late in life, and to a lesser extent, other complement deficiencies. For example, deficiency of the subunits of C1 (especially C1q) is associated with prominent cutaneous manifestations of either discoid or SLE, including renal disease, arthritis, Raynaud's phenomenon, and mucosal lesions. Recent observations from the Walport group (Botto et al. 1998, in press) have provided some understanding of the mechanisms accounting for this association (see below). Clinical laboratory data in C1-deficient patients are generally typical of those observed in SLE, except they are often antinuclear antibody-negative. Biopsy of affected organs often show Ig and complement (C3) deposition at sites of inflammation. Systemic or discoid lupus erythematosus and progressive immune complex renal disease (Hauptmann, Tappeiner, Schifferli, 1988) are also common in homozygous deficiency of C4 at *both* C4 genes (C4A and C4B). Deficiency at *one* of the C4 loci (partial C4 deficiency) is associated with SLE (Fiedler, Walport, Batchelor et al. 1983; Wilson and Perez 1988; Dunckley, Gatenby et al. 1987) and with other disorders (IgA nephropathy, type-I diabetes, etc.), especially in the context of specific extended major histocompatability complex haplotypes. SLE, discoid lupus, Schönlein-Hensch purpura (Einstein, Alper, Bloch, et al. 1975; Gelfand, Clarkson, Minta 1975), dermatomyositis (Leddy, Griggs et al. 1975), nonspecific vasculitis (Friend, Repine et al. 1975), and isolated glomerulonephritis (Kim and Friend et al. 1977) have also been reported in C2-deficient patients. It should be noted that many asymptomatic individuals totally deficient in either C2 or C4 have been identified during screening of family members in affected kindred or in mass population screening. These provide evidence for environmental factors and/or other genetic loci that are important in the expression of the clinical syndromes associated with genetic deficiencies of the classical complement pathway.

Over the past few years, the capacity to target complement genes for deletion has produced a more powerful probe to explore questions about complement-mediated inflammation. That is to say, specific deficits in complement effector or control functions can be generated and experimental animals can be manipulated in ways not ethical in humans. Unexpected interrelationships among the systems previously studied in isolation are revealed when produced in an intact experimental animal. For example, deficiency of the complement-derived peptide C5a and its receptor, a G protein-coupled receptor bearing seven transmembrane domains, has been most instructive in understanding pulmonary inflammation and host defenses. When bound to C5a receptor (c5aR), C5a, an 11-kDa cleavage product of the complement protein C5, causes smooth-muscle contraction, increased vascular permeability, the release of mediators from mast cells and promotes chemotaxis, adhesiveness, and the release of granule contents from granulocytes.

Ablation of the C5a receptor in mice by targeted gene deletion (Hopken, Lu et al. 1996) profoundly blocks immune-complex-mediated pulmonary inflammation (Bozic, Lu et al. 1996). This finding, coupled with similar results in mice rendered deficient in the NK-1R receptor (a receptor structurally similar to C5aR that mediates effects of the tachykinin, substance P), suggests a possible link between neurogenic and complement-dependent inflammatory mechanisms. That is, experiments in the NK-1R-knockout mice and the C5a-receptor-knockout mice indicate that a block in either the neurogenic tachykinin or the complement system protects against pulmonary inflammation. The price to be paid, however, is the compromise of the protective side of the inflammatory response. Challenge with live *Pseudomonas aeruginosa*, easily cleared by normal mice, causes overwhelming infection and death in the C5a-receptor-knockout mice (Hopken, Lu et al. 1996).

Evidence that complement plays a greater role in pulmonary than in cutaneous inflammation has been gleaned from comparison of the work cited above, with similar studies of the Arthus reaction in naturally deficient or knockout animals. In skin, the impact of complement on cutaneous inflammation is greatest in the immature host. For instance, studies of passive cutaneous anaphylaxis in C5-deficient and C5-sufficient mice (Ben-Efraim, Cinader 1964) show that, at low concentrations of antibody, no reaction can be elicited in the complement-deficient animals. When antibody is supplied in high concentration, the response is not primarily complement-dependent. In the adult or previously immunized animal, the cutaneous inflammatory response is both Fc receptor- and complement-dependent (Sylvestre et al. 1994; Takai et al. 1994; Colten 1994; Hazenbos et al. 1996; Sylvestre, Ravitch 1996). Likewise, the importance of complement in specific immunity (quantitative antibody response and isotype switch from IgM to IgG antibody) in complement-deficient animals is manifest only at low antigen doses (Burger R et al. 1986). The work of Carroll and colleagues (Croix et al. 1996; Fischer et al. 1996) has confirmed and extended these observations in C3 and C4 knockout mice. The conditions of limited antigen and antibody mimic the initial encounter of an immunologically virgin or minimally sensitized animal with a foreign antigen.

In nonimmune tissue injury, complement is also important. For instance, the size of experimental myocardial infarcts and other forms of post-ischemic reperfusion injury can be limited by blocking complement effector proteins, which in turn prevents inflammation-mediated propagation of tissue injury (Weiser et al. 1996). Walport and colleagues (Botto et al. 1998 in press) have observed a striking phenotype in C1q knockout mice that suggests a possible mechanism for complement-dependent propagation of nonimmune tissue injury. That is, the C1q-deficient mice developed glomerulonephritis, probably due to a failure in the clearance of apoptotic renal cells in the absence of C1q. Thus, mechanisms for the removal of dead cells may generate inflammation that in turn injures normal cells.

It is quite apparent that historical questions regarding complement-dependent inflammation will soon be answered using elegant methods for the dissection of the complex in vivo milieu. This review simply suggests that the promise of more interesting work is on the horizon.

References

Alper CA, Raum D, Awdeh Z, et al (1980) Studies of hepatic synthesis in vivo of plasma proteins including orosomucoid, transferrin, alpha-1-antitrypsin, C8 and factor B. Clin Immunol Immunopathol 16:84–89

Ahrenstedt O, Knutson L, Nilsson B, et al (1990) Enhanced local production of complement components in the small intestines of patients with Crohn's disease. N Engl J Med 322:1345–1349

Alper CA, Rosen FS (1967) Studies of the in vivo behavior of human C3 in normal subjects and patients. J Clin Invest 46:2021

Atkinson JP, Farries TJ (1987) Separation of self from non-self in the complement system. Immunol Today 8:212–215

Ault BH, Colten HR (1994) Cellular specificity of murine renal C3 expression in two models of inflammation. Immunology 81:655–660

Bartholomew RM, Esser AF (1980) mechanism of antibody-independent activation of the first component of complement (C1) on retrovirus membranes. Biochemistry 19:2847–2853

Ben-Efraim S, Cinader B (1964) The role of complement in the passive cutaneous reactions of mice. J Exp Med 120:925–942

Bozic CR, Lu B, Hopken UE, Gerard C, Gerard NP (1996) Neurogenic amplification of immune complex inflammation. Science 273:1722–1725

Botto M, Dell'Agnola C, Bygrave AE, Thompson EM, Cook HT, Petry F, Loos M, Pandolfi PP, Walport MJ (1998) Homozygous C1q deficiency causes glomerulonephritis associated with multiple apoptotic bodies. Nat Genet 19:56–59

Brooimans RA, Stegman APA, Daha MR, van der Ark AAJ, van der Woude JF, van Es LA, van Dorp WT (1991) Interleukin 2 mediates stimulation of complement C3 biosynthesis in human proximal tubular epithelial cells. J Clin Invest 88:379

Burger R, et al (1986) An inherited deficiency of the 3rd component of complement, C3, in guinea pigs. Eur J Immun 16:7–11

Colten HR (1994) News and Views: Drawing a double-edged sword. Nature 371:474–475

Cooper NR, Jensen FC, Welsh RM, Oldstone MBA (1976). Lysis of RNA tumor viruses by human serum: direct antibody-independent triggering of the classical complement pathway. J Exp Med 144:970–984

Cooper NR, Nemerow GR (1983) Complement, viruses, and virus-infected cells. Springer Semin Immunopathol 6:327–347

Croix DA, Ahearn JM, Carroll MC, Han S, Kelsoe G, Ma M, Rosengard AM (1996) Antibody response to a T-dependent antigen requires B cell expression of complement receptors. J Exp Med 183:1857–1864

Dunckley H, Gatenby PA, Hawkins B, Naito S, Serjeantson SW (1987) Deficiency of C4A is a genetic determinant of systemic lupus erythematosus in three ethnic groups. J Immunogenet 14:209–218

Einstein LP, Alper CA, Bloch KH, et al (1975) A biosynthetic defect in monocytes from humans with genetic deficiency of the second component of complement (C2). N Engl J Med 292:1169–1171

Falus A, Beuscher HU, Auerbach HS, Colten HR (1987) Constitutive and IL-1-regulated murine complement gene expression is strain and tissue specific. J Immunol 138:856

Fearon DT, Austen KF, Ruddy S (1973) Formation of a hemolytically active cellular intermediate by the interaction between proper din factors B and D and the activated third component of complement. J Exp Med 138:1305–1313

Fiedler AHL, Walport MJ, Batchelor JR, et al (1983) Family study of the MHC in patients with SLE: Importance of null alleles of C4A and C4B in determining disease susceptibility. Brit Med J 286:425–428

Fischer MB, Ma M, Carroll MC, Finco O, Goerg S, Han S, Howard RG, Kelsoe G, Kremmer E, Rosen FS, Rothstein TL, Xia J, Zhou X (1996) Regulation of the B cell response to T-dependent antigens by classical pathway complement. Immunol 157:549–556

Frank MM, Fries LF (1991) The role of complement in inflammation and phagocytosis. Immunol Today 12:322–326

Friend P, Repine J, Clawson CC, Kim Y, Michael AF (1975) Deficiency of the second component of complement (C2) with chronic vasculitis. Ann Int Med 83:813–816

Gelfand EW, Clarkson JO, Minta JO (1975) Selective deficiency of the second component of complement in a patient with anaphylactoid purpura. Clin Immunol Immunopathol 4:269–276

Hauptmann G, Tappeiner G, Schifferli JA (1988) Inherited deficiency of the fourth component of human complement. Immunodef Rev 1:3–22

Hazenbos WLW, Gessner JE, Capel PJA, Daeron M, Heijnen IAFM, Hofhuis FMA, Kuipers H, Meyer D, Sandor M, Schmidt RE, Van de Winkel JGJ, Verbeek JS (1996) Impaired IgG dependent anaphylaxis and Arthus reaction in FcGamma R111 (CD16) deficient mice. Immunity 5:181–188

Hopken UE, Lu B, Gerard C, Gerard NP (1996) The C5a chemoattractant receptor mediates mucosal defense to infection. Nature 383:86–89

Hourcade D, Holers VM, Atkinson JP (1989) The regulators of complement activation (RCA) gene cluster. Adv Immunol 45:381–416

Hugli TE (1986) Biochemistry and biology of anaphylatoxins. Complement 3:111–127

Kaplan MH, Volanakis JE (1974) Interaction of C-reactive protein complexes with the complement system. I. Consumption of human complement associated with the reaction of C-reactive protein with pneumococcal C-polysaccharide and with choline phosphatides, lecithin and sphingomyelin. J Immunol 112:2135–2147

Katz Y, Cole FS, Strunk RC (1988) Synergism between interferon-gamma and lipopolysaccharide for synthesis of factor B, but not C2, in human fibroblasts. J Exp Med 167:1–14

Kim Y, Friend PS, Dresner IG, Michael AF, Yunis EJ (1977) Inherited deficiency of the second component of complement (C2) deficiency with membranoproliferative glomerulonephritis. Am J Med 62:765–771

Kinoshita T, Medof ME, Silber R, Nussenzweig V (1985) Distribution of decay-accelerating factor in the peripheral blood of normal individuals and patients with paroxysmal nocturnal hemoglobinuria. J Exp Med 162:75–92

Kishimoto TK, Larson RS, Carabi AL, Dustin ML, et al (1989) The leukocyte integrins. In: Dixon FJ (ed) New York: Academic Press 46:149–182

Kubes P, Suzuki M, Granger DN (1991) Nitric oxide: an endogenous modulator of leukocyte adhesion. Proc Natl Acad Sci USA 88:4651–4655

Kushner I (1982) The phenomenon of the acute phase response. Ann NY Acad Sci 389:39–48

Leddy JP, Griggs RC, Frank MM, Klemperer MR (1975) Hereditary complement C3 deficient with dermatomyositis. Am J Med 58:83–91

Liszewski MJ, Tedja I, Atkinson JP (1994) Membrane cofactor protein (CD46) of complement. J Biol Chem 269:10776–10779

Lublin DM, Atkinson JP (1989) Decay-accelerating factor: Biochemistry, molecular biology, and function. Ann Rev Immunol 7:35–58

Mathew M, Bolten WK (1988) Linear C3 deposits on the tubular basement membrane in renal allograft biopsies. Amer J Kidney Dis 12:121

McEver RP (1991) Leukocyte interactions mediated by selectins. Thromb Haemost 66:80–87

Muller-Eberhard HJ (1975) Complement. Annu Rev Biochem 44:697–724

Muller-Eberhard HJ (1986) The membrane attack complex of complement. Ann Rev Immunol 4:503–528

Muller-Eberhard HJ (1988) Molecular organization and function of the complement system. Annu Rev Biochem 57:321–347

Naughton MA, Botto M, Carter MJ, Alexander GM, Goldman JM, Walport MJ (1996) Extrahepatic secreted complement C3 contributes to circulating C3 levels in humans. J Immunol 156:351

Naughton MA, Walport JM, Wurzner R, Carter MJ, Alexander GJM, Goldman JM, Botto M (1996) Organ-specific contribution to circulating C7 levels by the bone marrow and liver in humans. Eur J Immunol 26:2108–2112

Passwell J, Schreiner GF, Nonaka M, et al (1988) Local extrahepatic expression of complement genes C3, factor B, C2 and C4 is increased in murine lupus nephritis. J Clin Invest 82:1676–1684

Passwell JH, Schreiner GF, Wetsel RA, Colten HR (1990) Complement gene expression in hepatic and extrahepatic tissues of NZB and NZBxW (F1) mouse strains. Immunology 71:290–294

Pangburn MK, Muller-Eberhard HJ (1984) The alternative pathway of complement. Springer Semin Immunopathol 7:163–192

Patel KD, Zimmerman GA, Prescott SM, et al (1991) Oxygen radicals induce human endothelial cells to express GMP-140 and bind neutrophils. J Cell Biol 112:749–759

Perlmutter DH, Colten HR (1992) Complement: molecular genetics. Inflammation, 2nd edn, 81

Peters DK, Martin A, Weinstein A, et al (1972) Complement studies in membrano-proliferative glomerulonephritis. Clin Exp Immunol 11:311

Podack ER, Muller-Eberhard HJ (1985) Isolation of human S-protein, an inhibitor of the membrane attack complex of complement. J Biol Chem 254:9908–9914

Richards RL, Gewurz H, Alving CR, Osmand AP (1977) Interactions of C-reactive protein and complement with liposomes. Proc Natl Acad Sci USA 74:5672–5676

Rudofsky UH, Pollara B (1981) Experimental autoimmune renal tubulointerstitial disease. In: Cummings NB, Michael AF, Silson CB (eds) Immune mechanisms in renal disease. Plenum Medical Book Company, NY, p 261

Salvesen GS, Catanese JJ, Kress LF, Travis J (1985) Primary structure of the reactive site of human C1 inhibitor. J Biol Chem 260:2432–2436

Schifferli JA, Woo P, Peters DK (1982) Complement-mediated inhibition of immune precipitation. I. Role of the classical and alternative pathways. Clin Exp Immunol 47:555–562

Smith MJH, Ford-Hutchinson AW, Bray MA (1980) Leukotriene B: a potential mediator of inflammation. J Pharm Pharmacol 32:517–518

Springer TA (1990) Adhesion receptors of the immune system. Nature 346:425–434

Storrs SB, Kolb WP, Pinckard RN, Olson MS (1981) Characterization of the binding of purified human C1q to mitochondrial membranes. J Biol Chem 256: 10924–10929

Striker LJ, Olson JM, Striker GF (1990) The Renal Biopsy. W.B. Saunders Company, Philadelphia

Sylvestre DL, Ravetch JV (1994) Fc receptors initiate the Arthus reaction: redefining the inflammatory cascade. Science 265:1095–1098

Sylvestre DL, Ravetch JV (1996) A dominant role for mast cell Fc receptors in the Arthus reaction. Immunity 5:387–390

Takai T, Li M, Clynes R, Ravetch JV, Sylvestre D (1994) FcR gamma chain deletion results in pleiotrophic effector cell defects. Cell 76:519–529

Tillett WS, Francis T Jr (1930) Serological reactions in pneumonia with non-protein sumatic fraction of Pneumococcus. J Exp Med 52:561–571

Vogt W, Dames W, Schmidt G, Dieminger L (1997) Complement activation by the properdin system: formation of a stoichiometric C3 cleaving complex of properdin factor B with C3b. Immunochemistry 14:201–205

Weiser MR, Williams JP, Hechtman HB, Carroll MC, Kobzik L, Ma M, Moore FD Jr (1996) Reperfusion injury of ischemic skeletal muscle is mediated by natural antibody and complement. J Exp Med 183:2343–2348

Welsh RM, Cooper NR, Jensen FC, Oldstone MBA (1975) Human serum lyses RNA tumor viruses. Nature 257:612–614

Welch TR, Witte DP, Beischel LS (1991) Differential expression and cellular localization of messenger RNA for C3 and C4 in the human kidney. Complement Inflamm 8:141

Welch TR, Witte DP, Beischel LS (1991) Differential expression and cellular localization of messenger RNA for C3 and C4 in the human kidney. Complement Inflamm 8:241

Wilson WA, Perez MC (1988) Complete CC4B deficiency in black Americans with systemic lupus erythematosus. J Rheumatol 15:1855–1858

Winkelstein JA, Sullivan KE, Colten HR (1995) Genetically determined disorders of the complement system. In: Scriver CR, Beaudet AL, Sly WS, Alle D (eds) The metabolic and molecular bases of inherited disease, 7th ed. McGraw-Hill, New York, pp 3911–3941

Zipfel PF, Skerka C (1994) Complement factor H and related proteins: an expanding family of complement-regulatory proteins? Immunol Today 15:121–126

Role of Phospholipases A$_2$ in Inflammation

J. Pfeilschifter

Introduction

Phospholipase A$_2$ (PLA$_2$) comprises a group of lipolytic enzymes that specifically release fatty acids, often arachidonic acid, from the *sn*-2 position of membrane phospholipids for the production of important lipid mediators such as prostaglandins, leukotrienes, and platelet activating factor (van den Bosch, 1980; Glaser et al., 1993; Mayer and Marshall, 1993; Kudo et al., 1993). Arachidonic acid and its numerous metabolites act as intracellular and intercellular messengers, contributing to normal cellular physiology by modifying the activity of intracellular enzymes and ion channels. Moreover, PLA$_2$ and its products function as substrates for the generation of inflammatory lipid mediators that play an important role in the pathogenesis of inflammatory diseases (Vadas and Pruzanski, 1986; Pruzanski and Vadas, 1991). The level of free intracellular arachidonic acid is extremely low, and in most tissues and cells the synthesis of eicosanoids is limited by the availability of free arachidonic acid. The major mechanism usually considered to control the level of intracellular free arachidonic acid in most cell types is the activation of PLA$_2$ and the direct release of the fatty acid from membrane glycerophospholipids (Irvine, 1982; Burgoyne and Morgan, 1990). PLA$_2$ enzymes are ubiquitously expressed and thus can be found in nearly all cell types examined, as well as in bacteria and protozoa. In recent years, it has become evident that PLA$_2$s are a heterogeneous family of enzymes that can be divided into main classes based on their molecular mass and cellular distribution (Dennis, 1997). The class of low molecular weight secreted PLA$_2$s (sPLA$_2$s) and the high molecular weight cytosolic PLA$_2$s (cPLA$_2$s) which is subdivided into a Ca^{2+}-dependent and Ca^{2+}-independent group.

It has been described that cPLA$_2$ selectively liberates arachidonic acid and is responsible for eicosanoid synthesis seen after exposure of cells to Ca^{2+}-mobilizing hormones. The cPLA$_2$ is translocated by low concentrations of Ca^{2+} to the plasma membrane in a process using a Ca^{2+} dependent phospholipid-binding domain in the N-terminal part of the enzyme and is activated by phosphorylation. Phosphorylation recognition sites for protein kinase C (PKC), protein kinase A, mitogen-activated protein kinase (MAPK), and protein tyrosine kinases have been identified (Sharp et al., 1991).

Symposium in Immunology VIII
Eibl/Huber/Peter/Wahn (Eds.)
© Springer Verlag Berlin Heidelberg 1999

Secrectory PLA_2 ($sPLA_2$) enzymes are a rapidly growing family of distinct enzymes with low molecular masses of approximately 14 kDa. Presently, five mammalian $sPLA_2$ types have been identified and denoted as types I, IIA, IIC, V, and X (Dennis, 1997; Cupillard, 1997).

Mammalian group I PLA_2 comprises the pancreatic type of PLA_2 and is characterized by the presence of Cys11. Several nonpancreatic tissues contain group II PLA_2, which is found in soluble form at inflammatory sites such as peritoneal exudates or rheumatoid arthritis, is synthesized and secreted from many cell types, and is believed to play a role in the initiation and propagation of inflammatory processes (Vadas and Pruzanski, 1986; Pruzanksi and Vadas, 1991). Whereas mammals possess both types of $sPLA_2$ enzymes, snake venoms contain either group I PLA_2 (Elapidae and Hydrophidae) or group II PLA_2 (Crotalidae and Viperidae). Kuchler et al. (1989) have characterized another type of low molecular weight (14 kDa) PLA_2 from bee venom that has been referred to as group III PLA_2 (Dennis, 1997).

Recently, three additional mammalian types of $sPLA_2$ have been identified. Type IIC $sPLA_2$ has been observed in rats and mice. It has an extra disulfide bond and is abundantly expressed in testes, whereas it is a nonfunctional pseudogene in humans (Tischfield et al., 1996). The second type of $sPLA_2$ was reported in human, rat, and a murine-derived macrophage cell line (Chen et al., 1994a; 1994b; Balboa et al., 1996) and was designated type V $sPLA_2$. It has been suggested that this enzyme is primarily responsible for agonist-induced arachidonic acid release and subsequent eicosanoid synthesis in mast cells (Reddy et al., 1997) and mouse macrophages (Balboa et al., 1996). A third type of $sPLA_2$ was cloned and characterized by Cupillard et al. in 1997 and was denoted as type X $sPLA_2$. It is expressed in immune tissues like spleen thymus, and peripheral blood leukocytes and less abundantly in pancreas, lung, and colon. Essentially, nothing is known about physiological

Table 1. Comparison of the properties of selected PLA_2 subtypes

Group	Localization	Molecular mass	Disulfide bridges	Optimal Ca^{2+} requirement	Arachidonate preference	Regulatory phosphorylation
I	Secreted	≈ 14 kDa	7	$\approx$ mM	No	No
IIA	Secreted/ cell associated	≈ 14 kDa	7	$\approx$ mM	No	No
II C	Secreted	≈ 15 kDa	8	$\approx$ mM	No	No
IV	Cytosolic	≈ 85 kDa	–	$\approx$ µM	Yes	Yes
V	Secreted	≈ 14 kDa	6	$\approx$ mM	No	No
VI	Cytosolic	≈ 80 kDa	–	None	No	No
X	Secreted	≈ 14 kDa	8	$\approx$ mM	No	No

functions of the latter enzyme. The characteristic features of the different PLA$_2$s are summarized in Table 1.

A comprehensive review of the biochemistry and molecular biology of all phospholipases is not possible in this chapter, but the reader is referred to several excellent reviews of this general area that have been published recently (Glaser et al., 1993; Mayer and Marshall, 1993; Kudo et al., 1993; Dennis, 1997). The focus of this chapter is on the regulation of the synthesis and secretion of low molecular weight group IIA PLA$_2$ and the accumulating evidence that this enzyme contributes to the generation of inflammatory lipid mediators.

Regulation of sPLA$_2$ Type IIA Expression

Group IIA PLA$_2$ induces inflammatory reactions when injected into experimental animals. Furthermore, this type of PLA$_2$ has antimicrobial activity and decreases the vitality of bacteria when given in combination with the bactericidal/permeability-increasing protein and can even kill bacteria in vitro. The expression of group IIA PLA$_2$ has been reported in normal human tissue as well as in inflamed and neoplastic human tissues and is summarized in Table 2. These data demonstrate that many human tissue and cell types are capable of expression of group IIA PLA$_2$, but the functional roles of the enzyme are still poorly defined.

Group IIA PLA$_2$ is stored in secretory granules of platelets, mast cells, and neutrophils and is rapidly, within seconds or minutes, released upon stimulation with Ca^{2+} mobilizing agonists such as thrombin, adenosine diphos-

Table 2. Expression of group IIA PLA$_2$ in human tissues and cells

Tissue/cell	Method used	Reference
Normal tissues/cells		
Amnion	Immunoassay	Aitken et al., 1993
Amnionic epithelium	Immunohistochemistry	Nevalainen et al., 1993 a
Cartilage	Western blot, immuno-histochemistry	Nevalainen et al., 1993 b
	Protein sequence	Recklies et al., 1991
Colon	Immunohistochemistry	Kiyohara et al., 1992
Choriodecidua	Immunoassay	Aitken et al., 1993
Esophagus	Immunohistochemistry	Kiyohara et al., 1992
Female breast	Immunoassay	Yamashita et al., 1992
Gallbladder	Immunohistochemistry	Kiyohara et al., 1992

Table 2. Continued

Tissue/cell	Method used	Reference
Normal tissues/cells		
Kidney	Northern blot	Kramer et el., 1989
Lacrimal gland acinar cells	Immunohistochemistry	Nevalainen et al., 1994
Liver (hepatocytes, Kupffer cells)	Immunohistochemistry	Ying et al., 1994
Macrophages	Immunohistochemistry	Kiyohara et al., 1992
Pancreas (acinar cells, islet cells, duct cells)	Immunohistochemistry	Kiyohara et al., 1993
Paneth cells	Immunohistochemistry In situ hybridization	Nevalainen et al., 1995
Placenta	Immunohistochemistry, immunoassay	Crowl et al., 1990
	Cloning	Andersen et al., 1994
Platelets	Protein sequence	Kramer et al., 1989
Prostate gland cells	Immunoassay	Nevalainen et al., 1993c
Skin	Northern blot, immuno-histochemistry	Andersen et al., 1989
Spleen	Protein sequence, Northern blot	Kramer et al., 1989 Kanda et al., 1989
Small intestine	Immunohistochemistry	Kiyohara et al., 1992
Stomach	Immunohistochemistry	Kiyohara et al., 1992 Murata et al., 1993
Tonsil	Northern blot	Kramer et al., 1989
Neoplastic tissues		
Gastric carcinoma	Immunohistochemistry	Murata et al., 1993
Hepatocellular carcinoma	Western blot, Northern blot Immunoassay	Ying et al., 1994
Mammary carcinoma	Immunoassay	Yamashita et al., 1993
Pancreatic carcinoma	Immunohistochemistry	Kiyohara et al., 1993
Peritoneal effusions (various cancers)	Immunohistochemistry, Northern blot, in situ hybridization	Abe et al., 1997
Inflamed tissues		
Atherosclerotic carotic wall	Immunohistochemistry	Schäfer-Elinder et al., 1997
Pancreatitis (chronic form)	Immunohistochemistry	Kiyohara et al., 1993
Psoriatic skin	Northern blot, immuno-histochemistry	Andersen et al., 1994
Rheumatoid synovial cells	Northern blot	Kramer et al., 1989

Table 3. Modulatory factors of group IIA PLA_2 expression

Cells	Stimulators	Inhibitors	References
Alveolar macrophages	FCS	fMLP, dexamethasone	Hidi et al., 1993 Vial et al., 1997
Astrocytes	IL-1β, TNF-α, cAMP, LPS, phorbol ester	Dexamethasone, H-7	Oka et al., 1991
Chondrocytes	IL-1α, IL-1β	IGF-1, IGF–2	Lyons-Giordano et al., 1989 Kerr et al., 1989 Chang et al., 1986 Gilman, 1987 Berenbaum et al., 1994
Endothelial cells (HUVECs)	TNF-α		Murakami et al., 1993
Fibroblasts	IL-1β		Shinohara et al., 1992
Gastric cancer cells	IL-6		Yamashita et al., 1994
Hepatoma cells (Hep G_2)	IL-1α, TNF-α, IL-6		Crowl et al., 1991
Kupffer cells	LPS		Hatch et al., 1993
Macrophages (peritoneal)		TGFβ₁	Bolognese et al., 1995
Neutrophils	LPS, fMLP		Lanni et al., 1983 Forehand et al., 1993
Osteoblasts	IL-1α, TNF-α	TGFβ₁	Vadas et al., 1991 Ellies et al., 1991
Renal mesangial cells	IL-1α, IL-1β, TNF-α, cAMP	TGFβ₂, PDGF, dexamethasone cyclosporin, protein kinase inhibitors, tetra-nactin, bFGF, NF-κB inhibitor	Pfeilschifter et al., 1989a; 1989b; 1990; 1991; 1993 Schalkwijk et al., 1991a, 1991b; 1992a; 1992b Mühl et al., 1991; 1992 Walker et al., 1995; 1996; 1997; 1998 Vervoordeldonk et al., 1996
Synovial cells	IL-1β		Gilman et al., 1988
Tracheobronchial smooth muscle cells	IL-1β		Vadas et al., 1996
Vascular smooth muscle cells	IL-1β, TNF-α, LPS, cAMP	Dexamethasone, colchicine	Pfeilschifter et al., 1989c Nakano et al., 1990a,b Kurihara et al., 1991

FCS, fetal calf serum; IL, interleukin; TNF, tumor necrosis factor; cAMP, cyclic adenosine monophosphate; LPS, lipopolysaccharide; IGF, insulin-like growth factor; fMLP, formyl-methionyl-leucyl-phenylalanine; TGF, transforming growth factor; PDGF, platelet-derived growth factor; bFGF, basic fibroblast growth factor; NF, nuclear factor

phate (ADP), A23187, or formyl-methionyl-leucyl-phenylalanine (fMLP) (Kramer et al., 1989; Mizushima et al., 1989; Hayakawa et al., 1988; Lanni and Becker; 1983). In contrast, recent work on the regulation of group IIA PLA$_2$ expression has shown that a variety of cytokines can modulate gene expression and PLA$_2$ synthesis over a longer time period (hours) in several cellular systems. These data are summarized in Table 3.

Most prominent among the stimulatory factors are the inflammatory cytokines interleukin 1 (IL-1)α, IL-1β, and tumor necrosis factor (TNF)-α. Incubation of cells with these cytokines induces an enhanced synthesis and secretion of prostaglandins and group IIA PLA$_2$.

PLA$_2$s in Mesangial Cells

Many of the metabolites of arachidonic acid have important signaling functions and are involved in the cross-communication between cells. In the kidney, eicosanoids play crucial roles in the regulation of intrarenal vascular tone, the distribution of renal blood flow, and, in addition, they modulate salt and water transport. Besides these physiological functions, intrarenal eicosanoids, especially when derived from arachidonic acid lipoxygenation, are mainly proinflammatory and contribute to glomerular immune injury (Lianos et al., 1991). PLA$_2$ is the primary enzyme regulating arachidonic acid release and subsequent eicosanoid production in the kidney and in mesangial cells (Pfeilschifter, 1989, 1994). At least two forms of PLA$_2$ have been purified and characterized in rat kidney and mesangial cells: a cPLA$_2$ (Gronich et al., 1988) and a sPLA$_2$ (Pfeilschifter et al., 1989; Schalkwijk et al., 1991). Hormone-stimulated increases in intracellular free Ca^{2+} and activation of protein kinases are thought to regulate cPLA$_2$ activity by triggering the translocation of the enzyme from the cytosol to the membrane, thus mediating transient physiological eicosanoid synthesis. Notably, the cPLA$_2$ activity recovered from stimulated mesangial cells is increased compared with that extracted from unstimulated control cells, suggesting a stable modification of the enzyme (Gronich et al., 1988). The involvement of PKC in the regulation of cPLA$_2$ has been suggested for several cellular systems, including mesangial cells. Huwiler et al. (1991) have proposed that the ε-isoenzyme of PKC triggers cPLA$_2$ activation in mesangial cells. The cPLA$_2$ sequence contains consensus phosphorylation sites for various protein kinases, including PKC, protein kinase A, MAPK, and protein tyrosine kinases. At least in vitro, PKC and MAPK are able to directly phosphorylate cPLA$_2$ (Lin et al., 1993; Nemenoff et al., 1993). Whether PKC does so by directly phosphorylating cPLA$_2$ in vivo or by phosphorylating Raf-1 kinase and thus triggering the MAPK cascade, remains to be determined. More recently, it was shown that phosphorylation and activation of cPLA$_2$ can take place independently of the classical p42 and p44 MAPKs and that other proline-directed protein kinases may phosphorylate cPLA$_2$ (Kramer et al., 1995). The constitutive expression of cPLA$_2$, its exclusive intracellular localization, its high sensitivity to Ca^{2+}, and its regulation by protein kinases make this enzyme an obvious candidate for the physiological regulation of arachidonic acid release and subsequent eicosanoid synthesis. On the other hand, long-term exposure to inflammatory cytokines induces the expression of a sPLA$_2$ which is not present in unstimulated cells, which is mainly secreted and less sensitive to Ca^{2+}, and which is regulated on demand on a transcriptional level. It is tempting to call the latter enzyme an inflammatory PLA$_2$ that contributes to the excessive production of arachidonic acid metabolites found in cells exposed to cytokines like IL-1 or TNF.

Roles of sPLA$_2$ and cPLA$_2$ in Mesangial Cell Eicosanoid Synthesis

Under physiological conditions, i.e., in the absence of inflammatory cytokines and endotoxin, mesangial cells only express the high molecular weight cPLA$_2$. This enzyme is responsible for the small amounts of eicosanoids synthesized in response to calcium-mobilizing hormones like angiotensin II, vasopressin, or endothelin that trigger phosphoinositide turnover with a subsequent mobilization of calcium from intracellular stores and activation of PKC.

It remains difficult to discriminate between contributions of sPLA$_2$ and cPLA$_2$ activities in the liberation of arachidonic acid under pathological conditions. We and others have demonstrated that chronic treatment with IL-1β, TNF-α, or transforming growth factor (TGF)-β$_2$ not only increases sPLA$_2$ activity but also cPLA$_2$ activity in mesangial cells (Schalkwijk et al., 1992; Schalkwijk et al., 1993). We have reported that sPLA$_2$ in rat mesangial cells contributes in part to prostaglandin E$_2$ (PGE)$_2$ synthesis induced by IL-1β or TNF-α. Coincubation with an anti-sPLA$_2$ monoclonal antibody attenuates PGE$_2$ formation by about 50%, and incubation with the specific sPLA$_2$ inhibitor CGP 43182 reduces the response by about 70% (Pfeilschifter et al., 1993). But it also became clear that this sPLA$_2$ does not account for all of the arachidonic acid released or of the PGE$_2$ synthesized. An extracellularly acting sPLA$_2$ is of physiological significance in the activation process of cells leading to increased eicosanoid synthesis and thus may contribute to the pathogenesis of inflammatory reactions (Vadas et al., 1993).

Cross-Talk Between sPLA$_2$ and cPLA$_2$ in Mesangial Cells

We have obtained data demonstrating that there is not only a coexpression of sPLA$_2$ and cPLA$_2$ in mesangial cells in response to inflammatory cytokines but, in addition, there is a cross-talk between both types of enzyme. Addition of sPLA$_2$ to mesangial cells causes a rapid (within minutes) activation of PKC-δ and -ε isoenzymes and an activation of the MAPK module, i.e., Raf-1 kinase, mitogen-activated protein kinase kinase (MEK), and the p42 and p44 isoforms of MAPK. Finally, this causes phosphorylation and activation of cPLA$_2$ in mesangial cells (Huwiler et al., 1997). In this context it is worth noting that we have previously reported that PKC-ε mediates arachidonic acid release in hormone-stimulated mesangial cells (Huwiler et al., 1991) and, more recently, that a Ca^{2+}-independent PKC isoenzyme, most likely PKC-δ or -ε, mediates MAPK activation in angiotensin II- and extracellular nucleotide-stimulated mesangial cells (Huwiler and Pfeilschifter, 1994a). Thus, it is quite conceivable that sPLA$_2$-induced PKC-δ or -ε activation causes, either directly or by stimulation of the MAPK pathway, a phosphorylation and activation of cPLA$_2$. In order to establish such a crucial role of PKC and the MAPK cascade in mediating the cross-talk between sPLA$_2$ and cPLA$_2$, we have utilized two potent and selective low molecular weight inhibitors for PKC and MEK, respectively. Ro-318220 is a potent and highly selective inhibitor of PKC which can penetrate cells and which exhibits activity against PKC-driven responses in vitro and in vivo. PD 98059 can block the activity of MEK assayed both in vitro with recombinant enzyme and in a variety of intact cells and thus completely inhibits the activation of MAPK by several hormones and growth factors, presumably due to the blockade of its upstream activator. Both inhibitors completely block sPLA$_2$-induced cPLA$_2$ activation, thus arguing for an essential role of PKC and MEK in mediating the cross-communication between these two phospholipases (Huwiler et al., 1997). Another line of evidence supporting this view is the observation that the time course of IL-1β-stimulated PGE$_2$ synthesis closely parallels the induction of sPLA$_2$ in mesangial cells (Pfeilschifter et al., 1989). Although the addition of IL-1β to mesangial cells causes an immediate generation of ceramide, activation of the MAPK cascade, and phosphorylation of cPLA$_2$ (Huwiler and Pfeilschifter, 1994b, Huwiler et al., 1996), there is no immediate increase in cPLA$_2$ activity (Gronich et al., 1994) and only a minor generation of PGE$_2$ (Pfeilschifter et al., 1989, Huwiler et al., 1997). However, after expression of sPLA$_2$ (after 8–16 h) there is a dramatic increase in eicosanoid production. These results suggest that sPLA$_2$ is crucially involved in cytokine-induced PGE$_2$ production.

Activation of MAPK by sPLA$_2$ has recently also been reported by Sugiura et al. (1995). Concerning the mechanism of sPLA$_2$-triggered activation of

PKC and/or MAPK, at least two possibilities can be considered. First, in a simple mechanistic model, sPLA$_2$-triggered inflammatory reaction comprises the generation of arachidonic acid and lysophospholipids, which are subsequently metabolized into eicosanoids and platelet-activating factor. Moreover, arachidonic acid and lysophospholipids may themselves act as signaling molecules. An especially intriguing possibility is a sPLA$_2$-induced activation of PKC. Both products of PLA$_2$'s catalytic action, lysophosphatidylcholine (LPC) and cis-unsaturated fatty acids, including arachidonic acid, have previously been shown to amplify hormone-induced cellular responses by enhancing the 1,2-diacylglycerol-stimulated activation of PKC. Consistent with these observations, sPLA$_2$ has been reported to greatly intensify the activation of resting human T-lymphocytes exposed to membrane-permeant 1,2-diacylglycerol and Ca^{2+}-ionophore (Asaoka et al., 1993). Our observations are compatible with this model as addition of sPLA$_2$ or LPC and other lysophospholipids to mesangial cells causes a translocation and supposedly an activation of PKC-δ and -ε isoenzymes. It is well established that PKC stimulation leads to a sequential activation of Raf-1 kinase, MEK, and MAPKs and thus provides optimal conditions for subsequent phosphorylation and activation of cPLA$_2$. Moreover, arachidonic acid, the second split product of sPLA$_2$ action, has been reported to activate MAPKs in a variety of cell types.

A second alternative explanation is that sPLA$_2$ functions as a ligand for a specific receptor that in turn initiates the signaling cascades described in this paper. Some of the biological responses induced by sPLA$_2$ are thought to be mediated by high-affinity sPLA$_2$ receptors with molecular masses of 180–200 kDa which have been molecularly cloned and characterized (Lambeau et al., 1994; Ishizaki et al., 1994). Functional responses to sPLA$_2$ receptor activation includes eicosanoid synthesis and vascular smooth muscle cell migration and contraction and proliferation of rat chondrocytes. Most notably, mesangial cells have been described as expressing a single class of specific binding sites for sPLA$_2$ which have been shown to trigger sPLA$_2$ expression and prostaglandin synthesis (Kishino et al., 1994). Molecular cloning of rabbit, bovine, and human sPLA$_2$ receptors has recently been reported (Lambeau et al., 1994; Ishizaki et al., 1994; Higashino et al., 1994; Ancian et al., 1995). The binding properties show species-specific differences with varying affinities for the distinct members of the sPLA$_2$ family. The sPLA$_2$ receptor has sequence homologies to the macrophage mannose receptor, a membrane protein involved in the endocytosis of glycoproteins. The short cytoplasmic tail of the sPLA$_2$ receptor does not display any characteristic sequence motif that could be responsible for coupling to known signaling pathways. Thus it remains to be investigated whether this sPLA$_2$ receptor is able to link its occupancy to the delivery of an activating signal for the MAPK module. Very recently, Hanasaki et al. (1997) generated PLA$_2$ receptor mutant mice and reported that these mice were resistant to lethal effects of lipopolysaccharide, suggesting that PLA_2 receptor participates in promoting endotoxin shock.

In summary, these data support the notion that a sophisticated network of interactions between different PLA_2s may contribute to the progression of glomerular inflammatory processes and that mesangial cells are an important target and source for several types of PLA_2.

Conclusions

There is compelling evidence implicating PLA_2s in the pathogenesis of acute and chronic inflammatory processes. The recent discovery of distinct PLA_2 isoforms has promoted new research efforts in trying to define the roles of different types of PLA_2 in physiological and pathophysiological conditions. Furthermore, initial reports on differential inhibition of human secretory and cytosolic PLA_2s suggest that it will be possible to find isoenzyme-specific inhibitors for therapeutic intervention in inflammatory diseases. Traditionally, drug discovery has relied on the systematic screening of natural products and synthetic chemicals in order to identify specific and potent enzyme inhibitors. The identification of transcription factors as the key molecules regulating gene expression in eukaryotic cells, and the analysis of a set of factors involved in the regulation of specific gene products, e.g., PLA_2, make these proteins potential targets for pharmacological intervention. It may be possible to identify the transcription factors involved in cytokine-induced group IIA PLA_2 gene expression. Inhibition of nuclear factor (NF)-κB NF-IL6, or activator protein (AP)-2-mediated group IIA PLA_2 gene expression may provide a basis for the development of a transcription factor-based therapy of inflammatory diseases. This approach may lead to a totally new type of drug which challenges inflammation in a fundamentally new way.

Acknowledgments. This work was supported by a grant from the Wilhelm Sander-Stiftung, by the Deutsche Forschungsgemeinschaft (SFB 553), and by a grant from the Commission of the European Communities (Biomed 2, PL 950979).

References

Abe T, Sakamoto K, Kamohara H, Hirano Y, Kuwahara N, Ogawa M (1997) Group II phospholipase A$_2$ is increased in peritoneal and pleural effusions in patients with various types of cancer. Int J Cancer 74:245–250

Aitken MA, Farrugia W, Wong MH, Scott KF, Brennecke SP, Rice GE (1993) Type II phospholipase A$_2$ in human gestational tissues: Extractable immuno- and enzymatic activity in fetal membranes. Biochim Biophys Acta 1170:314–320

Ancian P, Lambeau G, Mattéi M-G, Lazdunski M (1995) The human 180-kDa receptor for secretory phospholipases A$_2$. J Biol Chem 270:8963–8970

Andersen S, Sjursen W, Laegreid A, Austgulen R, Johansen B (1994) Immunohistologic detection of non-pancreatic phospholipase A$_2$ (type II) in human placenta and its involvement in normal parturition at term. Prostaglandins Leukot Essent Fatty Acids 51:19–26

Andersen S, Sjursen W, Laegreid A, Volden G, Johansen B (1994) Elevated expression of human nonpancreatic phospholipase A$_2$ in psoriatic tissue. Inflammation 18:7–12

Balboa MA, Balsinde J, Winstead MV, Tischfield JA, Dennis EA (1996) Novel group V phospholipase A$_2$ involved in arachidonic acid mobilization in murine P388D1 macrophages. J Biol Chem 271:32381–32384

Berenbaum F, Thomas G, Poiraudeau S, Béréziat G, Corvol MT, Masliah J (1994) Insulin-like growth factors counteract the effect of interleukin 1β on type II phospholipase A$_2$ expression and arachidonic acid release by rabbit articular chondrocytes. FEBS Lett 340:51–55

Bolognese B, McCord M, Marshall LA (1995) Differential regulation of elicited-peritoneal macrophage 14 kDa and 85 kDa phospholipase A$_2$(s) by transforming growth factor-β. Biochim Biophys Acta 1256:201–209

Burgoyne RD, Morgan A (1990) The control of free arachidonic acid levels. Trends Biochem Sci 15:365–366

Chang J, Gillman SC, Lewis AJ (1986) Interleukin 1 activates phospholipase A$_2$ in rabbit chondrocytes: a possible signal for IL 1 action. J Immunol 136:1283–1287

Chen J, Engle SJ, Seilhamer JJ, Tischfield JA (1994a) Cloning and recombinant expression of a novel human low molecular weight Ca^{2+}-dependent phospholipase A$_2$. J Biol Chem 269:2365–2368

Chen J, Engle SJ, Seilhamer JJ, Tischfield JA (1994b) Cloning and characterization of novel rat and mouse low molecular weight Ca^{2+}-dependent phospholipase A$_2$s containing 16 cysteines. J Biol Chem 269:23018–23024

Crowl RM, Stoller TJ, Conroy RR, Stoner CR (1991) Induction of phospholipase A$_2$ gene expression in human hepatoma cells by mediators of the acute phase response. J Biol Chem 266:2647–2651

Cupillard L, Koumanov K, Mattéi M-G, Lazdunski M, Lambeau G (1997) Cloning, chromosomal mapping, and expression of a novel human secretory phospholipase A$_2$. J Biol Chem 272:15745–15752

Dennis, EA (1997) The growing phospholipase A$_2$ superfamily of signal transduction enzymes. Trends Biochem Sci 22:1–2

Ellies LG, Heersche JNM, Vadas P, Pruzanski W, Stefanski E, Aubin JE (1991) Interleukin-1α stimulates the release of prostaglandin E$_2$ and phospholipase A$_2$ from fetal rat calvarial cells in vitro. Relationship to bone nodule formation. J Bone Mineral Res 6:843 - 850

Forehand JR, Johnston RB, Bomalaski JS (1993) Phospholipase A$_2$ activity in human neutrophils. J Immunol 151:4918–4925

Gilman SC (1987) Activation of rabbit articular chondrocytes by recombinant human cytokines. J Rheumatol 14:1002–1007

Gilman SC, Chang J, Zeigler PR, Uhl J, Mochan E (1988) Interleukin-1 activates phospholipase A_2 in human synovial cells. Arthritis Rheumatism 31:126–130

Glaser KB, Mobilio D, Chang JY, Senko N (1993) Phospholipase A_2 enzymes: regulation and inhibition. Trends Pharmacol Sci 14:92–98

Gronich JH, Bonventre JV, Nemenoff RA (1988) Identification and characterization of a hormonally regulated form of phospholipase A_2 in rat renal mesangial cells. J Biol Chem 263:16645–16651

Gronich J, Konieczkowski M, Gelb MH, Nemenoff RA, Sedor JR (1994) Interleukin-1α causes rapid activation of cytosolic phospholipase A_2 by phosphorylation in rat mesangial cells. J Clin Invest 93:1224–1233

Hanasaki K, Yokota Y, Ishizaki J, Takeshi I, Arita H (1997) Resistance to endotoxic shock in phospholipase A_2 receptor-deficient mice. J Biol Chem 272:32792–32797

Hatch GM, Vance DE, Wilton DC (1993) Rat liver mitochondrial phospholipase A_2 is an endotoxin-stimulated membrane-associated enzyme of Kupffer cells which is released during liver perfusion. Biochem J 293:143–150

Hayakawa M, Kudo I, Tomita M, Nojima S, Inoue K (1988) The primary structure of rat platelet phospholipase A_2. Biochem J 104:767–772

Hidi R, Vargaftig BB, Touqui L (1993) Increased synthesis and secretion of a 14-kDa phospholipase A_2 by guinea pig alveolar macrophages: dissociation from arachidonic acid liberation and modulation by dexamethasone. J Immunol 151:5613–5623

Higashino K, Ishizaki J, Kishino J, Ohara O, Arita H (1994) Structural comparison of phospholipase A_2-binding regions in phospholipase-A_2 receptors from various mammals. Eur J Biochem 225:375–382

Huwiler A, Fabbro D, Pfeilschifter J (1991) Possible regulatory functions of protein kinase C α and -ε isoenzymes in rat renal mesangial cells. Stimulation of prostaglandin synthesis and feedback-inhibition of angiotensin II-stimulated phosphoinositide hydrolysis. Biochem J 279:441–445

Huwiler A, Pfeilschifter J (1994a) Stimulation by extracellular ATP and UTP of the mitogen-activated protein kinase cascade and proliferation of rat renal mesangial cells. Br J Pharmacol 113:1455–1463

Huwiler A, Pfeilschifter J (1994b) Transforming growth factor-β_2 stimulates acute and chronic activation of the mitogen-activated protein kinase cascade in rat renal mesangial cells. FEBS Lett 354:255–259

Huwiler A, Brunner J, Hummel R, Vervoordeldonk M, Stabel S, van den Bosch H, Pfeilschifter J (1996) Ceramide-binding and activation defines protein kinase c-Raf as a ceramide-activated protein kinase. Proc Natl Acad Sci USA 93:6959–6963

Huwiler A, Staudt G, Kramer R, Pfeilschifter J (1997) Cross-talk between secretory phospholipase A_2 and cytosolic phospholipase A_2 in rat renal mesangial cells. Biochim Biophys Acta 1348:257–272

Irvine RF (1982) How is the level of free arachidonic acid controlled in mammalian cells? Biochem J 204:3–16

Ishizaki J, Hanasaki K, Higashino K, Kishino J, Kikuchi N, Ohara O, Arita H (1994) Molecular cloning of pancreatic group I phospholipase A_2 receptor. J Biol Chem 269:5897–5904

Kanda A, Ono T, Yoshida N, Okamoto M (1989) The primary structure of a membrane-associated phospholipase A_2 from human spleen. Biochem Biophys Res Commun 163:42–48

Kerr JS, Stevens TM, Davis GL, McLaughlin JA, Harris RR (1989) Effects of recombinant interleukin 1 beta on phospholipase A$_2$ activity, phospholipase A$_2$ mRNA levels and eicosanoid formation in rabbit chondrocytes. Biochem Biophys Res Commun 165:1079–1084

Kishino J, Ohara O, Nomura K, Kramer RM, Arita H (1994) Pancreatic-type phospholipase A$_2$ expression and prostaglandin biosynthesis in rat mesangial cells. J Biol Chem 269:5092–5098

Kiyohara H, Egami H, Shibata Y, Murata K, Ohshima S, Ogawa M (1992) Light microscopic immunohistochemical analysis of the distribution of group II phospholipase A$_2$ in human digestive organs. J Histochem Cytochem 40:1659–1664

Kiyohara H, Egami H, Kako H, Shibata Y, Murata K, Ohshima S, et al (1993) Immunohistochemical localization of group II phospholipase A$_2$ in human pancreatic carcinomas. Int J Pancreatol 13:49–57

Kramer RM, Hession C, Johansen B, Hayes G, McGray P, Chow EP, Tizard R, Pepinsky RB (1989) Structure and properties of a human non-pancreatic phospholipase A$_2$. J Biol Chem 264:5768–5775

Kramer RM, Roberts EF, Hyslop PA, Utterback BG, Hui KY, Jakubowski JA (1995) Differential activation of cytosolic phospholipase A$_2$ by thrombin and thrombin receptor agonist peptide in human platelets. J Biol Chem 270:14816–14823

Kuchler K, Gmachl M, Sippl M, Kreil G (1989) Analysis of the cDNA for phospholipase A$_2$ from honeybee venom glands. Eur J Biochem 184:249–254

Kudo I, Murakami M, Hara S, Inoue K (1993) Mammalian non-pancreatic phospholipase A$_2$. Biochim Biophys Acta 117:217–231

Kurihara H, Nakano T, Takasu N, Arita H (1991) Intracellular localization of group II phospholipase A$_2$ in rat cultured astrocytes. Two distinct pathways of the gene expression. Biochim Biophys Acta 1082:285–292

Lambeau G, Ancian P, Barhanin J, Lazdunski M (1994) Cloning and expression of a membrane receptor for a secretory phospholipase A$_2$. J Biol Chem 269:1575–1578

Lanni C, Becker EL (1983) Release of phospholipase A$_2$ activity from rabbit peritoneal neutrophils by f-Met-Leu-Phe. Am J Pathol 113:90–94

Lianos EA, Bresnahan BA, Pan C (1991) Mesangial cell immune injury: Synthesis, origin and role of eicosanoids. J Clin Invest 88:623–631

Lin LL, Wartmann M, Lin AY, Knopf JL, Seth A, Davis RJ (1993) cPLA$_2$ is phosphorylated and activated by MAP kinase. Cell 72:269–278

Lyons-Giordano B, Davis GL, Galbraith W, Pratta MA, Arner EC (1989) Interleukin-1β stimulates phospholipase A$_2$ mRNA synthesis in rabbit articular chondrocytes. Biochem Biophys Res Commun 164:488–495

Mayer RJ, Marshall LA (1993) New insights on mammalian phospholipase A$_2$(s); comparison of arachidonoyl-selective and -nonselective enzymes. FASEB J 7:339–348

Mizushima H, Kudo I, Horigome K, Murakami M, Kayakawa M, Kim DK, Kondo E, Tomita M, Inoue K (1989) Purification of rabbit platelet secretory phospholipase A$_2$ and its characteristics. J Biochem 105:520–525

Mühl H, Geiger T, Pignat W, Märki F, van den Bosch H, Vosbeck K, Pfeilschifter J (1991) PDGF suppresses the activation of group II phospholipase A$_2$ gene expression by interleukin-1 and forskolin in mesangial cells. FEBS Lett 291:249–252

Mühl H, Geiger T, Pignat W, Märki F, van den Bosch H, Cerletti N, Cox D, Mc Master G, Vosbeck K, Pfeilschifter J (1992) Transforming growth factors type-β and dexamethasone attenuate group II phospholipase A$_2$ gene expression by interleukin-1 and forskolin in rat mesangial cells. FEBS Lett 301:190–194

Murakami M, Kudo I, Inoue K (1993) Molecular nature of phospholipase A$_2$ involved in prostaglandin I$_2$ synthesis in human umbilical vein endothelial cells: possible participation of cytosolic and extracellular type II phospholipase A$_2$. J Biol Chem 268:839–844

Murata K, Egami H, Kiyohara H, Ohshima S, Kurizaki T, Ogawa M (1993) Expression of group-II phospholipase A_2 in malignant and non-malignant human gastric mucosa. Br J Cancer 68:103–111

Nakano T, Ohara O, Teraoka H, Arita H (1990) Group II phospholipase A_2 mRNA synthesis is stimulated by two distinct mechanisms in rat vascular smooth muscle cells. FEBS Lett 261:171–174

Nakano T, Ohara O, Teraoka H, Arita H (1990) Glucocorticoids suppress group II phospholipase A_2 production by blocking mRNA synthesis and post-transcriptional expression. J Biol Chem 265:12745–12748

Nemenoff RA, Winitz S, Qian N-X, van Putten V, Johnson GL, Heasley LE (1993) Phosphorylation and activation of a high molecular weight form of phospholipase A_2 by p42 microtubule-associated protein 2 kinase and protein kinase C. J Biol Chem 268:1960–1964

Nevalainen TJ, Haapanen TJ (1993a) Distribution of pancreatic (group I) and synovial-type (group II) phospholipases A_2 in human tissues. Inflammation 17:453–464

Nevalainen TJ, Märki F, Kortesuo PT, Grütter M, DiMarco S, Schmitz A (1993b) Synovial-type (group II) phospholipase A_2 in cartilage. J Rheumatol 20:325–330

Nevalainen TJ, Meri K-M, Niemi M (1993c) Synovial-type (group II) phospholipase A2 in human seminal plasma. Andrologia 25:355–358

Nevalainen TJ, Aho HJ, Peuravuori H (1994) Secretion of group 2 phospholipase A_2 by lacrimal gland. Invest Ophtalmol Vis Sci 32:417–421

Nevalainen TJ, Grönrooss JM, Kallajoki M (1995) Expression of group II phospholipase A_2 in human gastrointestinal tract. Lab Invest 72:201–208

Oka S, Arita H (1991) Inflammatory factors stimulate expression of group II phospholipase A_2 in rat cultured astrocytes. Two distinct pathways of the gene expression. J Biol Chem 266:9956–9960

Pfeilschifter J, Pignat W, Vosbeck K, Märki F, Wiesenberg I (1989a) Susceptibility of interleukin 1- and tumour necrosis factor-induced prostaglandin E_2 and phospholipase A_2 release from rat renal mesangial cells to different drugs. Biochem Soc Transact 17:916–917

Pfeilschifter J, Pignat W, Vosbeck K, Märki F (1989b) Interleukin-1 and tumour necrosis factor synergistically stimulate prostaglandin synthesis and phospholipase A_2 release from rat renal mesangial cells. Biochem Biophys Res Commun 159:385–394

Pfeilschifter J (1989) Cross-talk between transmembrane signalling systems: a prerequisite for the delicate regulation of glomerular haemodynamics by mesangial cells. Eur J Clin Invest 19:347–361

Pfeilschifter J, Pignat W, Märki F, Wiesenberg I (1989c) Release of phospholipase A_2 activity from rat vascular smooth muscle cells mediated by cAMP. Eur J Biochem 181:237–242

Pfeilschifter J, Pignat W, Leighton J, Märki F, Vosbeck K, Alkan S (1990) Transforming growth factor β_2 differentially modulates interleukin-1β- and tumour-necrosis-factor-α stimulated phospholipase A_2 and prostaglandin E_2 synthesis in rat renal mesangial cells. Biochem J 270:269–271

Pfeilschifter J, Leighton J, Pignat W, Märki F, Vosbeck K (1991) Cyclic AMP mimics, but does not mediate, interleukin-1 and tumour-necrosis-factor-stimulated phospholipase A_2 secretion from rat renal mesangial cells. Biochem J 273:199–204

Pfeilschifter J, Mühl H, Pignat W, Märki F, van den Bosch H (1993a) Cytokine regulation of group II phospholipase A_2 expression in glomerular mesangial cells. Eur J Clin Pharmacol 44:S7–S9

Pfeilschifter J, Schalkwijk C, Briner VA, van den Bosch H (1993b) Cytokine-stimulated secretion of group II phospholipase A$_2$ by rat mesangial cells: Its contribution to arachidonic acid release and prostaglandin synthesis by cultured rat glomerular cells. J Clin Invest 92:2516–2523

Pruzanski W, Vadas P (1991) Phospholipase A$_2$ – a mediator between proximal and distal effectors of inflammation. Immunol Today 12:143–146

Recklies AD, White C (1991) Phospholipase A$_2$ is a major component of the salt-extractable pool of matrix proteins in adult human articular cartilage. Arth Rheum 34:1106–1115

Reddy ST, Herschman HR (1997) Prostaglandin synthase-1 and prostaglandin synthase-2 are coupled to distinct phospholipases for the generation of prostaglandin D$_2$ in activated mast cells. J Biol Chem 272:3231–3237

Schalkwijk C, Pfeilschifter J, Märki F, van den Bosch H (1991a) Interleukin-1β, tumour necrosis factor and forskolin stimulate the synthesis and secretion of group II phospholipase A$_2$ in rat renal mesangial cells. Biochem Biophys Res Commun 174:268–275

Schalkwijk C, Vervoordeldonk M, Pfeilschifter J, Märki F van den Bosch H (1991b) Cytokine- and forskolin-induced synthesis of group II phospholipase A$_2$ and prostaglandin E$_2$ in rat renal mesangial cells is prevented by dexamethasone. Biochem Biophys Res Commun 180:46–52

Schalkwijk C, de Vet E, Pfeilschifter J, van den Bosch H (1992a) Interleukin-1β and transforming growth factor-β$_2$ enhance cytosolic high molecular-mass phospholipase A$_2$ activity and induce prostglandin E$_2$ formation in rat mesangial cells. Eur J Biochem 210:69–176

Schalkwijk C, Pfeilschifter J, Märki F, van den Bosch H (1992b) Interleukin-1β and forskolin-induced synthesis and secretion of group II phospholipase A$_2$ and prostaglandin E$_2$ in rat renal mesangial cells is prevented by transforming growth factor-β$_2$. J Biol Chem 267:8846–8851

Schalkwijk C, Vervoordeldonk M, Pfeilschifter J, van den Bosch H (1993) Interleukin–1-β induced cytosolic phospholipase A$_2$ activity and protein synthesis is blocked by dexamethasone in rat mesangial cells. FEBS Lett 333:339–343

Schäfer-Elinder L, Dumitrescu A, Larsson P, Hedin U, Frostegard J, Claesson H-E (1997) Expression of phospholipase A$_2$ isoforms in human normal and atherosclerotic arterial wall. Arterioscler Thromb Vasc Biol 17:2257–2263

Sharp JD, White DL, Chiou X-G, Goodson T, Gamboa GC, McClure D, Burgett S, Hoskins J, Skatrud PL, Sportsman JR, Becker GW, Kang LH, Roberts EF, Kramer RM (1991) Molecular cloning and expression of human Ca(2 +)-sensitive cytosolic phospholipase A$_2$. J Biol Chem 266:14850–14853

Shinohara H, Amabe Y, Komatsubara T, Tojo H, Okamoto M, Wakano Y, Ishida H (1992) Group II phospholipase A$_2$ induced by interleukin-1β in cultured rat gingival fibroblasts. FEBS Lett 304:69–72

Sugiura T, Wada A, Itoh T, Tojo H, Okamoto M, Imai E, Kamada T, Ueda N (1995) Group II phospholipase A$_2$ activates mitogen-activated protein kinase in cultured rat mesangial cells. FEBS Lett 370:141–145

Tischfield JA, Xia Y-R, Shih DM, Klisak I, Chen J, Engle SJ, Siakotos AN, Winstead MV, Seilhamer JJ, Allamand V, Gyapay G, Lusis AJ (1996) Low-molecular weight, calcium-dependent phospholipase A$_2$ genes are linked and map to homologous chromosome regions in mouse and human. Genomics 32:328–333

Vadas P, Pruzanski W (1986) Biology of disease: role of secretory phospholipase A$_2$ in the pathobiology of disease. Lab Invest 55:391–404

Vadas P, Browning J, Edelson J, Pruzanski W (1993) Extracellular phospholipase A_2 expression and inflammation: the relationship with associated disease states. J Lipid Mediators 8:1–30

Vadas P, Stefanski E, Wloch M, Grouix B, van den Bosch H, Kennedy B (1996) Secretory nonpancreatic phospholipase A_2 and cyclooxygenase-1 expression by tracheobronchial smooth muscle cells. Eur J Biochem 235:557–563

Van den Bosch H (1980) Intracellular phospholipases A. Biochim Biophys Acta 604 : 191–246

Vervoordeldonk MJBM, Schalkwijk CG, Pfeilschifter J, van den Bosch H (1996) Effect of dexamethasone and transforming growth factor β_2 on group II phospholipase A_2 mRNA and activity levels in interleukin 1β- and forskolin-stimulated mesangial cells. Biochem J 315:435–441

Vial D, Senorale-Pose M, Havet N, Molio L, Vargaftig BB, Touqui L (1995) Expression of type II phospholipase A_2 in alveolar macrophages: down-regulation by an inflammatory signal. J Biol Chem 270:17327–17332

Walker G, Kunz D, Pignat W, van den Bosch H, Pfeilschifter J (1995) Pyrrolidine dithiocarbamate differently affects cytokine- and cAMP-induced expression of group II phospholipase A_2 in rat renal mesangial cells. FEBS Lett 364:218–222

Walker G, Kunz D, Pignat W, Wiesenberg I, van den Bosch H, Pfeilschifter J (1996) Tetranactin inhibits interleukin 1β and cAMP-induction of group II phospholipase A_2 in rat renal mesangial cells. Eur J Pharmacol 306:265–270

Walker G, Kunz D, Pignat W, van den Bosch H, Pfeilschifter J (1997) Suppression by cyclosporin A of interleukin 1β-induced expression of group II phospholipase A_2 in rat renal mesangial cells. Br J Pharmacol 121:787–793

Walker G, Kunz D, Pignat W, van den Bosch H, Pfeilschifter J (1998) Platelet-derived growth factor and fibroblast growth factor differentially regulate interleukin 1β- and cAMP-induced group II phospholipase A_2 expression in rat renal mesangial cells. Biochim Biophys Acta 1391:213–222

Yamashita S, Yamashita J, Sakamoto K, Inada K, Nakashima Y, Murata K, et al (1993) Increased expression of membrane-associated phospholipase A_2 shows malignant potential of human breast cancer cells. Cancer 71:3058–3064

Yamashita S, Ogawa M, Abe T, Yamashita J, Sakamoto K, Niwa H, Yamamura K (1994) Group II phospholipase A_2 in invasive gastric cancer cell line is induced by interleukin 6. Biochem Biophys Res Commun 198:878–884

Ying Z, Tojo H, Komatsubara T, Nakagawa M, Inada M, Kawata S, Masuzawa Y, Okamoto M (1994) Enhanced expression of group II phospholipase A_2 in human hepatocellular carcinoma. Biochim Biophys Acta 1226:201–205

Activation of NF-κB by Inflammatory Cytokines

M. Rothe

Introduction

Tumor necrosis factor (TNF), a pleiotropic cytokine produced mainly by activated macrophages, plays a central role in the generation of inflammatory responses (for review see Tracey, 1993). TNF activates the transcription of many genes encoding acute phase and proinflammatory proteins which bring about the dramatic changes that characterize the inflammatory phenotype. This function is mediated primarily by the transcription factor nuclear factor κB (NF-κB) whose binding motif is found in nearly all inflammatory response genes (for review see Barnes and Karin, 1997). NF-κB is composed of homo- and heterodimers of members of the Rel family of related transcription factors, and its activity is tightly regulated by cytokines and other stimuli (for review see Baeuerle and Henkel, 1994; Baeuerle and Baltimore, 1996; Baldwin, 1996; Lenardo and Baltimore, 1989; Siebenlist et al., 1994; Thanos and Maniatis, 1995; Verma et al., 1995). In most cell types, NF-κB is present as a heterodimer comprising a 50-kDa (p50) and 65-kDa subunit (p65) that is sequestered in the cytoplasm by a member of a family of inhibitory proteins termed IκB. IκB proteins mask the nuclear localization signal of NF-κB, thereby preventing NF-κB nuclear translocation. Conversion of NF-κB into an active transcription factor that translocates into the nucleus and binds to cognate DNA sequences entails the signal-induced phosphorylation of IκB proteins on specific serine residues, such as serines 32 and 36 of IκB-α and serines 19 and 23 of IκB-β. Subsequent to phosphoylation, IκB proteins are ubiquitinated and degraded through a proteasome-dependent pathway.

The past several years have seen intense research progress by numerous laboratories in delineating components of the TNF signal transduction pathway leading to NF-κB activation. These efforts have recently culminated in the identification of the elusive IκB kinase(s).

Symposium in Immunology VIII
Eibl/Huber/Peter/Wahn (Eds.)
© Springer Verlag Berlin Heidelberg 1999

TNF Receptor-Associated Proteins

Induction of the various cellular responses elicited by TNF is initiated by its interaction with two distinct cell surface receptors of approximately 55 kDa (TNF-R1) and 75 kDa (TNF-R2) which are independently capable of signaling NF-κB activation (for review see Tartaglia and Goeddel, 1992; Rothe et al., 1992; Vandenabeele et al., 1995). Both TNF receptors are members of the larger TNF receptor superfamily which also includes the Fas antigen, CD40, CD30, and the lymphotoxin-β receptor among others (for review see Smith et al., 1994). All of these diverse cell surface proteins share a characteristic repeating cysteine-rich motif in the extracellular region. The common structural framework of the extracellular domains is reflected in the ability of the TNF receptor superfamily members to interact with a parallel family of TNF-related cytokine ligands (for review see Smith et al., 1994; Gruss and Dower, 1995).

Signaling within the TNF receptor superfamily requires the aggregation of receptor monomers that is initiated by binding of the respective trimeric ligands (for review see Vandenabeele et al., 1995). The cytoplasmic domains of the TNF receptor superfamily members do not possess sequences indicative of catalytic activity, nor do they show homology among themselves. The only exception is a region of weak homology between the cytoplasmic domains of TNF-R1 and the Fas antigen which has been dubbed the "death domain" since it is responsible for promoting the signal for apoptotic cell death triggered by both receptors (Tartaglia et al., 1993; Itoh and Nagata, 1993). Recently, a number of additional TNF receptor family members have been characterized which also contain death domain motives in their cytoplasmic domains and transduce cell death signals (Kitson et al., 1996; Chinnaiyan et al., 1996a; Golstein, 1997).

Several families of TNF receptor-associated signaling proteins have been identified using biochemical purification and the yeast two-hybrid protein interaction cloning technique (Fields and Song, 1989) (Fig. 1). One family of adapter proteins contains death domain regions similar to those found in the cognate receptors. The TNF receptor-associated death domain (TRADD) protein associates directly with TNF-R1 in a TNF-dependent manner via interaction of its death domain with that of TNF-R1 and is required for NF-κB activation by TNF (Hsu et al., 1995; Shu et al., 1996). The receptor-interacting protein (RIP) is recruited indirectly into the TNF-R1 signaling complex by interaction of its death domain with the death domain of TRADD (Stanger et al., 1995; Hsu et al., 1996a). RIP mediates the TNF-induced NF-κB signal (Kelliher et al., 1998). However, an N-terminal serine-threonine kinase domain that is present in RIP appears dispensable for this activity (Ting et al., 1996). The Fas-associated death domain (FADD) protein

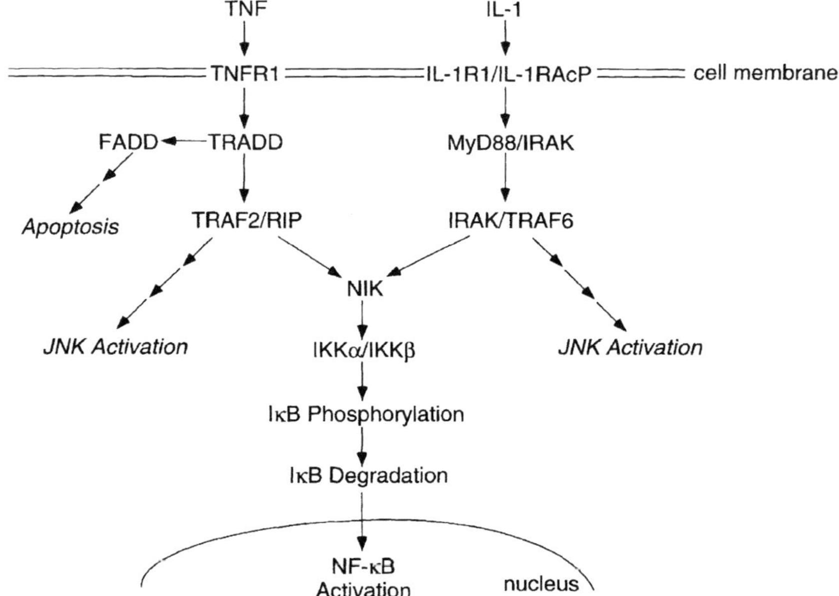

Fig. 1. A model for the nuclear factor κB (*NF-κB*) signal transduction pathways initiated by tumor necrosis factor (*TNF*) and interleukin 1 (*IL-1*). *FADD*, Fas-associated death domain; *TRADD*, TNF receptor-associated death domain; *RIP*, receptor-interacting protein; *JNK*, c-jun N-terminal kinase; *NIK*, NF-κB-inducing kinase; *IκB*, inhibitor of NF-κB; *IKKα/IKKβ*, IκB kinases α/β; *IRAK*, IL-1 receptor-associated kinase

binds directly to the death domain of Fas, where it propagates the cell death signal elicited by Fas ligand stimulation (Boldin et al., 1995; Chinnaiyan et al., 1995; Yeh et al., 1998; Zhang et al., 1998). FADD is also essential for TNF-induced apoptosis but not NF-κB activation through its association with TRADD (Chinnaiyan et al., 1996b; Hsu et al., 1996b; Yeh et al., 1998).

TNF receptor-associated factor (TRAF) proteins associate directly with the cytoplasmic domain of several members of the TNF receptor family, including TNF-R2, CD40, CD30, HVEM, and the lymphotoxin-β receptor (Rothe et al., 1994; Hu et al., 1994; Cheng et al., 1995; Mosialos et al., 1995; Song and Donner, 1995; Sato et al., 1995; Lee et al., 1996; Gedrich et al., 1996; Hsu et al., 1997; Marsters et al., 1997). In addition, TRAF proteins are recruited indirectly to TNF-R1 by interaction with the N-terminal region of TRADD located adjacent to the death domain (Hsu et al., 1996b; Shu et al., 1996). TRAF proteins also interact with RIP (Hsu et al., 1996b). They consist of a conserved C-terminal TRAF domain and an N-terminal region comprising a RING zinc finger motif (Freemont 1993; Saurin et al. 1996) and an additional array of zinc finger-like structures (Rothe et al., 1994; Hu et al., 1994;

Cheng et al., 1995). The zinc binding domains are involved in signaling downstream responses (Cheng et al., 1995; Rothe et al., 1995b). The TRAF domain mediates receptor association, homo- and heterooligomerization of TRAFs, and serves as a docking site for a number of other signaling proteins including TRADD and RIP (Rothe et al., 1994; Hu et al.,1994; Cheng et al., 1995; Rothe et al., 1995a; Hsu et al., 1996b; Song et al.,1996; Cheng and Baltimore, 1996; Rothe et al., 1996; Takeuchi et al., 1996; Lee et al., 1997a). The TRAF domain also mediates complex formation of TRAF1 and TRAF2 with cIAP1 and cIAP2, two closely related mammalian members of the inhibitor-of-apoptosis protein (IAP) family originally identified in baculoviruses (Rothe et al., 1995a; Clem and Miller, 1994). Like their baculovirus homologs, mammalian IAPs are involved in anti-apoptotic responses (Liston et al., 1996; Orth and Dixit, 1997).

Three of the six described TRAF family members have been implicated in NF-κB activation based on overexpression studies in mammalian cells. TNF-induced NF-κB activation requires TRAF2 (Rothe et al., 1995b; Hsu et al., 1996b). TRAF5 is also involved in NF-κB activation by members of the TNF receptor family (Nakano et al., 1996; Ishida et al., 1996; Hsu et al., 1997; Marsters et al., 1997). In contrast, TRAF6 participates in NF-κB activation by another important proinflammatory cytokine, interleukin-1 (IL-1) (Cao et al., 1996b) (see Fig. 1). TRAF6 associates with the serine-threonine kinase, IL-1 receptor-associated kinase (IRAK), following the IL-1-induced activation of IRAK in the IL-1 receptor complex (Cao et al., 1996a; Huang et al., 1997; Wesche et al., 1997; Muzio et al., 1997). Thus, although TNF and IL-1 initiate signaling cascades leading to NF-κB activation via distinct families of cell-surface receptors (for reviewed see Dinarello, 1996), both pathways utilize members of the TRAF family of adapter proteins as signal transducers.

Another prominent transcription factor responsible for the effects of TNF and IL-1 is activator protein 1 (AP1) (Brenner et al., 1989), which is activated through phosphorylation of the c-jun N-terminal kinase (JNK; also known as SAPK, stress activated protein kinase) (Minden et al., 1994). The JNK pathway is a mitogen-activated protein (MAP) kinase cascade composed of several kinases that sequentially phosphorylate and activate one another in response to inflammatory cytokines, growth factors, and environmental stress (for review see Kyriakis and Avruch, 1996). Similar to NF-κB activation, TRAF2, TRAF5, and TRAF6 have been implicated in activation of JNK by TNF and IL-1 (Liu et al., 1996; Natoli et al., 1997a; Reinhard et al., 1997; Song et al., 1997). Indeed, TNF signaling to JNK but not NF-κB is defective in vivo in TRAF2-deficient cells (Lee et al., 1997b; Yeh et al., 1997), suggesting that both TNF signaling pathways are distinct and diverge at the level of TRAF proteins.

Kinase Cascades

Recent studies have identified several serine-threonine protein kinases involved in TNF and IL-1 signal transduction (see Fig. 1). The NF-κB-inducing kinase (NIK) is a member of the MAP kinase kinase kinase (MAPKKK) family that was identified as a TRAF2-interacting protein (Malinin et al., 1997). NIK overexpression activates NF-κB, and kinase-inactive mutants of NIK comprising its TRAF2-interacting C-terminal domain or lacking the two lysine residues in its catalytic domain behave as dominant-negative inhibitors that suppress TNF-, IL-1-, TRADD-, RIP-, and TRAF2-induced NF-κB activation (Malinin et al., 1997). NIK also associates with other members of the TRAF family, including TRAF5 and TRAF6 (Song et al., 1997). Catalytically inactive mutants of NIK inhibit NF-κB activation by TRAF5 and TRAF6, similar to TRAF2 induced NF-κB activation. These observations provided a unifying concept for NIK as a common mediator in the NF-κB signaling cascades triggered by TNF and IL-1 downstream of TRAFs and other receptor-associated signaling proteins (Song et al., 1997). In contrast to NF-κB activation, NIK overexpression does not stimulate activation of JNK. Furthermore, a catalytically inactive NIK protein, which is a dominant-negative inhibitor of NF-κB activation, does not suppress TNF- or TRAF2-induced JNK activation (Song et al., 1997; Natoli et al., 1997b). Thus, NIK is not involved in JNK activation but is dedicated to the NF-κB pathway. However, NIK itself does not act as an IκB kinase (Régnier et al., 1997).

In yeast two-hybrid screen for targets of NIK-mediated NF-κB activation, a previously described serine-threonine kinase of orphaned function called CHUK [conserved helix-loop-helix ubiquitous kinase (Connelly and Marcu, 1995)] was identified as a NIK-interacting protein (Régnier et al., 1997). Search of an expressed sequence tag (EST) database revealed the existence of a CHUK-related kinase which displays 52% identity to CHUK on the amino acid level (Woronicz et al., 1997). Both kinases were identified independently by biochemical purification as 85-kDA and 87-kDA components of a high molecular mass complex ($\approx$ 500–900 kDA) that harbored IκB kinase activity (DiDonato et al., 1997; Mercurio et al., 1997; Zandi et al., 1997). Based on their functional properties described below, these novel serine-threonine kinases have been designated IκB kinase (IKK)-α (IKK-1; CHUK) and IKK-β (IKK-2).

Although the structures of IKK-α and IKK-β are similar to each other, they are unlike any other known serine-threonine kinase (Connelly and Marcu, 1995; Régnier et al., 1997; DiDonato et al., 1997; Mercurio et al., 1997; Woronicz et al., 1997; Zandi et al., 1997). IKK-α and IKK-β consist of 745 and 756 amino acids, respectively, and both kinases are composed of an N-terminal serine-threonine kinase domain, a central leucine zipper region, and a C-terminal helix-loop-helix domain. Both IKKs are expressed ubiquitously (Connelly and Marcu, 1995; Woronicz et al., 1997; Zandi et al., 1997), which is in agreement with the pleiotropic roles of NF-κB in many different cell types and tissues (reviewed in Lenardo and Baltimore, 1989; Baeuerle and Henkel, 1994; Baeuerle and Baltimore, 1996). Overexpression of each IKK is sufficient to cause the transactivation of NF-κB-dependent reporter genes in mammalian cells (Régnier et al., 1997; DiDonato et al., 1997; Mercurio et al., 1997; Woronicz et al., 1997; Zandi et al., 1997). However, differences exist between both kinases in their relative activities. IKK-β is constitutively active when transfected alone, whereas the activity of IKK-α is relatively low and requires costimulation by TNF to become fully active. Catalytically inactive mutants of IKK-α and IKK-β behave as dominant-negative inhibitors of TNF-, IL-1-, TRAF- and NIK-induced NF-κB activation (Régnier et al., 1997; Mercurio et al., 1997; Woronicz et al., 1997; Zandi et al., 1997). In addition, antisense IKKs block cytokine induction of NF-κB activity (DiDonato et al., 1997; Zandi et al., 1997).

IKK-α, and to a lesser extend IKK-ß, associate with NIK and IκB-α in mammalian cells (Régnier et al., 1997; Woronicz et al., 1997). Both IKK-α and IKK-β can self-associate, but heterodimer formation between both kinases occurs preferentially and has been detected endogenously in mammalian cells (Mercurio et al., 1997; Woronicz et al., 1997; Zandi et al., 1997). The interaction between IKK-α and IKK-β appears to be mediated through their leucine zipper motifs (Woronicz et al., 1997; Zandi et al., 1997). The IKK-α/β heterocomplex is able to form a ternary complex with NIK (Woronicz et al., 1997). Both IKKs can independently and specifically phosphorylate serines 32 and 36 in IκB-α, with IKK-β displaying more potent phosphorylation activity compared to IKK-α (Régnier et al., 1997; DiDonato et al., 1997; Mercurio et al., 1997; Woronicz et al., 1997; Zandi et al., 1997). Whereas IKK-β also phosphorylates serines 19 and 23 of IκB-β with equal efficiency, IKK-α has a marked preference for serine 23 over serine 19 of IκB-β, suggesting a subtle substrate specificity among both kinases (Régnier et al., 1997; DiDonato et al., 1997; Mercurio et al., 1997; Woronicz et al., 1997; Zandi et al., 1997). The ability of both kinases to phosphorylate IκB is augmented by addition of TNF, i.e., they represent cytokine-responsive IκB kinases (DiDonato et al., 1997; Mercurio et al., 1997; Woronicz et al., 1997; Zandi et al., 1997).

The phosphorylation of IκB-α by IKK-α is greatly enhanced by NIK costimulation (Régnier et al., 1997). In contrast, IκB-α phosphorylation by IKK-β is increased only slightly by NIK, presumably because NIK preferentially phosphorylates IKK-α over IKK-β (Woronicz et al., 1997; Ling et al., 1998). Both IKK-α and IKK-β contain canonical MAP kinase kinase (MAPKK) activation loops in their catalytic domains (Ser-X-X-X-Ser, where X can be any amino acid) which represent putative phosphorylation sites for upstream MAPKKKs such as NIK or MEKK1 (for review see May and Gosh, 1998). Mutational analysis revealed that, when the two serine residues (serines 177 and 181) of IKK-β are mutated to glutamates, a mutation that mimics phosphorylation, kinase activity is increased (Mercurio et al., 1997). Furthermore, replacement of the same residues with alanines creates a dominant-negative IKK-β mutant which inhibits TNF-induced NF-κB activation (Mercurio et al., 1997). Similarly, a mutant form of IKK-α containing glutamic acid instead of serine at residue 176 is constitutively active (Ling et al., 1998). A mutant IKK-α protein containing alanine at residue 176 cannot be phosphorylated or activated by NIK and acts as a dominant-negative inhibitor of cytokine-mediated NF-κB activation (Ling et al., 1998). Thus, the regulation of IKK activity is controlled through phosphorylation of specific serine residues in their kinase domains.

Conclusion

The identification of components of the signal transduction pathways initiated by the cytokines TNF and IL-1 has provided important insights into the mechanisms of action of these proinflammatory mediators. The newly deciphered signaling pathways consist of cascades of contiguous protein–protein interactions which delineate a functional hierarchy among the components (see Fig. 1). Importantly, the TNF- and IL-1-induced NF-κB activation pathways merge into the same kinase cascade leading to IκB phosphorylation and subsequent degradation. On the other hand, several other responses triggered by these cytokines utilize certain components of the NF-κB pathway but diverge at discrete levels, such as the TNF-induced apoptosis pathway and the JNK pathway activated by TNF and IL-1 (see Fig. 1).

The recently reported IKKs represent catalytic subunits of a large IκB kinase complex that links the TNF- and IL-1-induced kinase cascades to NF-κB activation. Future efforts will be directed to characterize other components of the IκB kinase complex and to examine its regulation in response to cytokines and other stimuli that are known to activate NF-κB. An exciting task which remains to be elucidated is the identification of kinases that mediate the signal for JNK activation that is initiated at the proximal receptor complexes for IL-1 and TNF.

TNF and IL-1 exert key roles in the cytokine network with regard to the pathogenesis of many infectious and inflammatory diseases (for review see Dinarello, 1996; Eigler et al., 1997). TNF neutralizing antibodies have been efficacious in the treatment of rheumatoid arthritis and Crohn's disease (Feldman et al., 1996; Stack et al., 1997; Targan et al., 1997). Similar results were obtained for a recombinant human TNF receptor-Fc fusion protein for treatment of rheumatoid arthritis (Moreland et al., 1997). Thus, beneficial effects of inhibiting TNF responses in chronic inflammatory diseases have been demonstrated in clinical settings. Based on this proof of concept, elucidation of the TNF and IL-1 signaling pathways provides a number of attractive novel targets for therapeutic intervention and drug discovery approaches in the area of inflammation research.

References

Baeuerle PA, Baltimore D (1996) NF-κB: Ten years after. Cell 87:13–20

Baeuerle PA, Henkel T (1994) Function and activation of NF-κB in the immune system. Annu Rev Immunol 12:141–179

Baldwin AS (1996) The NF-κB and IκB proteins: new discoveries and insights. Annu Rev Immunol 14:649–681

Barnes PJ, Karin M (1997) Nuclear factor-κB – a pivotal transcription factor in chronic inflammatory diseases. N Engl J Med 336:1066–1071

Boldin MP, Varfolomeev EE, Pancer Z, Mett IL, Camonis JH, Wallach D (1995) A novel protein that interacts with the death domain of Fas/APO1 contains a sequence motif related to the death domain. J Biol Chem 270:7795–7798

Brenner DA, O'Hara M, Angel P, Chojkier M, Karin M (1989) Prolonged activation of jun and collagenase genes by tumor necrosis factor-alpha. Nature 337:661–663

Cao Z, Henzel WJ, Gao X (1996a) IRAK: a kinase associated with the interleukin-1 receptor. Science 271:1128–1131

Cao Z, Xiong J, Takeuchi M, Kurama T, Goeddel DV (1996b) TRAF6 is a signal transducer for interleukin-1. Nature 383:443–446

Cheng G, Baltimore D (1996) TANK, a co-inducer with TRAF2 of TNF- and CD40L-mediated NF-κB activation. Genes Dev 10:963–973

Cheng G, Cleary AM, Ye Z-S, Hong D, Lederman S, Baltimore D (1995) Involvement of CRAF1, a relative of TRAF, in CD40 signaling. Science 267:1494–1498

Chinnaiyan AM, O'Rourke K, Yu G-L, Lyons RH, Garg M, Duan DR, Xing L, Gentz R, Ni J, Dixit VM (1996a) Signal transduction by DR3, a death domain-containing receptor related to TNFR-1 and CD95. Science 274:990–992

Chinnaiyan AM, O'Rourke K, Tewari M, Dixit VM (1995) FADD, a novel death domain-containing protein, interacts with the death domain of Fas and initiates apoptosis. Cell 81:505–512

Chinnaiyan AM, Tepper CG, Seldin MF, O'Rourke K, Kischkel FC, Hellbardt S, Krammer PH, Peter ME, Dixit VM (1996b) FADD/MORT1 is a common mediator of CD95 (Fas/APO-1) and tumor necrosis factor rector-induced apoptosis. J Biol Chem 271:4961–4965

Clem RJ, Miller LK (1994) Control of programmed cell death by the baculovirus genes p35 and iap. Mol Cell Biol 14:5212–5222

Connelly MA, Marcu KB (1995) CHUK, a new member of the helix-loop-helix and leucine zipper families of interacting proteins, contains a serine-threonine kinase catalytic domain. Cell Mol Biol Res 41:537–549

DiDonato JA, Hayakawa M, Rothwarf DM, Zandi E, Karin M (1997) A cytokine-responsive IκB kinase that activates the transcription factor NF-κB. Nature 388:548–554

Dinarello CA (1996) Biologic basis for interleukin-1 in disease. Blood 87:2095–2147

Eigler A, Sinha B, Hartmann G, Endres S (1997) Taming TNF: strategies to restrain this proinflammatory cytokine. Immunol Today 19:487–492

Feldman M, Brennan FM, Maini RN (1996) Rheumatoid arthritis. Cell 85:307–310

Fields S, Song O-K (1989) A novel genetic system to detect protein-protein interactions. Nature 340:245–246

Freemont PS (1993) The RING finger: a novel protein sequence motif related to the zinc finger. Ann NY Read Sci 684:174–192

Gedrich RW, Gilfillan MC, Duckett CS, Van Dongen JL, Thompson CB (1996) CD30 contains two binding sites with different receptor specificities for members of the tumor necrosis factor receptor-associated factor family of signal transducing proteins. J Biol Chem 271:12852–12858

Golstein P (1997) Cell death: TRAIL and its receptors. Curr Biol 7:R750-R753

Gruss H-J, Dower SK (1995) Tumor necrosis factor ligand superfamily: involvment in the pathology of malignant lymphomas. Blood 85:3378–3404

Hsu H, Huang J, Shu H-B, Baichwal V, Goeddel DV (1996a) TNF-dependent recruitment of the protein kinase RIP to the TNF receptor-1 signaling complex. Immunity 4:387–396

Hsu H, Shu H-B, Pan M-G, Goeddel DV (1996b) TRADD-TRAF2 and TRAD-FADD interactions define two distinct TNF receptor-1 signal transduction pathways. Cell 84:299–308

Hsu H, Solovyev I, Colombero A, Elliott R, Kelley M, Boyle WJ (1997) ATAR, a novel tumor necrosis factor receptor family member, signals through TRAF2 and TRAF5. J Biol Chem 272:13471–13474

Hsu H, Xiong J, Goeddel DV (1995) The TNF receptor-1 associated protein TRADD signals cell death and NF-κB activation. Cell 81:495–504

Hu HM, O'Rourke K, Boguski MS, Dixit VM (1994) A novel RING finger protein interacts with the cytoplasmic domain of CD40. J Biol Chem 269:30069–30072

Huang J, Gao X, Li S, Cao Z (1997) Recruitment of IRAK to the interleukin 1 receptor complex requires interleukin 1 receptor accessory protein. Proc Natl Acad Sci USA 94:12829–12832

Ishida T, Tojo T, Aoki T, Kobayashi N, Ohishi T, Watanabe T, Yamamoto T, Inoue J-I (1996) TRAF5, a novel tumor necrosis factor receptor-associated factor family protein, mediates CD40 signaling. Proc Natl Acad Sci USA 93:9437–9442

Itoh N, Nagata S (1993) A novel protein domain required for apoptosis. J Biol Chem 268:10932–10937

Kelliher MA, Grimm S, Ishida Y, Kuo F, Stanger BZ, Leder P (1998) The death domain kinase RIP mediates the TNF-induced NF-κB signal. Immunity 8:297–303

Kitson J, Raven T, Jiang Y-P, Goeddel DV, Giles KM, Pun K-T, Grinham CJ, Brown R, Farrow SN (1996) A death-domain-containing receptor that mediates apoptosis. Nature 384:372–375

Kyriakis JM, Avruch J (1996) Protein kinase cascades activated by stress and inflammatory cytokines. Bioassays 18:567–577

Lee SY, Lee SL, Kandala G, Liou M-L, Liou H-C, Choi Y (1996) CD30-TRAF interaction: NF-κB activation and binding specificity. Proc Natl Acad Sci USA 93: 9699–9703

Lee SY, Lee SY, Choi Y (1997a) TRAF-interacting protein (TRIP): a novel component of the tumor necrosis factor (TNFR)- and CD30-TRAF signaling complexes that inhibits TRAF2-mediated NF-κB activation. J Exp Med 185:1275–1285

Lee SY, Reichlin A, Santana A, Sokol KA, Nussenzweig MC, Choi Y (1997b) TRAF2 is essential for JNK but not NF-κB activation and regulates lymphocyte proliferation and survival. Immunity 7:703–713

Lenardo M, Baltimore D (1989) NF-κB: a pleiotropic mediator of inducible and tissue-specific gene control. Cell 58:227–229

Ling L, Cao Z, Goeddel DV (1998) NF-κB-inducing kinase activates IKK-α by phosphorylation of Ser-176. Proc Natl Acad Sci USA 95:3792–3793

Liston P, Roy N, Tamai K, Lefebvre C, Baird S, Cherton-Horvat G, Farahani R, McLean M, Ikeda J-E, MacKenzie A, Korneluk RB (1996) Suppression of apoptosis in mammalian cells by NAIP and a related family of IAP genes. Nature 379: 349–353

Liu Z-G, Hsu H, Goeddel DV, Karin M (1996) Dissection of TNF receptor 1 effector functions: JNK activation is not linked to apoptosis while NF-κB activation prevents cell death. Cell 87:565–576

Malinin NL, Boldin MP, Kovalenko AV, Wallach D (1997) MAP3K-related kinase involved in NF-κB induction by TNF, CD95 and IL-1. Nature 385:540–544

Marsters SA, Ayres TM, Skubatch M, Gray CL, Rothe M, Ashkenazi A (1997) Herpesvirus Entry Mediator, a member of the tumor necrosis factor receptor (TNFR) family, interacts with members of the TNFR-associated factor family and activates the transcription factors NF-κB and AP-1. J Biol Chem 272:14029–14032

May MJ, Gosh S (1998) Signal transduction through NF-κB. Immunol Today 19: 80–88

Mercurio F, Zhu H, Murray BW, Shevchenko A, Bennett BL, Li JW, Young DB, Barbosa M, Mann M, Manning A, Rao A (1997) IKK-1 and IKK-2: Cytokine activated IκB kinases essential for NF-κB activation. Science 278:860–866

Minden A, Lin A, Claret F-X, Lange-Carter C, Dérijard B, Davis RJ, Johnson GL, Karin M (1994) Differential activation of ERK and JNK mitogen-activated protein kinases by RAF-1 and MEKK. Science 266:1719–1723

Moreland LW, Baumgartner SW, Schiff MH, Tindall EA, Fleischmann RM, Weaver AL, Ettlinger RE, Cohen S, Koopman WJ, Mohler K, Widmer MB, Blosch CM (1997) Treatment of rheumatoid arthritis with a recombinant human tumor necrosis factor receptor (p75)-Fc fusion protein. N Engl J Med 337:141–147

Mosialos G, Birkenbach M, Yalamanchill R, VanArsdale T, Ware C, Kieff E (1995) The Epstein-Barr virus transforming protein LMP1 engages signaling proteins for the tumor necrosis factor receptor family. Cell 80:389–399

Muzio M, Ni J, Feng P, Dixit VM (1997) IRAK (Pelle) family member IRAK-2 and MyD88 as proximal mediators of IL-1 signaling. Science 278:1612–1615

Nakano H, Oshima H, Chung W, Williams-Abbott L, Ware CF, Yagita H, Okumura K (1996) TRAF5, an activator of NF-κB and putative signal transducer for the lymphotoxin-β receptor. J Biol Chem 271:14661–14664

Natoli G, Costanzo A, Ianni A, Templeton DJ, Woodgett JR, Balsano C, Levrero M (1997a) Activation of SAPK/JNK by TNF receptor 1 through a noncytotoxic TRAF2-dependent pathway. Science 275:200–203

Natoli G, Costanzo A, Moretti F, Fulco M, Balsano C, Levrero M (1997b) Tumor necrosis factor (TNF) receptor 1 signaling downstream of TNF receptor-associated factor 2. Nuclear factor κB (NF-κB)-inducing kinase requirement for activation of activating protein 1 and NF-κB but not c-Jun N-terminal kinase/stress-activated protein kinase. J Biol Chem 272:26079–26082

Orth K, Dixit VM (1997) Bik and Bak induce apoptosis downstream of CrmA but upstream of inhibior of apoptosis. J Biol Chem 272:8841–8844

Régnier CH, Song HY, Gao X, Goeddel DV, Cao Z, Rothe M (1997) Identification and characterization of an IκB kinase. Cell 90:373–383

Reinhard C, Shamoon B, Shyamala V, Williams LT (1997) Tumor necrosis factor α-induced activation of c-jun N-terminal kinase is mediated by TRAF2. EMBO J 16:1080–1092

Rothe J, Gehr G, Loetscher H, Lesslauer W (1992) Tumor necrosis factor receptors – structure and function. Immunol Res 11:81–90

Rothe M, Pan M-G, Henzel WJ, Ayres TM, Goeddel DV (1995a) The TNF receptor 2-TRAF signaling complex contains two novel proteins related to baculoviral inhibitor of apoptosis proteins. Cell 83:1243–1252

Rothe M, Sarma V, Dixit VM, Goeddel DV (1995b) TRAF2-mediated activation of NF-κB by TNF receptor 2 and CD40. Science 269:1424–1427

Rothe M, Wong SC, Henzel WJ, Goeddel DV (1994) A novel family of putative signal transducers associated with the cytoplasmic domain of the 75 kDa tumor necrosis factor receptor. Cell 78:681–692

Rothe M, Xiong J, Shu H-B, Williamson K, Goddard A, Goeddel DV (1996) I-TRAF is a novel TRAF-interacting protein that regulates TRAF-mediated signal transduction. Proc Natl Acad Sci USA 93:8241–8246

Sato T, Irie S, Reed JC (1995) A novel member of the TRAF family of putative signal transducing proteins binds to the cytosolic domain of CD40. FEBS Lett 358:113–118

Saurin AS, Borden KLB, Boddy MN, Freemont PS (1996) Does this have a familiar RING? Trends Biochem Sci 21:207–214

Shu H-B, Takeuchi M, Goeddel DV (1996) The tumor necrosis factor recetor 2 signal transducers TRAF2 and c-IAP1 are components of the tumor necrosis factor receptor 1 signaling complex. Proc Natl Acad Sci USA 93:13973–13978

Siebenlist U, Franzoso G, Brown K (1994) Structure, regulation and function of NF-κB. Annu Rev Cell Biol 10:405–455

Smith CA, Farrah T, Goodwin RG (1994) The TNF receptor superfamily of cellular and viral proteins: activation, costimulation, and death. Cell 76:959–962

Song HY, Donner DB (1995) Association of a RING finger protein with the cytoplasmic domain of the human type-2 tumour necrosis factor receptor. J Biochem 809:825–829

Song HY, Régnier CH, Kirschning CJ, Goeddel DV, Rothe M (1997) Tumor necrosis factor (TNF)-mediated kinase cascades: bifurcation of nuclear factor-κB and c-jun N-terminal kinase (JNK/SAPK) pathways at TNF receptor-associated factor 2. Proc Natl Acad Sci USA 94:9792–9796

Song HY, Rothe M, Goeddel DV (1996) The tumor necrosis factor-inducible zinc finger protein A20 interacts with TRAF1/TRAF2 and inhibits NF-κB activation. Proc Natl Acad Sci USA 93:6721–6725

Stack WA, Mann SD, Roy AJ, Heath P, Sopwith M, Freemann J, Long R, Forbes A, Kamm MA (1997) Randomised controlled trial of CDP571 antibody to tumor necrosis factor-α in Crohn's disease. Lancet 1997:521–524

Stanger BZ, Leder P, Lee T-H, Kim E, Seed B (1995) RIP: a novel protein containing a death domain that interacts with Fas/APO-1 (CD95) in yeast and causes cell death. Cell 81:513–523

Takeuchi M, Rothe M, Goeddel DV (1996) Anatomy of TRAF2: distinct domains for NF-κB activation and association with TNF signaling proteins. J Biol Chem 271:19935–19942

Targan SR, Hanauer SB, van Deventer SJ, Mayer L, Present DH, Braakman T, DeWoody KL, Schaible TF, Rutgeerts PJ (1997) A short-term study of chimeric monoclonal antibody cA2 to tumor necrosis factor α for Crohn's disease. Crohn's disease cA2 study group. N Eng J Med 337:1029–1035

Tartaglia LA, Ayres TM, Wong GHW, Goeddel DV (1993) A novel domain within the 55 kd TNF receptor signals cell death. Cell 74:845–853

Tartaglia LA, Goeddel DV (1992) Two TNF receptors. Immunol Today 13:151–153

Thanos D, Maniatis T (1995) NF-κB: a lesson in family values. Cell 80:529–532

Ting AT, Pimentel-Muiños FX, Seed B (1996) RIP mediates tumor necrosis factor receptor 1 activation of NF-κB but not Fas/APO-1-initiated apoptosis. EMBO J 15:6189–6196

Tracey KJ, Cerami A (1993) Tumor necrosis factor, other cytokines and disease. Annu Rev Cell Biol 9:317–343

Vandenabeele P, Declercq W, Beyaert R, Fiers W (1995) Two tumor necrosis factor receptors: structure and function. Trends Cell Biol 5:392–399

Verma IM, Stevenson JK, Schwarz EM, Van Antwerp D, Miyamoto S (1995) Rel/ NF-κB/IκB family: intimate tales of association and dissociation. Genes Dev 9: 2723–2735

Wesche H, Henzel WJ, Shillinglaw W, Li S, Cao Z (1997) MYD88: an adapter that recruits IRAK to the IL-1 receptor complex. Immunity 7: 837–847

Woronicz JD, Gao X, Cao Z, Rothe M, Goeddel DV (1997) IκB Kinase-β: NF-κB activation and complex formation with IκB kinase-α and NIK. Science, in press

Yeh W-C, Pompa JL, McCurrach ME, Shu HB, Elia AJ, Shahinian A, Ng M, Wakeham A, Khoo W, Mitchell K, El-Deiry WS, Lowe SW, Goeddel DV, Mak TW (1998) FADD: essential for embryo development and signaling from some, but not all, inducers of apoptosis. Science 279:1954–1958

Yeh W-C, Shahinian A, Speiser D, Kraunus J, Billia F, Wakeham A, de la Pompa JL, Ferrick D, Hum B, Iscove N, Ohashi P, Rothe M, Goeddel DV, Mak TW (1997) Early lethality, functional NF-κB activation, and increased sensitivity to TNF-induced cell death in TRAF2-deficient mice. Immunity 7:715–725

Zandi E, Rothwarf DM, Delhase M, Hayakawa M, Karin M (1997) The IκB kinase complex (IKK) contains two kinase subunits, IKKα and IKKβ, necessary for IκB phosphorylation and NF-κB activation. Cell 91:243–252

Zhang J, Cado D, Chen A, Kabra NH, Winoto A (1998) Fas-mediated apoptosis and activation-induced T-cell proliferation are defective in mice lacking FADD/Mort1. Nature 392:296–300

Interaction of the Parasite *Echinococcus granulosus* with Host Innate Immunity

A. J. Díaz, A. M. Ferreira, F. Irigoin, M. Breijo, and R. B. Sim

Introduction: The Parasite

The larval stages of the parasites belonging to the genus *Echinococcus* (phylum Platyhelminthes; subclass Cestoda; order Cyclophyllidea; family Taeniidae) cause hydatid disease. There are four recognised species in this genus, of which only two are important for human health and economic welfare. These are *E. multilocularis* and *E. granulosus*, agents of alveolar and cystic (or unilocular) hydatid disease, respectively. In these organisms, the adult worms parasitise dogs and other canids (the definitive hosts) and the larvae (metacestodes) parasitise a wide range of mammalian species, including humans (the intermediate hosts). The life cycle requires a predator–prey relationship between the definitive and intermediate hosts. Human hydatid disease does not therefore normally lead to completion of the parasite cycle: humans are said to be accidental intermediate hosts. The general biology of *Echinococcus* has been reviewed by Thompson (1995).

E. granulosus is adapted to an environment in which livestock farming plays a central role, completing its cycle through dogs and a variety of livestock species, mainly sheep, cattle, pigs, horses, goats and camels. Dogs become infected as they feed on infected livestock offal which harbours cysts, each of which may contain several thousand protoscoleces, each with the potential to become an adult worm. Protoscoleces are around 100 μm in diameter, and possess four suckers and a crown of hooks which allow them to attach to the dog's gut wall. Establishment of the protoscoleces takes place in the crypts of Lieberkün of the dog's small intestine, where they develop in around 1 month into 5-mm long adult worms. The adult worms are hermaphroditic. Between 34 and 58 days postinfection, adults begin to release, every 1 or 2 weeks, a new gravid proglottid, which passes out with the dog's faeces, and carries some 1500 eggs. The eggs (35 μm in diameter) are protected by a tough keratin-type layer, and can withstand adverse conditions for long periods. The intermediate hosts become infected through ingestion of eggs in contaminated food or water. The host digestive enzymes dissolve the egg's shell, releasing the oncosphere, which burrows through the host's gut wall and is transported via blood or lymph to the target organs, which are

Symposium in Immunology VIII
Eibl/Huber/Peter/Wahn (Eds.)
© Springer Verlag Berlin Heidelberg 1999

mainly, but not solely, liver and lungs. Within 14 days the parasite forms a cyst: this is a bladder-like structure made turgid by the fluid it contains (hydatid cyst fluid) and bound by two parasite-derived layers. The inner, cellular, germinal layer, is only a few cell bodies wide. The outer layer, called the laminated layer, is a thick, modified glycocalix which endows the cyst with mechanical resistance. The germinal layer is capable of asexual reproduction. It buds inwards towards the cyst cavity, giving rise to brood capsules, which produce the protoscoleces; brood capsules with protoscoleces eventually detach and float in the cyst fluid. Protoscoleces are not just the infecting stage for the definitive host, but are also capable of reverse development towards cysts when released by rupture of the mother cyst into the peritoneal cavity of the intermediate host. This phenomenon of secondary infection (as opposed to primary infection by oncospheres) can be experimentally reproduced by injection of protoscoleces in a wide range of experimental animals.

E. granulosus has a wide geographical distribution, being most prevalent in Southern South America, Northern and East Africa, the Middle East, China, South Asia, Australasia, and Southern and South-Eastern Europe. Infection of humans is rare in western Europe: only 43 human cases were reported in the UK in 1997. There is a minor concern that the rise in European fox populations, due partly to measures taken against rabies, may increase transmission via foxes. *E. granulosus* infection of livestock is associated with pastoral economies (Schantz et al., 1995). The disease is important both from the veterinary point of view, because of the losses of meat, milk and wool production, and from the point of view of human health (Schwabe, 1986). Pathology in human hydatidosis is associated mainly with the pressure exerted by the cyst on the organ inside which it is growing. Frequent complications include cyst rupture and spillage through trauma or surgery, which give rise to the growth of multiple daughter cysts (secondary infection) and, on occasion, also to anaphylactic shock. Therapy almost always involves surgery, often combined with chemotherapy with benzimidazole anthelmintic agents. Diagnosis is done by non-specific imaging techniques, usually in combination with serological tests (reviewed by Amman and Eckert, 1995).

A commercial veterinary or human vaccine against hydatid disease is not available. The control of the disease is feasible and has been achieved in some countries. Successful control campaigns have been based on the restriction of the slaughter of livestock at farm sites (Iceland, New Zealand, Tasmania), the elimination of stray dogs, along with a very strict control of dogs (Cyprus), and on the regular administration of the echinococcicidal drug praziquantel to dogs (Schantz et al., 1995).

In spite of the importance of cystic hydatid disease in many areas of the world and of the lethality of alveolar hydatid disease caused by *E. multi-*

locularis, research on *Echinococcus* lags well behind that on most other important human pathogens, including the helminths of the genus *Schistosoma*, and the filarial nematodes. The *E. granulosus* life cycle cannot be completed in vitro (reviewed by Howell and Smyth, 1995). Genetically defined parasite material is not available and, in fact, most research is carried out on material recovered from natural infections. The two stages of the life cycle which are available for study include: (a) The fully-developed cyst, containing protoscoleces obtained from natural infections (e.g., of cattle), (b) the early cystic stages retrieved from experimental infections (e.g., of mice), (c) worms and eggs obtained from infected dogs, which pose safety problems.

A recent advance in (b) has come from the use of inert diffusion chambers which can be inserted into mouse peritoneum, and protoscoleces subsequently inserted into the chambers. These procedures permit recovery from the chambers of various stages in the differentiation towards cysts, and study of the infiltration of host cells or humoral factors into the chambers (Breijo et al, 1998).

Immunology of the Infection

Various aspects of the immunology of the infection have been reviewed by Rickard and Williams (1982), Craig (1988), Lightowlers (1990, 1996), Nieto et al. (1994), Thompson (1995), Heath (1995) Dixon and Jenkins (1995a,b) and Dixon (1997). The main feature of the host-parasite relationship in hydatid disease is the chronic nature of the infection, which may last nearly as long as the host's lifespan. This chronic infection coexists with readily detectable antibody and cellular responses against parasite antigens. Hydatid disease is an example of the phenomenon known as concomitant immunity. This means that established cysts induce in the host immunity to newly incoming parasites of the same species, while remaining themselves unharmed. Concomitant immunity is not entirely effective, as protoscoleces released by cyst rupture or surgical intervention can establish secondary infections in humans. The most important factor allowing the established cyst to survive the host response is that the laminated membrane acts as a barrier against the infiltration by host cells. The immunology of the disease has been conceptually divided into the immunology of the establishment phase and that of the established cyst: the laying down of the protective laminated layer, thought to take place within the first 2 weeks of infection, sets these two phases apart.

The establishment phase is when the parasite is most susceptible to host attack. Little information is available on the initial events in primary infection; it is known that degeneration of host tissue occurs at the site where the oncosphere penetrates the gut epithelium, and that the parasite then migrates by either blood or lymph to the target organs. Both in primary and in secondary infection, the establishment phase is characterised by cellular infiltration and killing of a significant proportion of the invading parasites. Neutrophils, macrophages and eosinophils can be seen adhering to dying parasites. These latter are too large to allow classical phagocytosis, but once the parasites are killed, phagocytic cells penetrate and ingest their remnants. Surviving parasites in the inoculum are free of host cellular attachment; rather, they cause necrosis of host cells around them. The race between the initial host cellular reaction and the development of the parasite evasion mechanisms determines the success of the infection. Non-specific activation of the host cellular response by inoculation with BCG results in protection against experimental secondary infection. Parasite evasion mechanisms which are likely to be important at this stage, in addition to the evasion of complement discussed below, are the release of molecules which are cytotoxic to host cells and the interference with chemotaxis; some evidence for both of these mechanisms based on in vitro experiments exists.

Priming of the host by an existing infection or by immunisation results in enhanced killing of the parasites during the establishment phase. Impressive degrees of protection, exceeding a 95% reduction in the number of cysts, can be obtained. In primary infection, both in sheep and in a mouse model, the crude extracts most effective at evoking protective immunity are those derived from the oncosphere stage. Immunity can be conferred by passively transferred antibodies. It is thought that complement-fixing antibody, assisted by effector cells, possibly neutrophils, is responsible for immune attrition in primed hosts. Recently, a recombinant protein from a cDNA library of activated *E. granulosus* oncospheres was shown to evoke very high protection in sheep against an oral challenge with oncospheres (Lightowlers et al., 1996).

In the established cyst phase the parasite is much less susceptible to the host immune system. In addition to the protection afforded by the laminated layer, a range of other evasion mechanisms may be in operation. There is evidence for considerable interference with the regulation of the host immune system, including polyclonal activation of B-cells, with hypergammaglobulinemia and lack of antibody avidity maturation. Nevertheless, established cysts can be harmed by the host: the destruction of well developed cysts is not uncommon. Morphologically, cyst destruction is seen as the degeneration of the germinal layer, and sometimes the collapse of the cyst wall into the cyst cavity or the calcification of the lesion. The parasite structures, in particular the laminated layer, never seem to be completely resorbed by the host. Immunologically, the killing of the established cyst has not been traced to any particular immune status, and in fact thriving and degenerated cysts often coexist in the same individual host. There is strong circumstantial evidence that the killing of the established cyst is associated with the lack of resolution of the host local inflammatory response, as discussed below. There is also circumstantial evidence that the live parasite exerts some control over local inflammatory response. This stems from the observations that: (a) *E. granulosus elicits* a relatively weak local host response in comparison, for example, with the *Schistosoma* ovum, another structure of helminth origin lodged in an organ parenchyma; and (b) the local response becomes much more marked when the parasite dies. Various types of interference with the host cytokine system have been documented for several parasites (Riffkin et al. 1996). This may involve abnormal stimulation of host cytokine-secreting cells, or synthesis by the parasite of cytokine or cytokine receptor mimics or antagonists. There is not yet any conclusive evidence for this type of control in *E. granulosus*, but Dixon (1997) has reviewed evidence for two types of cytokine-like activities associated with cysts of related Taeniidae species. One activity appears to mediate the reported mitogenic effects of hydatids. The other impairs the accessory effects of macrophages in lymphoproliferative responses.

The Host-Parasite Interface in the Metacestode (Cyst) Stage

The Hydatid Cyst Wall

The cyst wall consists mainly of the inner germinal layer which can be up to 65µm thick, being generally less developed in sterile cysts (Bortoletti and Ferreti, 1978). The germinal layer tegument is the outermost structure consisting of live parasite tissue. It is a syncytium, connected by cytoplasmic projections to the tegumentary cell bodies situated towards the interior. These cell bodies, which are multinucleated, are intermingled with several other cell types including muscle, glycogen-storing, and undifferentiated cells. The latter give rise to brood capsules and protoscoleces (reviewed by Thompson, 1995).

The outer laminated layer, a structure only found in the genus *Echinococcus,* is considered to be an exaggerated version of the glycocalix found in other cestodes (Richards et al., 1983). It is produced by the germinal layer, apparently by secretion of carbohydrate-rich vesicles generated in the Golgi complex of tegumentary cells, transported up to the tegument, and subsequently released (Richards et al., 1983; Lascano et al., 1975; Richards, 1984; Rogan and Richards, 1989). The laminated layer is composed of dense, irregularly arranged, microfibrillar material in which irregularly shaped, electron-dense bodies are embedded. The structure of the laminated layer is basically the same throughout its depth and the striations observed under optical microscopy, along which the structure is often seen to break up upon manipulation, result from different degrees of compaction of the same components (Morseth, 1967; Rodriguez-Caabeiro and Casado, 1988). Both the fibrillar matrix and the electron-dense bodies stain for carbohydrate histochemically; the fibrillar material also contains protein (Richards, 1984), some of which originates from the host. The mode of assembly of the structure is not understood, but useful clues are the observations by conventional histochemistry that: (a) The protein components appear as mostly basic, while the carbohydrates, though mostly neutral, seem to contain acid (mostly carboxylated) groups, and (b) disulphide bonds are detectable (Richards, 1984). It has been suggested that the structure has a low turnover, a factor which may allow (non-enzymatic) polymerisation to occur (Kilejian et al., 1962). The presence of disulphide bridges has also been proposed to explain the resistance and elasticity of the structure, much as in chitin (Richards, 1984). Excised pieces of the laminated layer can be seen to curve with the opposite concavity as they had in the intact cyst (our unpublished observations), suggesting that the outer strata of the structure are under mechanical tension in vivo.

The laminated layer is permeable to macromolecules. Coltorti and Varela-Díaz (1974) observed that, in vitro, peroxidase (40 kDa) and immunoglobulin G (IgG) penetrated the structure. Hustead and Williams (1977) observed limited and variable uptake of macromolecules into the cyst fluid in vitro (possibly coupled with degradation). Extensive evidence shows that host macromolecules find their way into hydatid cyst fluid in vivo, and do so in an apparently non-specific way. The concentrations of host IgG and albumin are much lower in cyst fluid than in host plasma (by between three and four orders of magnitude; Coltorti and Varela-Díaz, 1972). Total protein concentrations in hydatid cyst fluid vary over a wide range but are much lower than those of host plasma (typically by between two and three orders of magnitude; Benex 1970; Khorsandi and Tabibi, 1978; Hurd, 1988). The overall picture is one of non-selective but restricted passage of proteins across the tegument, perhaps in combination with protein degradation.

It can be assumed that both faces of the parasite germinal layer are exposed to host plasma molecules. However, while the inner face seems to be exposed to low concentrations of host factors, the outer face is probably exposed to concentrations which are very close to those in extracellular fluid. The syncytial tegument of the germinal layer, which is bound by a single unit membrane, is a crucial element of the host–parasite interface.

The polysaccharides of the laminated layer are known to be composed of galactose and amino sugars in approximately equimolar amounts. Within the amino sugars, galactosamine is preponderant over glucosamine (Kilejian et al., 1962; Korc et al., 1967; Kilejian and Schwabe, 1971). A mucopolysaccharide fraction, thought to be represented in the main component of the laminated layer, showed an infrared spectrum similar in some respects to those of chitin, some types of pneumococcal polysaccharide and some blood group carbohydrates (Kilejian et al., 1962). A di-galactosylated carbohydrate epitope reacting with antibodies against the P1 blood group antigen is known to be present in the laminated layer; it is carried both on glycoproteins (Russi et al., 1974) and on glycolipids (Dennis et al., 1993). A detailed analysis of the N-glycans found in the hydatid cyst wall has recently been published (Khoo et al., 1997); the glycans were found to be mostly neutral, and in some respects to be more reminiscent of "conventional" mammalian structures than of those found in some other invertebrates.

The Host Local Response Outside the Laminated Layer

The hydatid cyst is often described, simplistically, as being surrounded by a host collagenous capsule ("adventitious layer"), outside which mild local inflammation may occur. This picture arises mostly from studies in human infection (see for example Muffarij et al., 1990). However, the local reaction to the cyst shows, across different hosts, organs and cyst sizes and shapes, a continuous spectrum of morphologies, which ranges from a fairly intense granulomatous-type response to a reaction limited to the non-infiltrated collagenous capsule (reviewed by Smyth and Heath, 1970, and by Thompson, 1995). The latter type of situation is the product of the resolution of inflammation. Resolution takes place nearly always in humans, less generally in sheep and pigs, and least often in cattle. Across the spectrum of host responses, cyst fertility correlates with resolution of inflammation, while intense responses are associated with infertility and, more extremely, degeneration of the cysts.

The inflammatory response is typically three-layered. The innermost layer is composed of epithelioid cells and giant multinucleated cells, disposed radially with respect to the cyst. These cells are in close contact with the laminated layer, but sometimes an area of necrosis is observed in between (Thomas and Khotare, 1975). The second layer out, commonly referred to as "microcellular infiltrate", is composed of lymphocytes, small numbers of eosinophils and possibly monocytes. On the outside is the collagenous layer, in which fibroblasts lay down what may, upon resolution of inflammation, become the collagenous capsule. The two outer layers are not always separated by a sharp boundary. On the outside of the area of inflammation, the host organ parenchyma is generally minimally disrupted.

A recent biochemical survey of the major host or parasite proteins and glycoproteins localised in the hydatid cyst wall of cysts derived from cattle provided extensive information on the major biosynthetic activities and secretions of the host cells surrounding the cyst (Díaz, 1997; Díaz et al., 1997; 1998 a, b). Cysts were obtained from cattle and host tissue dissected away. The cyst laminated layer and germinal layer were subjected to a series of extraction procedures, including detergents and acidic and denaturing washes to extract strongly-bound macromolecules (Díaz et al., 1997). Among several proteins and glycoproteins extracted, four host proteins were particularly abundant. These included host IgG, complement Factor H (discussed below), cathepsin K and annexin II.

The recently cloned cysteine proteinase cathepsin K has aroused great interest as the main effector in the digestion of extracellular matrix during bone resorption by osteoclasts. The enzyme has strong digestive activity against extracellular matrix components and is a highly regulated effector, rather than a "housekeeping" lysosomal enzyme. It is expressed in osteoclasts in all the mammalian species where it has been studied. Díaz et al. (1998a) have shown that cathepsin K is associated with a superficially very different process: the granulomatous reaction against persistent pathogens or foreign bodies. Cathepsin K is produced in vivo in cattle in the reaction against *Echinococcus granulosus.* It is associated with the outer wall of the parasite cyst and was identified by N-terminal sequencing and Western blotting. Cathepsin K was shown by immunohistochemistry to derive from the epithelioid and giant multinucleated cells elicited by the parasite. These inflammatory cells are specialised types of activated macrophages which are the hallmarks of granuloma; inflammatory giant cells have long been noted to be related to osteoclasts. This strongly suggests that the mechanism by which the body attempts to digest persistent unwanted material is closely related to the physiological mechanism employed in bone resorption. Cathepsin K may be a major effector in the tissue destruction often associated with uncontrolled granulomatous inflammation.

Annexin II is a 36-kDa, mostly intracellular protein composed of a 3-kDa N-terminal domain and a 33-kDa C-terminal core composed of four annexin repeats, (reviewed by Raynal and Pollard, 1994; Moss, 1997). Annexin II, identified as an abundant protein in the hydatid cyst wall by N-terminal sequencing and Western blotting (Díaz et al., 1998 b), most probably derives from the local host inflammatory reaction as it is not an abundant plasma protein (Raynal and Pollard, 1994). The striking amount of annexin II found in the hydatid cyst wall may play a role in the host–parasite relationship. Annexin II has been shown to have antiinflammatory and anticoagulant activities (reviewed by Raynal and Pollard, 1994), associated with the sequestration of phospholipids. The amounts of annexin II present in the hydatid cyst wall could be locally antiinflammatory in vivo, provided that the phospholipid-binding site was left vacant by the mode of binding of the protein to the cyst wall components. Low-affinity IgG-Fc receptor activity in the human placenta has also been reported for extracellular annexin II (Kristoffersen et al., 1994). It is conceivable that part of the IgG found to be associated with the hydatid cyst wall may be bound through its Fc region to annexin II. Extracellular annexin II also plays an important role in the calcification of cartilage (Genge et al., 1992) by virtue of its Ca^{2+}-binding properties. The release of this protein by the host inflammatory reaction and its retention by the parasite hydatid cyst wall may contribute to calcification, an outcome often associated with an intense local response to the cysts (Rao and Mohiyuddin, 1974; Slais and Vanek, 1980).

Thus, the presence of both cathepsin K and annexin II in the hydatid cyst wall extracts suggest that the host uses mechanisms related to bone resorption and deposition as a response to a persistent foreign body.

Echinococcus granulosus and the Host Complement System

The complement system is a very important component of immune defense against infection (for review see Sim and Malhorta, 1994; Law and Reid, 1995). It is part of the innate (non-adaptive) immune system and can respond to challenges by microorganisms before an adaptive immune response has developed. Complement promotes and regulates the phagocytosis or lysis of foreign cells, particles or macromolecules and host tissue breakdown products.

The human complement system is composed of more than 30 proteins, both soluble (in blood plasma and other body fluids) and membrane-bound (on blood cells and other tissues), that interact with each other when the system is activated by various stimuli (Fig. 1). The cell-surface proteins act either as receptors for fragments of soluble complement proteins, or as regulatory proteins which control the activities of soluble complement proteins and protect the host cells on which they are situated from attack by complement.

In addition to its role in innate immunity, complement interacts with the adaptive immune system in several ways. These include recognition and activation of complement by antibody–antigen complexes, roles in regulating B-lymphocyte activity and participation in localisation of some antigens to antigen-presenting cells.

Various proteins of the complement system detect "targets" and bind to these targets, usually by mechanisms which involve recognition of patterns of distribution of charge or of carbohydrate on the surface of the target. There are two major routes of recognition and activation, referred to as the classical and alternative pathways. Binding of complement proteins to the targets results in activation of the complement system and to the formation, on the target, of unstable protease complexes (the C3 convertases). The C3

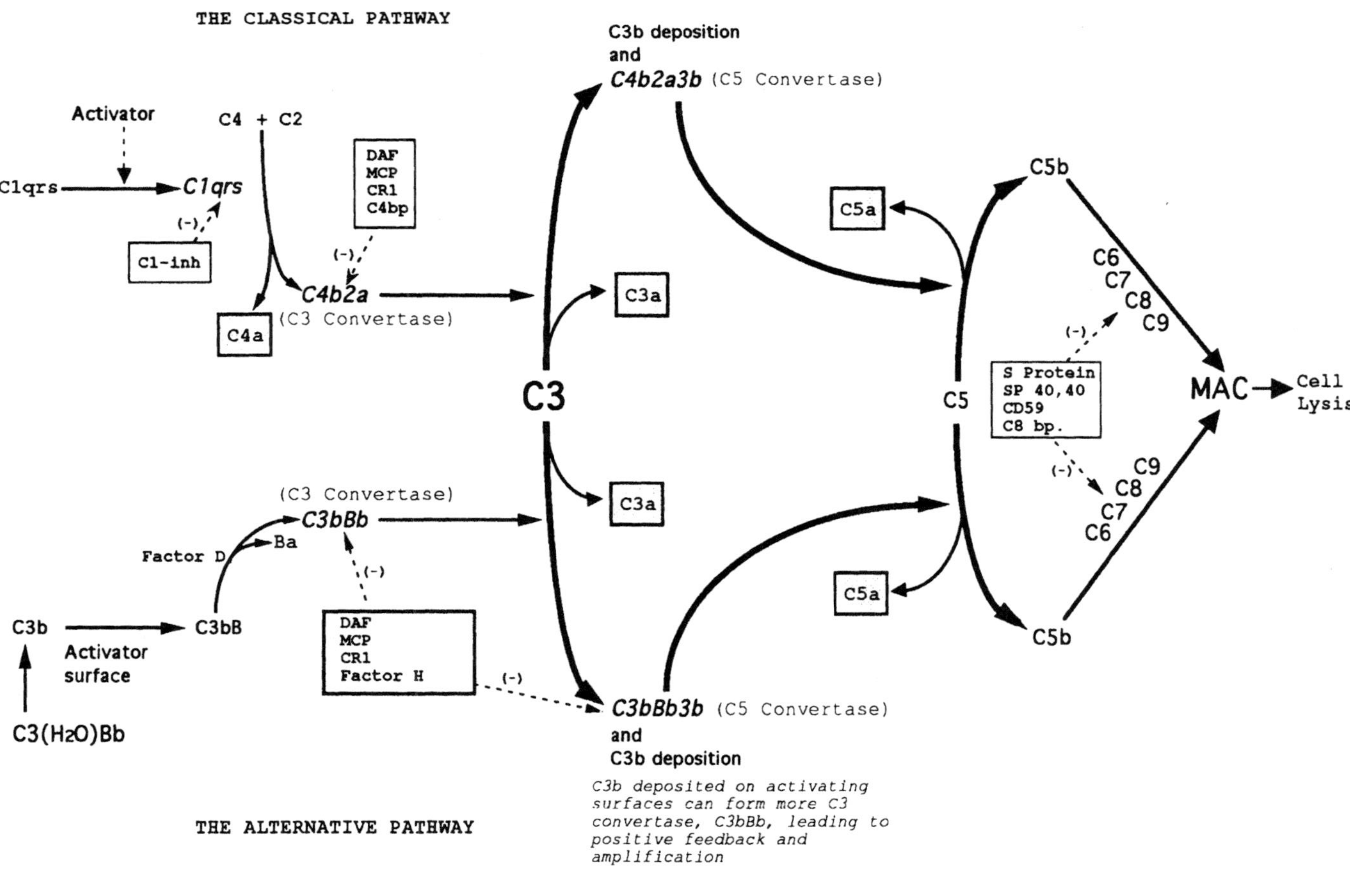
THE CLASSICAL PATHWAY
Activator
C4 + C2
C3b deposition
and
C4b2a3b (C5 Convertase)
C1qrs
C1qrs
(-)
C1-inh
DAF
MCP
CR1
C4bp
(-)
C4b2a
(C3 Convertase)
C4a
C3a
C5a
C5b
C6
C7
C8
C9
(-)
S Protein
SP 40,40
CD59
C8 bp.
MAC
Cell Lysis
C3
C5
(-)
C9
C8
C7
C6
(C3 Convertase)
C3bBb
C3a
Factor D
Ba
(-)
C3b
Activator
surface
C3bB
DAF
MCP
CR1
Factor H
(-)
C5a
C5b
C3(H2O)Bb
C3bBb3b (C5 Convertase)
and
C3b deposition
C3b deposited on activating
surfaces can form more C3
convertase, C3bBb, leading to
positive feedback and
amplification
THE ALTERNATIVE PATHWAY

convertases (named C4b2a or C3bBb) of both complement pathways are each made up of two protein components. One component is covalently bound to the surface of the complement activator and the other is a serine protease which is able to cleave and activate C3, the most abundant complement component. The major fragment of activated C3, C3b, binds covalently to complement-activating surfaces (e.g. cells, viruses, immune complexes). When large amounts of C3b or its proteolytic breakdown product, iC3b, have been deposited on activating surfaces, phagocytosis of the coated substance is greatly enhanced. This occurs partly through the interaction of the surface-bound C3 fragments with C3 receptors located on phagocytic cells. If the complement activator has a lipid bilayer, lysis can also occur through interaction with the membrane of components C5–9, which bind together to form the membrane attack complex (MAC). The major, well-established in vivo activities of complement are opsonisation/phagocytosis and cell lysis as well as roles in the control of vascular permeability and neutrophil chemotaxis. A complement system similar to the human system occurs in all mammals examined, and variants of the system occur in all other vertebrate classes. Since complement has the capacity to damage host tissues if inappropriately activated, the system has many down regulatory control proteins to prevent prolonged activation. Particularly important among these is a group of homologous proteins encoded in the "regulation of complement activation" gene cluster on human chromosome 1. These include Factor H, CR1, MCP, DAF and C4bp, which all down-regulate C3 turnover by destabilising the C3bBb and C4b2a enzymes which cleave C3.

As a tissue-dwelling pathogen, *E. granulosus* is exposed to complement for almost all its existence in the intermediate host. Before cyst establishment, all the main recognised effects of complement activation, i.e. opsonisation, damage to cell membranes and induction of inflammation, are likely to be detrimental to the parasite. Once the laminated layer is laid down, opsonisation may be of little significance, but cell membrane attack and induction of inflammation have the potential to damage the parasite. From evidence for a major role of covalently deposited C3d in enhancing the immunogenicity of T-cell-dependent antigens (Dempsey et al., 1996), complement deposition on parasite molecules could have major effects on the acquired immune response.

◀ **Fig. 1.** The complement system. Complement is activated by various stimuli which trigger either the classical or alternative pathway, or both. A third activation mechanism, sometimes called the lectin pathway, is very similar to the classical pathway, except that the protein mannose-binding lectin replaces C1q and the serine proteases, MASP-1 and MASP-2, replace C1r and C1s. The complement system is highly regulated, to prevent damage to host tissue. Host regulatory proteins (*Factor H, DAF, CD59*, etc.) are shown in *boxes*. *MAC*, membrane attack complex

In vitro, protoscoleces (Herd, 1976; Kassis and Tanner, 1976a; Rickard et al., 1977) and adult worms (Herd, 1976) are readily destroyed by complement in normal serum from humans and various other mammalian species. Killing, which results from extensive tegumental damage, follows alternative pathway activation by the parasite surface (Herd, 1976; Rickard et al., 1977; Ferreira et al., 1992). Recent in vivo experiments on secondary infection in normal mice (Ferreira et al., 1998) and mice deficient in the complement protein C5 showed that the normal mice exhibited greater resistance to infection, and larger cysts developed in the C5-deficient mice. This suggests that C5-mediated mechanisms are detrimental to the growth of establishing cysts. Analysis of cell types recovered from the peritoneal cavity of mice showed that by day 10 post infection only C5-sufficient mice exhibited a significant infiltration of eosinophils. These results suggest that C5a-mediated eosinophil infiltration may contribute to restrict the establishment of infection and could also be involved in controlling cyst growth. Similarly, complement depletion causes exacerbated parasite burdens in secondary *E. multilocularis* infection in cotton rats (Kassis and Tanner, 1977). Oncospheres are also sensitive to complement-mediated killing.

Protoscoleces seem to develop resistance to lysis as they lose their hooks and vesiculate in vitro, developing into cysts (Kassis and Tanner, 1976a). It has been suggested (Rickard et al., 1977) that this is the result of shedding of the protoscolex glycocalix, which is known to be denser at the posterior end of the organism, where complement lysis is seen to start in vitro (Rau and Tanner, 1976). Protoscoleces inside brood capsules are still lysed when incubated with serum, but those inside intact cysts are protected (Kassis and Tanner, 1976a). Substitution of the cyst fluid by 20% normal host serum in vivo does not kill the cysts, showing that the inside-facing cell surfaces of the germinal layer are resistant to complement attack. The survival of the cyst in vivo requires that the outward-facing germinal layer tegument is also resistant to near-physiological concentrations of complement, as well as specific antibodies.

As noted above, the host complement regulatory protein Factor H becomes concentrated in the hydatid cyst wall of cysts isolated from cattle (Díaz et al., 1997). Factor H is a powerful down-regulator of complement activation, as it destabilises the complex protease, C3bBb, which cleaves C3. Limiting the cleavage of C3 limits the generation of opsonic capacity and, perhaps more importantly in this system, the generation of inflammatory and chemotactic peptides (C3a and C5a). Thus, the parasite makes use of the host's own complement regulators to control complement activation on the parasite surface. There are several known examples of sequestration or mimicry of host complement control proteins by microrganisms (Fishelson, 1991, 1994; Joiner, 1988). Further studies are required to elucidate why Factor H localises in the hydatid cyst wall: it may interact with glycosaminoglycan-like structures or other macromolecules.

In a wide-ranging survey of potential mechanisms of complement control by cysts (Díaz, 1997; Díaz et al., 1998c), no evidence was obtained for a serpin-like control protein (like the complement regulator C1-inhibitor), but a further mechanism controlling formation of the protease C3bBb was found. This is a potent activity which prevents interaction of complement Factor B with C3b.

Overall, the available information is compatible with the existence of parasite mechanisms of evasion of complement which may be poorly or not expressed in the infective stages and may be upregulated during the development towards the cyst stage.

There may be further regulatory mechanisms at various stages of parasite development which interfere with the membrane attack complex (C5b–9) as suggested by Irigoín et al. (1996). There is considerable further information on possible complement evasion molecules in *E. granulosus* which may work by complement depletion: that is, they activate complement at sites not immediately adjacent to the parasite surface, thereby depleting complement without damaging the parasite. This type of activity was first observed in lysed protoscoleces (Kassis and Tanner, 1976a) and is present in hydatid cyst fluid, where it is mostly associated with parasite-derived high molecular weight carbohydrate-rich components (Hammerberg et al., 1977; Ferreira and Nieto 1992; Ferreira et al., 1995). Activation takes place mostly through the alternative pathway and generates C5b6 complex and membrane attack complex in solution (Ferreira et al., 1992, 1995). In addition, part of the complement-activating capacity of hydatid cyst fluid is due to immune complexes (Ferreira and Nieto, 1992). Activation by protoscolex products is also associated with very high molecular weight, neutral carbohydrate-rich components (Irigoín et al., 1997). The host's systemic complement levels are not significantly depressed during infection, either in humans (Bajeva et al., 1995), or in mice inoculated with protoscoleces (Díaz et al., 1995). However, it seems likely that local depletion in the vicinity of an infective inoculum or within hydatid cyst fluid plays a role in vivo, as proposed by Kassis and Tanner (1976 a, b). Soluble extracts of the hydatid cyst wall obtained by sonication were, in contrast, found to be very poor activators of complement compared to similar extracts from protoscoleces and to hydatid cyst fluid (Irigoín et al., 1996). Thus upon development into a cyst, the parasite deploys a host-exposed surface structure (cyst wall) which in inert towards complement.

Acknowledgements. The authors' work was funded by the European Union International Scientific Cooperation programme through grant CI1*-CT93-0307, and by the UK Medical Research Council. A.D. was additionally supported by scholarships from the Consejo Nacional de Investigaciones Científicas y Técnicas (CONICYT, Ministry of Education, Uruguay) and the Comisión Sectorial de Investigación Científica (CSIC, University of Uruguay).

References

Ammann R, Eckert J (1995) Clinical diagnosis and treatment of echinococcosis in humans. In: Thompson RCA, Lymbery AJ (eds) Echinococcus and hydatid disease. CAB International, Wallingford, UK, pp 411–464

Baveja UK, Basak S, Thusoo TK (1995) A study of immune profile in human hydatid diseases. Journal of Communicable Diseases 27:61–69

Benex J (1970) Analyse et évaluation de divers antigènes extraits de kystes d'Echinococcus granulosus. Annals de l'Institut Pasteur 118:49–60

Bortoletti G, Ferreti G (1978) Ultrastructural aspects of fertile and sterile cysts of Echinococcus granulosus developed in hosts of different species. International Journal for Parasitology 8:421–431

Breijo M, Spinelli P, Sim RB, Ferreira AM (1998) Echinococcus granulosus: an intraperitoneal diffusion chamber model of secondary infection in mice. Experimental Parasitology, in press

Coltorti EA, Varela-Díaz VM (1972) IgG levels and host specificity in hydatid cyst fluid. Journal of Parasitology 58:753–756

Coltorti EA, Varela-Díaz VM (1974) Echinococcus granulosus: penetration of macromolecules and their localization on the parasite membranes of cysts. Experimental Parasitology 35:225–231

Craig PS (1988) Immunology of human hydatid disease. In: ISI Atlas of Science: Immunology:95–100. Institute for Scientific Information, Philadelphia, p 95

Dempsey PW, Allison MED, Akkaraju S, Goodnow CC, Fearon DT (1996) C3d of complement as a molecular adjuvant: bridging innate and acquired immunity. Science 271:348–350

Dennis RD, Baumeister S, Irmer G, Gasser RB, Geyer E (1993) Chromatographic and antigenic properties of Echinococcus granulosus hydatid cyst-derived glycolipids. Parasite Immunology 15:669–681

Díaz AJ (1997) A search for mechanisms restricting activation of the host complement system in Echinococcus granulosus. D Phil thesis, University of Oxford, UK

Díaz A, Ferreira AM, Nieto A (1995) Echinococcus granulosus: Interactions with host complement in secondary infection in mice. Experimental Parasitology 80:473–482

Díaz A, Ferreira AM, Sim RB (1997) Complement evasion by Echinococcus granulosus: sequestration of host factor H in the hydatid cyst wall. J Immunol 158:3779–3786

Díaz A, Willis AC, Sim RB (1998a) Evidence that physiological bone resorption and pathological granulomatous inflammation make use of common degradative mechanisms. Submitted

Díaz A, Willis AC, Sim RB (1998b) Host annexin II in the Echinococcus granulosus hydatid cyst wall. Submitted

Díaz A, Irigoín F, Sim RB (1998c) A heat-stable inhibitor of factor B activation from the parasite Echinococcus granulosus. (Abstract) Molecular Immunology, in press

Dixon JB, Jenkins P (1995a) Immunology of mammalian metacestode infections. II. Antigens, protective immunity and immunopathology. Helminthological Abstracts 64:533–542

Dixon JB, Jenkins P (1995b) Immunology of mammalian metacestode infections. II. Immune recognition and effector function. Helminthological Abstracts 64:599–613

Dixon JB (1997) Echinococcosis. Comparative Immunology and Microbiology of Infectious Diseases. 20:87–94

Ferreira A, Nieto A (1992) Preliminary characterisation of anticomplementary components of hydatid cyst fluid. International Journal for Parasitology 22:113–115

Ferreira A, Trecu T, Reisin I (1992) Echinococcus granulosus: Study of the in vitro complement activation by protoscoleces by measuring the electric potential difference across the tegumental membrane. Experimental Parasitology 75:259–268

Ferreira AM, Würzner R, Hobart MJ, Lachmann PJ (1995) Study of the in vitro activation of the complement alternative pathway by Echinococcus granulosus hydatid cyst fluid. Parasite Immunology 17:245–251

Ferreira A, Breijo M, Sim RB, Nieto A (1998) Contribution of C5-mediated mechanisms to host defense against the parasite Echinococcus granulosus. (Abstract) Molecular Immunology, in press

Fishelson Z (1991) Complement evasion by parasites: search for "Achilles heel". Clinical and Experimental Immunology 86 (Suppl 1):47–52

Fishelson Z (1994) Complement-related proteins in pathogenic organisms. Springer Seminars in Immunopathology 15:345–368

Genge BR, Cao X, Wu LNY, Buzzi WR, Showman RW, Arsenault AL, Ishikawa Y, Wuthier RE (1992) Establishment of the primary structure of the major lipid and calcium-ion binding proteins of chicken growth plate cartilage vesicles; identity with annexin V and annexin II. J Bone Mineral Res 7:807–819

Hammerberg B, Musoke AJ, Williams JF (1977) Activation of complement by hydatid cyst fluid of Echinococcus granulosus. Journal of Parasitology 63:327–331

Heath DD (1995) Immunology of Echinococcus infections. In: Thompson RCA, Lymbery AJ (eds) Echinococcus and hydatid disease. CAB International, Wallingford, UK, pp 183–200

Herd RP (1976) The cestoicidal effect of complement in normal and immune sera in vitro. Parasitology 72:3225–3234

Howell MJ, Smyth JD (1995) Maintenance and cultivation of Echinococcus species in vivo and in vitro. In: Thompson RCA, Lymbery AJ (eds) Echinococcus and hydatid disease. CAB International, Wallingford, UK, pp 201–232

Hurd H (1988) Echinococcus granulosus: a comparison of free amino acid concentration in hydatid fluid from primary and secondary cysts and host plasma. Parasitology 98:135–143

Husted ST, Williams JF (1977) Permeability studies on taeniid metacestodes: I. Uptake of proteins by larval stages of Taenia taeniaeformis, T. crassiceps, and Echinococcus granulosus. Journal of Parasitology 63:314–321

Irigoín F, Würtzner R, Sim RB, Ferreira A (1996) Comparison of complement activation in vitro by different Echinococcus granulosus extracts. Parasite Immunology 18:371–375

Irigoín F, Dell A, Nieto A, Sim RB, Ferreira A (1997) Preliminary characterisation of complement activator carbohydrates from the metacestode of Echinococcus granulosus. Abstr Ninth European Carbohydrate Symp, p 419

Joiner KA (1988) Complement evasion by bacteria and parasites. Annual Review of Microbiology 42:201–230

Kassis AI, Tanner CE (1976a) The role of complement in hydatid disease: in vitro studies. International Journal for Parasitology 6:25–35

Kassis AI, Tanner CE (1976b) Novel approach to the treatment of hydatid disease. Nature 262:588

Kassis AI, Tanner CE (1977) Echinococcus multilocularis: Complement's role in vivo in hydatid disease. Experimental Parasitology 43:390–395

Khoo K-H, Nieto A, Morris HR, Dell A (1997) Structural characterisation of the N-glycans from Echinococcus granulosus hydatid cyst membrane and protoscoleces. Molecular and Biochemical Parasitology 86:237–248

Khorsandi HO, Tabibi V (1978) Similarities of human hydatid cyst fluid components and the host serum. Acta Medica Iranica 21:161–172

Kilejian A, Schwabe CW (1971) Studies on the polysaccharides of the Echinococcus granulosus cyst, with observations on a possible mechanism for laminated membrane formation. Comparative Biochemistry and Physiology 40B:25–36

Kilejian A, Sauer K, Schwabe CW (1962) Host-parasite relationship in echinococcosis. VIII. Infrared spectra and chemical composition of the hydatid cyst. Experimental Parasitology 12:377–392

Korc I, Hierro J, Lasalvia E, Falco M, Calcagno M (1967) Chemical characterisation of the polysaccharide of the hydatid membrane of Echinococcus granulosus. Experimental Parasitology 20:219–224

Kristoffersen EK, Ulvestad E, Bjørge L, Aarli A, Matre R (1994) Fcγ-Receptor activity of placental annexin II. Scandinavian Journal of Immunology 40:237–242

Lascano EF, Coltorti EA, Varela-Díaz VM (1975) Fine structure of the germinal membrane of Echinococcus granulosus cysts. Journal of Parasitology 61:853–860

Law SKA, Reid KBM (1995) Complement. IRL Press at Oxford University Press, Oxford, UK

Lightowlers MW (1990) Immunology and molecular biology of Echinococcus infections. International Journal for Parasitology 20:471–478

Lightowlers MW (1996) Vaccination against cestode parasites. International Journal for Parasitology 26:819–824

Lightowlers MW, Lawrence SB, Gauci CG, Young J, Ralston MJ, Maas D, Heath DD (1996) Vaccination against hydatidosis using a defined recombinant antigen. Parasite Immunology 18:457–462

Morseth DJ (1967) Fine structure of the hydatid cyst and protoscolex of Echinococcus granulosus. Journal of Parasitology 53:312–325

Moss SE (1997) Annexins. Trends Cell Biol 7:87–89

Mufarrij AA, Arnaut A, Meshefedjian G, Matossian RM (1990) Comparative histopathological study in the hepatic and pulmonary human hydatidosis. Helminthologia 27:279–290

Nieto A, Fernández C, Ferreira AM, Díaz A, Baz A, Bentancor A, Casabó L, Dematteis S, Irigoín F, Marco M, Míguez M (1994) Mechanisms of evasion of host immune response by E. granulosus. In: Ehrlich R, Nieto A (eds) Biology of Parasitism. Ediciones Trilce, Montevideo, Uruguay, pp 85–98

Rao DG, Mohiyuddin S (1974) Incidence of hydatid cyst in bovines and histopathological changes of pulmonary tissue in hydatidosis. Indian Journal of Animal Science 44:437–440

Rau ME, Tanner CE (1976) Echinococcus multilocularis in the cotton rat. The in vitro protoscolecidal activity of peritoneal exudate cells. International Journal for Parasitology 6:195–198

Raynal P, Pollard HB (1994) Annexins: the problem of assessing the biological role for a gene family of multifunctional calcium- and phospholipid-binding proteins. Biochimica et Biophysica Acta 1197:63–93

Richards KS (1984) Echinococcus granulosus equinus: the histochemistry of the laminated layer of the hydatid cyst. Folia histochemica et Cytobiologia 22:21–23

Richards KS, Arme C, Bridges JF (1983) Echinococcus granulosus equinus: an ultrastructural study of the laminated layer, including changes on incubating cysts in various media. Parasitology 86:399–405

Rickard MD, Williams JF (1982) Hydatidosis/Cysticercosis: Immune mechanisms and immunization against infection. Advances in Parasitology 21:229–296

Rickard MD, Davies C, Bout DT, Smyth JD (1977) Immunohistological localisation of two hydatid antigens (antigen 5 and antigen B) in the cyst wall, brood capsules and protoscoleces of Echinococcus granulosus (ovine and equine) and E. multilocularis using immunoperoxidase methods. Journal of Helminthology 51:359–364

Riffkin M, Seow HF, Jackson D, Brown L, Wood P (1996) Defence against the immune barrage. Helminth survival strategies. Immunol Cell Biol 74:564–574

Rodríguez-Caabeiro F, Casado N (1988) Evidence of in vitro germinal layer development in Echinococcus granulosus cysts. Parasitology Research 74:558–562

Rogan MT, Richards KS (1989) Development of the tegument of Echinococcus granulosus (Cestoda) protoscoleces during cystic differentiation in vivo. Parasitology Research 75:299–306

Russi S, Siracusano A, Vicari G (1974) Isolation and characterization of a blood P_1 active carbohydrate antigen of Echinococcus granulosus cyst membrane. Comparative Biochemistry and Physiology 40B:25–36

Schantz PM, Chai J, Craig PS, Eckert J, Jenkins DJ, McPherson CNL, Thakur A (1995) Epidemiology and control of hydatid disease. In: Thompson RCA, Lymbery AJ (eds) Echinococcus and Hydatid Disease. CAB International, Wallingford, UK, pp 233–332

Schwabe CW (1986) Current status of hydatid disease: a zoonosis of increasing importance. In: Thompson RCA (ed) The Biology of Echinococcus and hydatid disease. Allen and Unwin, London, UK, pp 81–113

Sim RB, Malhotra R (1994) Interactions of carbohydrates and lectins with complement. Biochem Soc Trans 22:106–111

Slais J, Vanek M (1980) Tissue reaction to spherical and lobular hydatid cysts of Echinococcus granulosus (Batsch, 1786). Folia Parasitologica (Praha) 27:135–143

Smyth JD, Heath DD (1970) Pathogenesis of larval cestodes in mammals. Helminthological Abstracts 39:1–22

Thomas JA, Kothare SN (1975) Tissue response in hydatidosis. Indian Journal of Medical Research 63:1761–1766

Thompson RCA (1995) Biology and systematics of Echinococcus. In: Thompson RCA, Lymbery AJ (eds) Echinococcus and Hydatid Disease. CAB International, Wallingford, UK, pp 1–50

Endo- and Exotoxins and Soluble Receptors

Nitric Oxide, Systemic Inflammatory Response Syndrome and Circulatory Shock

C. THIEMERMANN

Systemic Inflammatory Response Syndrome (SIRS) and Septic Shock

The medical syndrome of shock can be defined as a "progressive failure of the circulation to provide blood and oxygen to vital organs of the body". In clinical practice, the key symptom of shock is a severe fall in blood pressure which is often associated with the dysfunction or failure of several important organs including lung, kidney, liver and brain. The most common cause of shock is the contamination of blood with bacteria (bacteremia), viruses, fungi or parasites, resulting in systemic infection and ultimately shock (septic shock). Other causes of shock include severe hemorrhage (hemorrhagic shock), trauma (traumatic shock), failure of the heart to maintain a sufficient cardiac output (cardiogenic shock), interruption of the innervation of blood vessels (neurogenic shock) and severe allergic reactions (anaphylactic shock). Septic shock, regardless of its aetiology, is defined as sepsis (systemic response to infection) with hypotension despite adequate fluid replacement, resulting in impaired tissue perfusion and oxygen extraction (Parrillo, 1990). The definition of septic shock is independent of the presence or absence of a multiple organ dysfunction syndrome (MODS), which is defined as impaired organ function such that homeostasis cannot be maintained without intervention (Baue, 1993). Primary MODS is a direct result of a well-defined insult to a specific organ. Secondary MODS occurs as a consequence of an exaggerated host response, termed systemic inflammatory response syndrome (SIRS). Current therapeutic approaches to septic shock include antimicrobial chemotherapy, volume replacement, inotropic and vasopressor support, oxygen therapy and mechanical ventilation, as well as hemodialysis and hemofiltration. These, however, have failed to make a substantial impact on the high mortality associated with septic shock (Nathanson et al., 1994) and, hence, septic shock remains the major cause of death in non-coronary intensive care units with an estimated mortality ranging between 50% and 80%. As shock is also by far the most common cause of prolonged admission to an intensive care unit, the clinical and socio-economic importance of this illness is substantial. Numerous clinical trials which have evaluated the effects of potential novel therapeutic interventions in patients

Symposium in Immunology VIII
Eibl/Huber/Peter/Wahn (Eds.)
© Springer Verlag Berlin Heidelberg 1999

with septic shock have (at best) demonstrated a 5% reduction in 28-day mortality. Interestingly, in trials with more than 300 patients, this benefit has consistently been demonstrated using a variety of drugs which interfere with different aspects of the pathophysiology of septic shock [e.g. antibodies against tumor necrosis factor (TNF)α, interleukin (IL)-1 receptor antagonist, platelet activating factor receptor antagonists, to name but a few] (Charles Nathanson, personal communication). This chapter reviews the role of endogenous nitric oxide (NO) in the pathophysiology of SIRS and septic shock and discusses the effects and side effects of inhibitors of the formation of NO in animals and man.

Physiological Roles of Nitric Oxide

Nitric oxide is generated from L-arginine by a family of enzymes collectively called NO synthases. The synthesis of NO from L-arginine and molecular oxygen involves, firstly, the generation of N^G-hydroxy-L-arginine and water and, subsequently, the oxidation of N^G-hydroxy-L-arginine in the presence of molecular oxygen to form NO, L-citrulline and water. When generated, NO diffuses to adjacent cells where it activates soluble guanylate cyclase, resulting in the formation of cyclic guanosine monophosphate (cGMP), which in turn mediates many (but not all) of the effects of NO. NO is generated by many mammalian cells by at least three different isoforms of nitric oxide synthase (NOS). The NOS in endothelial cells (eNOS or NOS III) and neuronal cells (nNOS or NOS I) are expressed constitutively, and both enzymes require an increase in intracellular calcium for activation. Activation of macrophages and many other cells with pro-inflammatory cytokines or endotoxin results in the expression of a distinct isoform of NOS (inducible NOS; iNOS or NOS II), the activity of which is functionally independent of changes in intracellular calcium (see Nathan, 1992; Dinerman et al., 1993; Moncada and Higgs, 1993; Morris and Billiar, 1993; Thiemermann, 1994; Szabo and Thiemermann, 1995 for review). Thus, it is not surprising that NO has many biological functions in the cardiovascular, nervous and immune systems. For instance, activation of eNOS by shear stress results in a continuous release of picomolar amounts of NO which helps to regulate blood pressure and organ blood flow by causing vasodilatation and opposing the effects of circulating catecholamines. NO also reduces the adhesion of platelets and polymorphonuclear leukocytes (PMNs) to the endothelium (Moncada and Higgs, 1993). The latter effect of NO is, at least in part, due to the prevention by NO of the expression of the adhesion molecules P-selectin and intercellular adhesion molecule (ICAM-1) on the surface of endothelial cells (see Loscalzo and Welch, 1995).

Role of Nitric Oxide in the Pathophysiology of Septic Shock

In 1990, we reported that the hypotension caused by endotoxin in the rat was attenuated by the NOS inhibitor N^G-methyl-L-arginine (L-NMMA). In this publication we concluded that an enhanced formation of NO contributes to the hypotension caused by endotoxin and proposed that inhibitors of NO formation may be useful in the therapy of circulatory shock (Thiemermann and Vane, 1990). Similarly, Dr Kilbourn and colleagues reported that an enhanced formation of NO also contributes to the hypotension caused by TNF and endotoxin in the dog (Kilbourn et al., 1990 a, b). In addition, an enhanced formation of NO also accounts for the vascular hyporesponsiveness to vasoconstrictor agents (also termed vasoplegia) caused by endotoxin (Julou-Schaeffer et al., 1990; Rees et al., 1990). The finding that NOS inhibitors caused liver injury in certain models of endotoxemia provided the first evidence that inhibition of NOS activity may also lead to the generation of side effects (Billiar et al., 1990). We know today that an enhanced formation of NO not only contributes to the circulatory failure, but also to many other aspects of the pathophysiology of circulatory shock (Fig. 1). The overproduction of NO in animal models of circulatory shock is due to an early activation of eNOS (which is transient) and the delayed induction of iNOS activity in macrophages (host defense), vascular smooth muscle (hypotension, vascular hyporeactivity, maldistribution of blood flow) and parenchymal cells

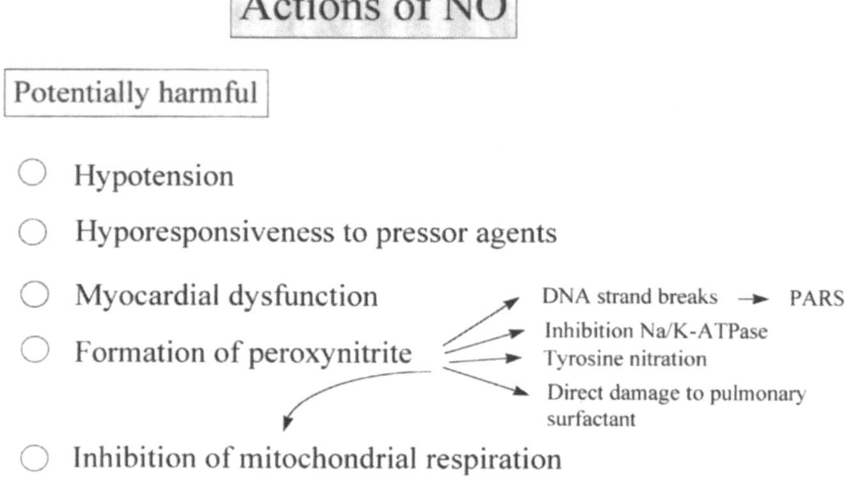

Fig. 1. Potentially harmful effect of nitric oxide (*NO*) in animals and man with systemic inflammatory response syndrome and septic shock

Table 1. The possible beneficial and adverse effects of inhibitors of nitric oxide synthase in septic shock

Beneficial	Adverse
Increased blood pressure	Excessive vasoconstriction
Restores responsiveness to pressor agents	Pulmonary hypertension
Cardiac output return to baseline values	Fall in cardiac output
Decreased production of peroxynitrite	Increased platelet adhesiveness
Attenuation of inhibition of mitochondrial respiration	Increased neutrophil adhesion
Improved organ function	Worsened organ function
Improved survival	

(see Thiemermann, 1997). The finding that mice in which the iNOS gene has been inactivated by gene-targeting (iNOS knockout mice) exhibit only a minor fall in blood pressure when challenged with endotoxin (MacMicking et al., 1995; Wei et al., 1995) also supports the hypothesis that an overproduction of NO by iNOS contributes to the circulatory failure in septic shock. It is less clear whether increased formation of NO also contributes to the organ injury and dysfunction caused by endotoxin. The formation of NO by eNOS (and potentially also by iNOS) also exerts beneficial effects in shock including vasodilatation, prevention of platelet and leukocyte adhesion, maintenance of microcirculatory blood flow and augmentation of host defence. Thus, it is not surprising that basic and clinical scientists have advocated the use of contrasting therapeutic approaches including inhibition of NOS activity, enhancement of the availability of NO (NO donors, NO inhalation) or a combination of both approaches. The following paragraphs highlight some of the effects and side effects of inhibitors of NOS activity (Table 1) in animal models of septic shock. For a more detailed review of: (a) the many roles of NO in the pathophysiology of septic (or other forms of shock), (b) the mechanisms leading to the induction of iNOS (Fig. 2) and (c) a more detailed account of the chemistry and pharmacology (iso-enzyme selectivity) of NOS inhibitors, the interested reader is referred to recent reviews of these topics (Thiemermann, 1995; Morris and Billiar, 1994; Szabo and Thiemermann, 1995; Southan and Szabo, 1996).

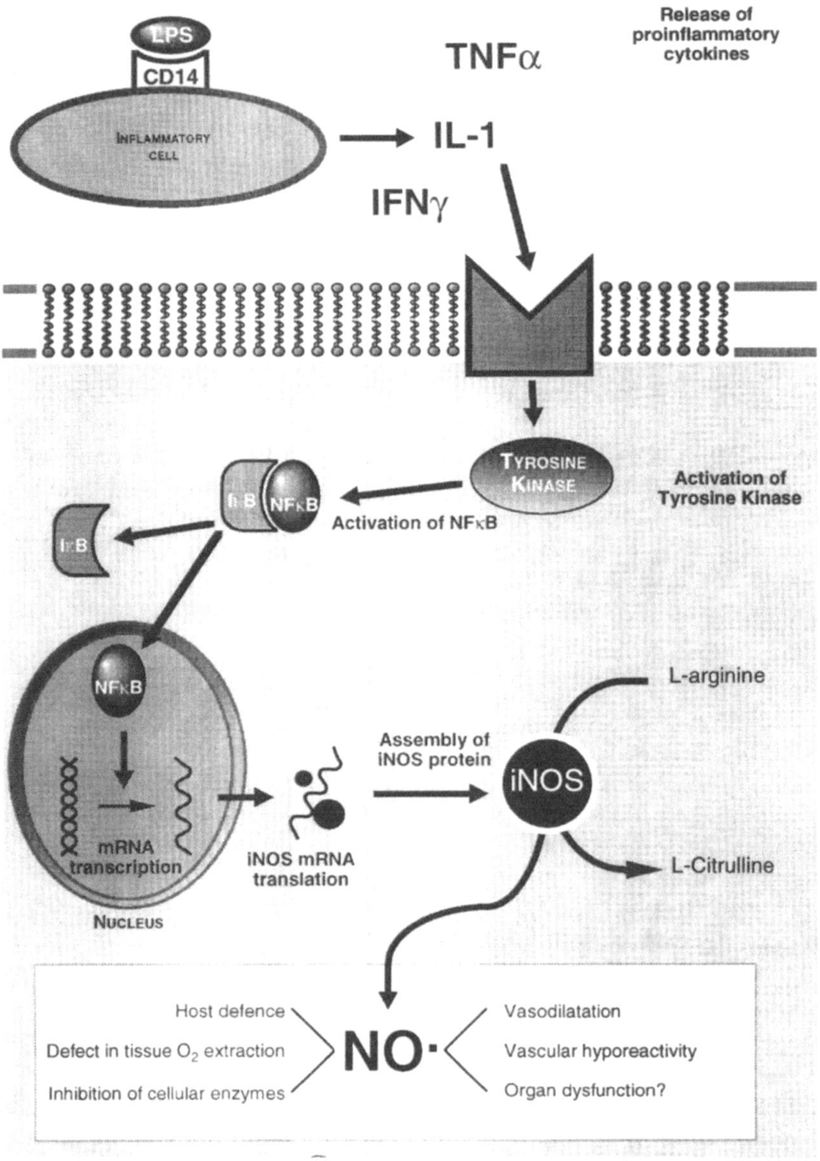

Fig. 2. Mechanisms leading to the induction of the inducible isoform of nitric oxide (*NO*) synthase in shock. *LPS*, lipopolysaccharide; *TNF*, tumor necrosis factor; *IL*, interleukin; *IFN*, interferon; *NFκB*, nuclear factor κB; *IκB*, inhibitor of NFκB; *iNOS*, inducible nitric oxide synthase

Inhibition of NOS Activity in Animal Models of Septic or Endotoxic Shock

Although there is strong evidence that endotoxemia or sepsis in rodents results in the induction of iNOS (in various tissues) leading to an increase in the plasma levels of nitrite/nitrate (from 20 to up to 600 µM), there is limited information regarding the time course of iNOS induction, the degree of iNOS activity (in tissues) or even the plasma levels of nitrite/nitrate in large animal models (pig, dog, sheep, baboon) of shock or in humans with sepsis and septic shock. Clearly, sepsis (or endotoxemia) results in an increase in the plasma levels of nitrite/nitrate in these species. However, it appears that the rise in the plasma levels of nitrite/nitrate in e.g. humans with septic shock is much smaller than in rodents. When evaluating the role of NO or elucidating the effects of NOS inhibitors in animal models of shock, one needs to remember that: (a) many of the models used are non-resuscitated, hypodynamic models of shock, (b) the effects (and side effects) of non-selective inhibitors of NOS activity (see below) will greatly vary depending upon the degree of iNOS induction in the species, and (c) any observed effects of the respective NOS inhibitor used will obviously depend on the chosen dose regimen and timing of the intervention.

N^G-methyl-L-arginine

The N-substituted L-arginine analogue L-NMMA was the first agent reported to inhibit NOS activity. L-NMMA is an endogenous substance present in the urine of both animals and man (Park et al., 1988; Carnigie et al., 1977). Although L-NMMA inhibits all isoforms of NOS to a variable degree, it is a more potent inhibitor of iNOS than eNOS activity in cultured cells (Gross et al., 1990) and in the rat (Thiemermann et al., 1995). L-NMMA is a competitive inhibitor of the binding of L-arginine to NOS and, hence, excess of L-arginine reverses the inhibition of NOS activity by L-NMMA. As L-NMMA is only a moderately selective inhibitor of iNOS activity, it is not entirely surprising that the effects of L-NMMA in models of shock vary from "very beneficial" (inhibition of iNOS activity) to "moderately beneficial with some adverse effects" (inhibition of eNOS activity masks the beneficial effects of iNOS inhibition) to "detrimental" (marked inhibition of eNOS activity). Clearly, the observed result is very dependent on the dose of L-NMMA as well as the model of shock (e.g. species, degree of iNOS induction etc.) used. When given after the onset of hypotension, infusions of relatively low doses of L-NMMA (3–10 mg/kg per hour) have been convincingly demonstrated to exert beneficial hemodynamic effects in rodent (Thiemermann and Vane,

1990), sheep (Booke, 1996), canine (Kilbourn et al., 1990) and baboon (see below) models of endotoxemia and sepsis. In contrast to rodents, sheep are very sensitive to small doses of endotoxin in a manner similar to humans. Indeed, infusion of either endotoxin or bacteria into sheep leads to a hyperdynamic circulation with a fall in peripheral vascular resistance, an increase in cardiac output and increases in organ blood flow associated with a reduction in oxygen extraction. In this model, prolonged periods of endotoxemia or bacteremia (*Pseudomonas aeruginosa*) are also associated with increases in total renal blood flow and the development in precapillary arterio-venous shunts resulting in regional maldistribution of renal blood flow, fall in glomerular filtration pressure and, ultimately, glomerular filtration rate. Interestingly, administration (at 24 h after the onset of endotoxemia) of L-NMMA increased urine output and reversed the impairment in creatinine clearance caused by infusion of bacteria, without causing a significant fall (below baseline) of renal blood flow. In addition to these beneficial effects on renal blood flow and function, NOS inhibition also resulted in an increase in oxygen extraction, a fall in organ blood flow from elevated to normal levels (in brain, heart, jejunum, ileum), an increase in peripheral vascular resistance, but no significant increase in lactate, indicating a normalisation of hemodynamic parameters in the absence of excessive vasoconstriction (Booke et. al., 1996 a, b). In conscious baboons, administration of live *Escherichia coli* bacteria resulted in a significant increase in the serum levels of biopterin, neopterin and nitrate, suggesting induction of guanosine triphosphate (GTP) cyclohydrolase I and iNOS (Strohmeier et al., 1995). In this model, infusion of L-NMMA (5 mg/kg per hour) attenuated the rise in the serum levels of nitrate and creatinine, the hypotension and fall in peripheral vascular resistance and the substantial 7-day mortality caused by severe sepsis in this species (Daryl Rees and Heinz Redl, personal communication). These findings clearly document that the circulatory failure caused by septic shock in baboons is largely mediated by an enhanced formation of NO by iNOS and that inhibition of iNOS with L-NMMA improves outcome in this model. In conclusion, L-NMMA (currently developed by Glaxo Wellcome, Stevenage, UK, 546C88, for use in septic shock; see below) is a non-toxic (e.g. LD_{50} in the rat: > 1–2 g/kg) inhibitor of NOS activity which exerts beneficial hemodynamic effects in animals and man with septic shock.

N^G-nitro-L-arginine methylester

Following early findings in 1990 that L-NMMA exerted beneficial hemodynamic effects in animal models of endotoxemia, many subsequent studies aimed at elucidating the role of NO in septic shock have used the NOS inhibitor N^G-nitro-L-arginine methylester (L-NAME) rather than L-NMMA, as

L-NAME is cheap and readily available. In contrast to L-NMMA, L-NAME is a relatively selective inhibitor of eNOS rather than iNOS activity (Southan et al., 1995) and, hence, higher doses of this agent may cause excessive vasoconstriction (particularly in the pulmonary, renal and myocardial vascular bed) and enhance the incidence of both microvascular thrombosis and neutrophil adhesion to the endothelium. Thus, L-NAME reduces oxygen delivery (Walker et al., 1995; Waurick et al., 1997) and exacerbates organ injury in many, but not all animal models of endotoxic or septic shock (see Thiemermann, 1997). These results are not necessarily solely due to the use of very large amounts of L-NAME, but rather a reflection of the fact that L-NAME is a more selective inhibitor of eNOS than iNOS activity. In rats with endotoxemia, infusion of a very low dose L-NAME (e.g. 0.03–0.3 mg/kg per hour) results in a dose-related increase in blood pressure (due to inhibition of eNOS activity) without reducing the rise in the plasma levels of nitrite/nitrate (an indicator of iNOS activity) or the organ injury caused by endotoxin (Wu et al., 1996). The notion that L-NAME is a very potent (and fairly selective) inhibitor of eNOS activity is highlighted by the findings that infusions of very low doses (30–50 µg/kg per minute) of L-NAME cause: (a) a reduction in renal cortical blood flow without causing an increase in blood pressure in the rat (Walder et al., 1991), and (b) a significantly enhanced increase in pulmonary vascular resistance caused by endotoxin in the pig (Robertson et al., 1994). Thus, L-NAME is a relatively selective inhibitor of eNOS activity which, with very few exceptions (see Meyer et al., 1994), exerts detrimental effects in animals with septic shock. In our opinion, this compound is not an appropriate pharmacological tool when aimed at modulating NO biosynthesis in shock in order to improve organ dysfunction or survival.

Aminoguanidine and Derivatives

Aminoguanidine was the first relatively selective inhibitor of iNOS activity to be discovered (Corbett et al., 1992). Although aminoguanidine is a more potent inhibitor of iNOS than eNOS activity in vitro and in vivo, aminoguanidine is not a very potent inhibitor of iNOS activity (IC_{50}: approximately 100–150 µM) (see Thiemermann, 1997). The inhibition of NOS by aminoguanidine becomes greater with increasing incubation time, indicating that aminoguanidine is a mechanism-based inhibitor (Wolff and Lubeskie, 1995). Aminoguanidine attenuates the delayed hypotension in rats (Wu et al., 1995) and rabbits (Seo et al., 1996) with endotoxin shock and improves survival in mice challenged with endotoxin (Wu et al., 1995). Aminoguanidine and its analogue, 1-hydroxy-2-guanidine, also attenuate the liver injury and hepatocellular dysfunction caused by endotoxin in the rat (Wu et al., 1996; Ruetten et al., 1996). In rats with endotoxic shock, aminoguanidine also decreases the degree of bacterial translocation, presumably by preventing the injury to the gut mucosal barrier, attenuates the disruption of the blood brain barrier (Boje, 1996) and reduces the increase in pulmonary transvascular flux (Arkovitz et al., 1996). The interpretation of the mechanism(s) by which aminoguanidine exerts these beneficial effects is difficult, as aminoguanidine is not a specific inhibitor of iNOS activity. Indeed, aminoguanidine has many other pharmacological properties including inhibition of: (a) histamine metabolism, (b) polyamine catabolism, (c) the formation of advanced glycosylation end products, and of (d) catalase activity (as well as other copper- or iron-containing enzymes). Interestingly, aminoguanidine also prevents the expression of iNOS protein by a hitherto unknown mechanism (see Thiemermann, 1997). Thus, aminoguanidine has to be regarded as an agent which: (a) is a relatively selective, but not very potent, inhibitor of iNOS activity, (b) reduces the formation of NO by two distinct mechanisms, namely prevention of the expression of iNOS protein and inhibition of iNOS activity, and (c) exerts many other effects, which appear to be unrelated to the inhibition of iNOS activity (non-specific effects).

Aminoethyl-isothiourea and Other *S*-Substituted Isothioureas

S-substituted isothioureas (ITUs) are non-amino acid analogues of L-arginine and also potent inhibitors of iNOS activity with variable isoform selectivity (Garvey et al., 1994; Szabo et al., 1994; Southan et al., 1995). The most potent isothioureas are those with only short alkyl chains on the sulphur atom and no substituents on the nitrogen atoms. For instance, S-ethyl-ITU is a potent competitive inhibitor of all isoforms of human NOS, while S-ethyl-ITU, aminoethyl-ITU and S-methyl-ITU are more selective inhibitors of iNOS than of eNOS activity (Southan et al., 1995). In 1994, we demonstrated that S-methyl-ITU reverses the circulatory failure caused by endotoxin in the rat. This beneficial hemodynamic effect of S-methyl-ITU was associated with an attenuation of the liver injury and hepatocellular dysfunction caused by endotoxin in rats, as well as an increase in the survival rate of mice challenged with a high dose of endotoxin (Szabo et al., 1994). Similarly, administration of aminoethyl-ITU (1 mg/kg per hour commencing 2 h after injection of endotoxin) results in beneficial hemodynamic effects and attenuates the degree of liver injury/dysfunction caused by endotoxin in the rat (Thiemermann et al., 1995). In pigs with endotoxemia, injection of aminoethyl-ITU (10 mg/kg i.v. at 3 h after endotoxin) restores hepatic arterial blood flow (from reduced to normal levels) and increases hepatic oxygen consumption, without affecting cardiac output (Saetre et al., 1997). Having stressed that some of the beneficial effects of aminoguanidine in shock may not be due to its ability to inhibit iNOS activity (e.g. non-specific effects), it should be noted that *S*-substituted ITUs are also likely to elicit effects which are unrelated to inhibition of NOS activity. For instance, aminoethyl-ITU is a scavenger of peroxynitrite and exerts beneficial effects in models of disease/pathology known to be mediated by oxygen-derived free radicals (see Thiemermann, 1997). Interestingly, dimethyl-ITU (which does not inhibit iNOS activity) is a weak radical scavenger which inhibits the activation of the transcription factor, nuclear factor (NF)-κB. In rats challenged with either endotoxin or live *Salmonella typhimurium*, dimethyl-ITU attenuates the formation of tumor necrosis factor (TNF)-α and improves survival (Sprong et al., 1997). It is conceivable that other *S*-substituted ITUs will also prevent the activation of NF-κB. This may well explain why aminoethyl-ITU prevents the expression of iNOS protein caused by endotoxin in cultured macrophages and in the rat in vivo (Ruetten and Thiemermann, 1996).

Highly Selective Inhibitors of iNOS Activity: 1400 W and L-NIL

S-substituted ITUs and guanidines contain the amidine function ($-CH(=NH)NH_2$), a feature which they have in common with *O*-substituted isoureas and amidines themselves. In 1996, we reported that certain amidines (e.g. 2-iminopiperidine, butyramine, 2-aminopyridine, propioamidine and acetamidine) inhibit NOS activity (Southan et al., 1996). Recently, an analogue of acetamidine termed 1400 W [N-(3-(aminomethyl)benzyl)acetamidine] has been reported to be a slow, tight binding inhibitor of human iNOS. The inhibition by 1400 W of the activity of human iNOS is potent (kDa value ~ 7 nM), dependent on the co-factor nicotinamide adenine dinucleotide phosphate, reduced (NADPH) and either irreversible or extremely slowly reversible. Most notably, 1400 W was approximately 5000-fold more potent as an inhibitor of iNOS activity than of eNOS activity (human). In a rat model of vascular injury caused by endotoxin, 1400 W is 50-fold more potent as an inhibitor of iNOS than eNOS activity and attenuates the vascular leak syndrome (Garvey et al., 1997). We have recently shown that selective inhibition of iNOS activity with 1400 W attenuates the circulatory failure, but not the liver injury/dysfunction caused by endotoxin in the rat (Wray et al., 1998). In addition to 1400 W, L-N^G-(L-iminoethyl)lysine (L-NIL) is a highly selective and potent inhibitor of iNOS activity in the rat (Faraci et al., 1996) and mouse (Moore et al., 1994). Like 1400 W, L-NIL (3 mg/kg i.v. at 2 h after administration of endotoxin) attenuates the delayed hypotension, but does not reduce the degree of renal dysfunction, liver dysfunction or hepatocellular injury caused by endotoxin in the rat (Fig. 3). These findings support the view that selective inhibition of iNOS activity might be a useful approach in the restoration of blood pressure in patients with shock. Most notably, however, our data are also consistent with the notion that – as in the case of iNOS

Urea

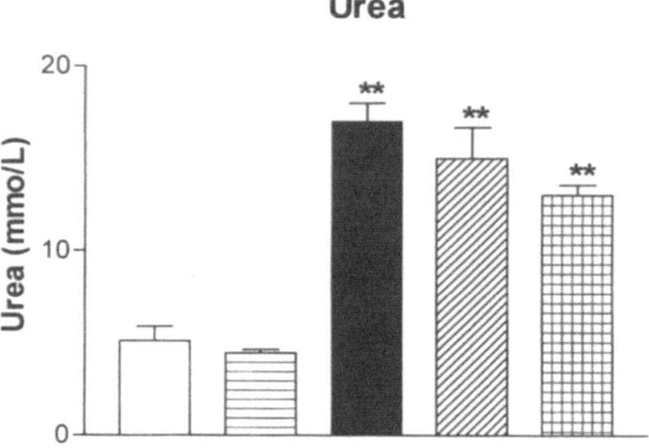

Aspartate aminotransferase

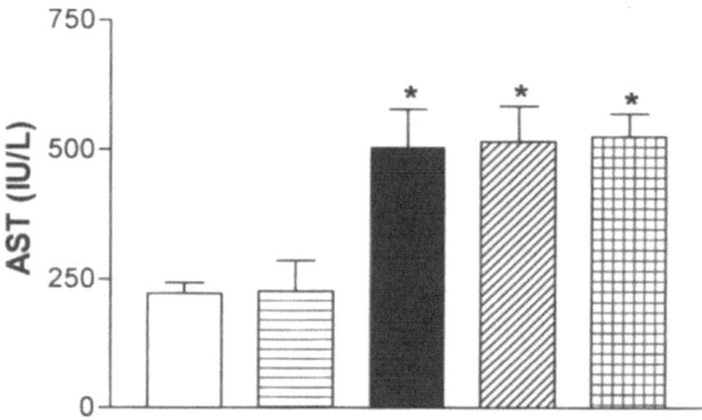

Fig. 3. This figure shows the effects of the selective inducible nitric oxide synthase (*iNOS*) inhibitor 1400 W on the rise in the serum levels of urea (an indicator of the development of renal dysfunction) and aspartate aminotransferase (*AST*) (an indicator of hepatocellular injury) in anaesthetised rats challenged with endotoxin [lipopolysaccharide (LPS), 6 mg kg^{-1} i.v.]. Animals received injections of saline rather than LPS and were treated with infusions of either saline (vehicle for 1400 W, *open columns, n* = 10) or 1400 W (10 mg kg^{-1} bolus plus 10 mg kg^{-1} h^{-1} (*horizontal stripes, n* = 3). Different groups of LPS rats were treated with (starting 2 h after LPS): (a) vehicle (saline control, *black columns, n* = 10) 1400 W 3 mg kg^{-1} bolus + 3 mg kg^{-1} h^{-1} (*diagonal stripes, n* = 8), (b) 1400 W 10 mg kg^{-1} bolus + 10 mg kg^{-1} h^{-1} (*checked column, n* = 5). * p < 0.01, ** p < 0.001 when compared by analysis of variance to rats which had received vehicle rather than LPS. There were no differences in urea or AST between the LPS controls and 1400 W-treated rats

knockout mice challenged with endotoxin (MacMicking et al., 1995) – enhanced formation of NO by iNOS primarily contributes to the circulatory failure, but not to the liver injury or dysfunction caused by endotoxin.

Nitric Oxide Synthase Inhibition in Humans with Septic Shock

There is evidence that endotoxin and cytokines (when given in combination) cause the expression of iNOS as well as the formation of NO in various human cells (primary or cell lines) including hepatocytes, mesangial cells, retinal pigmented epithelial cells and lung epithelial cells (Morris and Billiar, 1993; Preiser and Vincent, 1996). Elevated plasma and urine levels of nitrite/nitrate have been reported in adults and children with severe septic shock, as well as in patients with burn injuries who subsequently developed sepsis. Taken together, these studies support the view that septic shock in man is associated with an enhanced formation of NO. It should be stressed, however, that the increase in the plasma levels of nitrite/nitrate elicited by endotoxin, cytokines or bacteria in rodents (ten-fold) is substantially higher than the observed increases in the plasma levels of these metabolites of NO in other animal species (pig, sheep, etc.) or humans. Moreover, our understanding of: (a) the biosynthesis of NO, (b) the regulation of and the mechanism involved in the expression of iNOS and (c) the role of NO in MODS in shock are largely based on animal experiments of endotoxic shock in rodents. In contrast, we know relatively little about the role of NO in patients with septic and other forms of circulatory shock.

Early reports of the beneficial hemodynamic effects of L-NMMA in humans with septic shock (Petros et al., 1991; Schilling et al., 1993; Lorente et al., 1993; Petros et al., 1994) stimulated a phase-1, multilcentre, open-label, dose-escalation (1, 2.5, 5, 10 or 20 mg/kg per hour for up to 8 h) study using L-NMMA (546C88) in 32 patients with septic shock. In this study, L-NMMA sustained blood pressure and enabled a reduction in vasopressor (norepinephrine) support. The cardiac index fell to baseline values (possibly due to an increase in peripheral vascular resistance) and left ventricular function was well maintained. Moreover, L-NMMA increased oxygen extraction, while pulmonary shunt was not worsened (Watson et al., 1995). A recent, placebo-controlled multicentre study involving 312 patients with septic shock has evaluated the effects of L-NMMA on the resolution of shock at 72 h (primary endpoint). The severity of illness according to the SAPS II score was similar between the placebo and L-NMMA groups. Infusion of L-NMMA enhanced mean arterial blood pressure and systemic vascular resistance index and decreased cardiac output (from elevated towards normal levels). L-NMMA had no effect on left ventricular systolic work index, indicating that the fall in cardiac output was not due to an impairment in cardiac contractility. In septic patients treated with L-NMMA, in whom pulmonary vascular resistance was already elevated, there was a transient further increase in mean pulmonary artery pressure. Interestingly, L-NMMA did not affect the thrombocytopenia or the renal dysfunction caused by sepsis. Most notably, 41% of patients treated with L-NMMA, but only 21% of patients treated with placebo, recovered from shock within 72 h. There was also a strong trend towards a reduction in mortality (at day 14) in patients treated with L-NMMA. A phase-3 clinical trial to evaluate the effects of L-NMMA on outcome is currently being conducted.

Concluding Remarks

Since 1990, numerous studies have documented an enhanced formation of NO in various animal models of endotoxin and septic shock. Similarly, patients with septic shock and IL-2 immunotherapy exhibit elevated plasma levels of nitrite/nitrate. Although the enhanced formation of NO in animals and man with septic shock contributes to hypotension and hyporeactivity of the vasculature to vasoconstrictor agents (vasoplegia), it is still unclear whether NO (from iNOS) contributes to the organ dysfunction/failure syndrome associated with severe septic shock. Our finding that highly selective inhibitors of iNOS activity, such as 1400 W or L-NIL, attenuate the delayed hypotension, but do not affect the multiple organ dysfunction caused by endotoxin in the rat, supports the view that an enhanced formation of NO within the vasculature contributes to circulatory failure (vasodilatation, vasoplegia and possibly vascular leak), but does not directly contribute to the development of organ injury. This notion is supported by the finding that mice in which the iNOS gene has been deleted by gene targeting, elicit less hypotension (but do develop liver injury) when challenged with endotoxin.

Although there is some evidence that human cells/tissues can, in principle, induce iNOS protein and activity (when challenged with endotoxin and cytokines), the degree of iNOS activity in patients with septic shock appears to be substantially lower than in some animal species (e.g. rodents). Nevertheless, inhibition of NOS activity with L-NMMA exerted beneficial hemodynamic effects (e.g. resolution of shock) without causing significant side effects. Whether any beneficial hemodynamic effects elicited by L-NMMA in patients with septic shock will be sufficient to attenuate 28-day mortality is currently being determined in a large (more than 2000 patients) phase-3 multicentre trial.

References

Arkovitz MS, Wispe JR, Garcia VF, Szabo C (1996) Selective inhibition of the inducible isoform of nitric oxide synthase prevents pulmonary transvascular flux during acute endotoxemia. J Pediatr Surg 31:1009–1015

Baue AE (1993) The multiple organ or systems failure syndrome. In: Schlag G, Redl H (eds) Pathophysiology of shock, sepsis and organ failure, Springer, Berlin, pp 1004–1018

Billiar TR, Curran RD, Harbrecht BG, Stuehr DJ, Demetris AJ, Simmons RL (1990) Modulation of nitrogen oxide synthesis in vivo: N^G-monomethyl-L-arginine inhibits endotoxin-induced nitrite/nitrate biosynthesis while promoting hepatic damage. J Leukoc Biol 48:565–569

Boje KM (1996) Inhibition of nitric oxide synthase attenuates blood-brain barrier disruption during experimental meningitis. Brain Res 720:75–83

Booke M, Hinder F, McGuire R, Traber LD, Traber DL (1996a) Nitric oxide synthase inhibition versus norepinephrine for the treatment of hyperdynamic sepsis in sheep. Crit Care Med 24:835–844

Booke M, Hinder F, McGuire R, Traber LD, Traber DL (1996b) Nitric oxide synthase inhibition versus norepinephrine in ovine sepsis: effects on regional blood flow. Shock 5:362–370

Carnigie PR, Fellows FCI, Symington GR (1977) Urinary excretion of methylarginine in human disease. Metabolism 26:531–537

Corbett JA, Tilton RG, Chang K, Hasan KS, Ido Y, Wang JL, Sweetland MA, Lancaster JR, Williamson JR, McDaniel ML (1992) Aminoguanidine, a novel inhibitor of nitric oxide formation, prevents diabetic vascular dysfunction. Diabetes 41:552–558

Dinerman JL, Lowenstein CJ, Snyder SH (1993) Molecular mechanism of nitric oxide regulation: potential relevance to cardiovascular disease. Circ Res 73:217–222

Faraci WS, Nagel AA, Verdries KA, Vincent LA, Xu H, Nichols LE, Labasi JM, Salter ED, Pettipher ER (1996) 2-Amino-4-methylpyridine as a potent inhibitor of inducible NO synthase activity in vitro and in vivo. Br J Pharmacol 119:1101–1108

Garvey EP, Oplinger JA, Furfine ES, Kiff RJ, Laszlo F, Whittle BJR, Knowles RG (1997) 1400W is a slow, tight binding, and highly selective inhibitor of inducible nitric oxide synthase in vitro and in vivo. J Biol Chem 272:4959–4963

Garvey PE, Oplinger JA, Tanoury GJ, Sherman PA, Fowler M, Marshall S, Marmon MF, Paith JE, Furfine ES (1994) Potent and selective inhibition of human nitric oxide synthases. Inhibition by non-amino acid isothioureas. J Biol Chem 269:26669–26676

Gross SS, Stuehr DJ, Aisaka K, Jaffe EA, Levi R, Griffith OW (1990) Macrophage and endothelial nitric oxide synthesis: cell-type selective inhibition by N^G-aminoarginine, N^G-nitroarginine and N^G-methyl-arginine. Biochem Biophys Res Commun 170:96–103

Julou-Schaeffer G, Gray GA, Fleming I, Schott C, Parratt JR, Stoclet JC (1990) Loss of vascular responsiveness induced by endotoxin involves the L-arginine pathway. Am J Physiol 259:H1038–1043

Kilbourn RG, Gross SS, Jubran A, Adams J, Griffith OW, Levi R, Lodato RF (1990) N^G-methyl-L-arginine inhibits tumour necrosis factor-induced hypotension: implications for the involvement of nitric oxide. Proc Natl Acad Sci USA 87:3629–3632

Kilbourn RG, Juburan A, Gross SS, Griffith OW, Levi R, Adams J (1990) Reversal of endotoxin-mediated shock by N^G-monomethyl-L-arginine, an inhibitor of nitric oxide synthesis. Biochem Biophys Res Commun 172:1132–1138

Lorente JA, Landin L, De Pablo R, Renes E, Liste D (1993) L-arginine pathway in the sepsis syndrome. Crit Care Med 21:1287–1295

Loscalzo J, Welsch G (1995) Nitric oxide and its role in the cardiovascular system. Proj Cardiovascular Dis 38:87–104

MacMicking JD, Nathan C, Hom G (1995) Altered responses to bacterial infection and endotoxic shock in mice lacking inducible nitric oxide synthase. Cell 82:641–650

Meyer J, Lentz CW, Stothert JC, Traber LD, Herndon DN, Traber DL (1994) Effects of nitric oxide synthesis inhibition in hyperdynamic endotoxemia. Crit Care Med 22:306–312

Moncada S, Higgs A (1993) The L-arginine-nitric oxide pathway. N Eng J Med 329:2202–2212

Moore WM, Webber RK, Jerome GM, Tjoeng FS, Misko TP, Currie MD (1994) L-N6-(1-iminoethyl)lysine: a selective inhibitor of inducible nitric oxide synthase. J Med Chem 37:3886–3888

Morris SM, Billiar TR (1994) New insights into the regulation of inducible nitric oxide synthase. Am J Physiol 266:E829–E839

Nathan C (1992) Nitric oxide as a secretory product of mammalian cells. FASEB J 6:3051–3064

Nathanson C, Hoffmann WD, Suffredini EF, Eichacker PQ, Danner RL (1994) Selected treatment strategies for septic shock based on proposed mechanism of pathogenesis. Ann Intern Med 120:771–783

Park KS, Lee HW, Hong SY (1988) Determination of methylated amino acids in human serum by high-performance liquid chromatography. J Chromatography 440:225–230

Parillo JE (1990) Septic shock in humans. Advances in the understanding of pathogenesis, cardiovascular dysfunction and therapy. Ann Intern Med 113:227–242

Petros A, Bennett D, Vallance P (1991) Effect of nitric oxide synthase inhibitors on hypotension in patients with septic shock. The Lancet 338:1557–1558

Petros A, Lamb G, Leone A, Moncada S, Bennett D, Vallance P (1994) Effects of a nitric oxide synthase inhibitor in humans with septic shock. Cardiovasc Res 28:34–39

Preiser JC, Vincent JL (1996) Nitric oxide involvement in septic shock: Do human beings behave like rodents? In: Vincent JL (ed) 1996 Yearbook of Intensive Care and Emergency Medicine Springer, Berlin, pp 358–365

Rees DD (1995) Role of nitric oxide in the vascular dysfunction in septic shock. Biochem Soc Trans 23:1025–1029

Rees DD, Cellek S, Palmer RMJ, Moncada S (1990) Dexamethasone prevents the induction of nitric oxide synthase and the associated effects on the vascular tone: an insight into endotoxic shock. Biochem Biophys Res Commun 173:541–547

Robertson FM, Offner PJ, Ciceri DP, Becker WK, Pruitt BA Jr (1994) Detrimental hemodynamic effects of nitric oxide synthase inhibition in septic shock. Arch Surg 129:149–155

Ruetten H, Southan GJ, Abate A, Thiemermann C (1996) Attenuation of the multiple organ dysfunction caused by endotoxin by 1-amino-2-hydroxy-guanidine, a potent inhibitor of inducible nitric oxide synthase. Br J Pharmacol 118:261–270

Saetre T, Gundersen Y, Thiemermann C, Lilleansen P, Aasen AO (1998) Aminoethyl-isothiourea, a selective inhibitor of inducible nitric oxide synthase activity, improves liver circulation and oxygen metabolism in a porcine model of endotoxaemia. Shock; in press

Schilling J, Cakmakci M, Battig U, Geroulanos S (1993) A new approach in the treatment of hypotension in human septic shock by N^G-monomethyl-L-arginine, an inhibitor of the nitric oxide synthetase. Intensive Care Med 19:227–231

Seo HG, Fujiwara N, Kaneto H, Asashi M, Fujii J, Taniguchi N (1996) Effect of the nitric oxide synthase inhibitor, S-ethyl-isothiourea, on cultured cells and cardiovascular functions of normal and lipopolysaccharide-treated rabbits. J Biochem 119:553–558

Southan G, Szabo C, Thiemermann C (1995) Isothioureas: potent inhibitors of nitric oxide synthases with variable isoform selectivity. Br J Pharmacol 114:510–516

Southan GJ, Szabo C (1996) Selective pharmacological inhibition of distinct nitric oxide synthase isoforms. Biochem Pharmacol 51:383–394

Southan GJ, Szabo C, O'Conner MP, Salzman AC, Thiemermann C (1996) Amidines are potent inhibitors of constitutive and inducible nitric oxide synthases: Preferential inhibition of the inducible isoform. Eur J Pharmacol 291:311–318

Sprong RC, Aarsman CJM, Oirschot JFLM, Asbeck BS (1997) Dimethylthiourea protects rats against gram-negative sepsis and decreases tumour necrosis factor and nuclear factor κB activity. J Lab Clin Med 129:470–481

Strohmeier W, Werner ER, Redl H, Wachter H, Schlag G (1995) Plasma nitrate and pteridine levels in experimental bacteremia in baboons. Pteridines 6:8–11

Szabo C, Southan G, Thiemermann C (1994) Beneficial effects and improved survival in rodent models of septic shock with S-methyl-isothiourea sulfate, a novel, potent and selective inhibitor of inducible nitric oxide synthase. Proc Natl Acad Sci USA 91:12472–12476

Szabo C, Thiemermann C (1995) Regulation of the expression of the inducible isoform of nitric oxide synthase. Adv Pharmacol 34:113–154

Thiemermann C (1994) The role of L-arginine: nitric oxide pathway in circulatory shock. Adv Pharmacol 28:45–79

Thiemermann C (1998) The use of selective inhibitors of inducible nitric oxide synthase in septic shock. Sepsis, in press

Thiemermann C, Ruetten H, Wu CC, Vane JR (1995) The multiple organ dysfunction syndrome caused by endotoxin in the rat: Attenuation of liver dysfunction by inhibitors of nitric oxide synthase. Br J Pharmacol 116:2845–2851

Thiemermann C, Vane JR (1990) Inhibition of nitric oxide synthesis reduces the hypotension induced by bacterial lipopolysaccharide in the rat. Eur J Pharmacol 182:591–595

Walder CE, Thiemermann C, Vane JR (1991) The involvement of endothelium-derived relaxing factor in the regulation of renal cortical blood flow in the rat. Br J Pharmacol 102:967–973

Walker TA, Curtis SE, King-VanVlack CE, Chapler CK, Vallet B, Cain SM (1995) Effects of nitric oxide synthase inhibition on regional hemodynamics and oxygen transport in endotoxic dogs. Shock 4:415–420

Waurick R, Bone HG, Meyer J, Booke M, Meissner A, Prien T, Van Aken H (1997) Haemodynamic effects of dopexamine and nitric oxide synthase inhibition in healthy and endotoxaemic sheep. Eur J Pharmacol 333:181–186

Wei X, Charles IG, Smith A (1995) Altered immune responses in mice lacking inducible nitric oxide synthase. Nature 375:408–411

Wolff DJ, Lubeskie A (1995) Aminoguanidine is an isoform-selective, mechanism-based inactivator of nitric oxide synthase. Arch Biochem Biophys 316:290–301

Wu CC, Chen SJ, Szabo C, Thiemermann C, Vane JR (1995) Aminoguanidine attenuates the delayed circulatory failure and improves survival in rodent models of endotoxic shock. Br J Pharmacol 114:1666–1672

Wu CC, Ruetten H, Thiemermann C (1996) Comparison of the effects of aminoguanidine and N^G-nitro-L-arginine methylester on the multiple organ dysfunction caused by endotoxaemia in the rat. Eur J Pharmacol 300:99–104

Intracellular Protein Modification and Signal Transduction in Response to Lipopolysaccharide

S. HAUSCHILDT and H. HEINE

Introduction

Post-translational covalent modifications are powerful tools to regulate protein functions. Modifications may occur e.g. via acylation, hydroxylation, methylation, thiolation, glycosylation, ADP (adenosine diphosphate) ribosylation and phosphorylation. Among these modifications, protein phosphorylation seems to be a principal mechanism involved in signal transduction processes. There is increasing evidence that other modifications like mono-ADP-ribosylation also contribute to signaling events (Wang et al. 1996; Vedia et al. 1992). Mono-ADP-ribosylation catalyzed by ADP-ribosyltransferases involves the transfer of the ADP-ribose moiety of nicotinamide adenine dinucleotide $(NAD)^+$ to a specific amino acid in a target protein while the nicotinamide moiety is released. The best understood ADP-ribosyltransferases are bacterial toxins including cholera and pertussis toxin that interfere with signal transduction in human host cells by ADP-ribosylating regulatory G-proteins.

It is now apparent that eukaryotic cells use analogue mechanisms to regulate intracellular events (Mc Manon et al. 1993; Zolkiewska and Moss 1993; Schuman et al. 1994). Recently, endogeneous ADP-ribosyltransferases have been identified and characterized (Zolkiewska et al. 1992; Tsuchiya et al. 1994). One effective way to investigate the involvement of ADP-ribosylation in cellular events is to modulate ADP-ribosyltransferase activity with a specific inhibitor and analyze the ensuing changes in cellular functions.

Inhibitors of ADP-Ribosylation Suppress LPS-Induced Cytokine Release

Monocytes $(4 \times 10^6/ml)$ isolated from peripheral blood mononuclear cells (PBMC) by counter flow elutriation were pretreated with inhibitors of ADP-ribosylation, namely metaiodobenzylguanidine (MIBG), nicotinamide, and novobiocin for 15 min before they were exposed to lipopolysaccharide (LPS)

Symposium in Immunology VIII
Eibl/Huber/Peter/Wahn (Eds.)
© Springer Verlag Berlin Heidelberg 1999

(10 ng/ml). After 4 h of incubation, supernatants were collected for measurement of interleukin (IL)-1, IL-6, and tumor necrosis factor (TNF)-α. The inhibitors belong to different chemical classes: nicotinamide is a vitamin, MIBG is a functional analogue of the neurotransmitter norepinephrine, and novobiocin is an inhibitor of DNA-gyrase, used as an antibiotic. All three compounds inhibited LPS-induced TNF-α and IL-6 production, whereas only novobiocin blocked IL-1 synthesis.

Complete TNF-α and IL-6 inhibition was achieved by 25 mM nicotinamide and by 0.5 mM MIBG and novobiocin (Fig. 1). A total of 0.5 mM novobiocin was needed to prevent IL-1 production. Not only cytokine production but also nitrite formation has been shown to be suppressed by inhibitors of ADP-ribosylation (Hauschildt et al. 1991). The inhibitors block protein and/or RNA synthesis – biosynthetic processes that may require ADP-ribosylation-dependent reactions (Hauschildt et al. 1991; Heine et al. 1995).

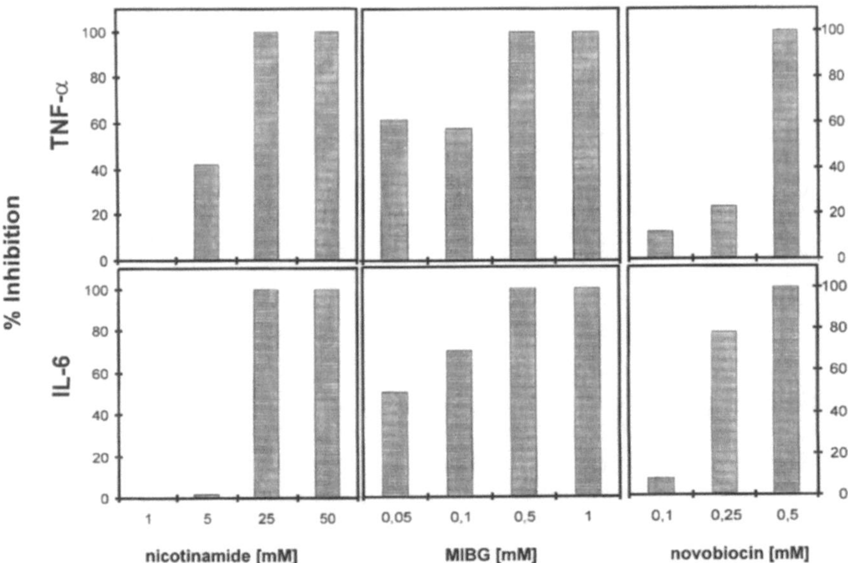

Fig. 1. Effect of nicotinamide, metaiodobenzylguanidine (*MIBG*) and novobiocin on lipopolysaccharide (LPS)-induced cytokine production. Monocytes (4×10^6/ml) were incubated in the absence or in the presence of different concentrations of nicotinamide, MIBG or novobiocin 15 min before the addition of LPS (10 ng/ml) for 4 h. Supernatants were harvested and analyzed for cytokine content. Control, LPS-stimulated cells. *IL*, interleukin; *TNF-α*, tumor necrosis factor-α

Inhibitors of ADP-Ribosylation Prevent LPS-Induced Phosphorylation of p36/38

The role of phosphorylation in the regulation of LPS-induced cytokine biosynthesis is far better understood than that of ADP-ribosylation. LPS has been shown to rapidly increase tyrosine phosphorylation of a number of substrates including mitogen-activated protein (MAP) kinases (Dong et al. 1993). Inhibition of this pathway by tyrosine kinase inhibitors appears to block TNF-α synthesis and inhibitors of phosphatases, which effectively increase protein phosphorylation, stimulate TNF-α production (Novogrodsky et al. 1994; Sung et al. 1992).

Since phosphorylation and ADP-ribosylation both interfere with cytokine production, we tested whether phosphorylation of proteins may be regulated by ADP-ribosylation. Monocytes (4×10^6/ml) were suspended in RPMI 1640 supplemented with 10% (v/v) human serum and antibiotics and incubated with LPS (10 ng/ml). After 4 h, cells were pelleted and resuspended in ice-cold permeabilizing buffer containing 10 mM Tris HCl, pH 7.8, 1 mM EDTA, 4 mM $MgCl_2$, 30 mM 2-ME, and 1 mM vanadate. After sonification, the homogenate was centrifuged for 1 h at 100 000 g. Aliquots of the cytosolic supernatant containing about 30 µg of protein in a volume of 50 µl of buffer were added to 25 µl of a phosphorylation reaction mixture. The mixture contained: 100 mM Tris/HCl, pH 7.8, 120 mM $MgCl_2$, 0.01% leupeptin, 0.1 mM phenylmethylsulfonyl fluoride (PMSF) and [γ-^{32}P] ATP (5 µCi/aliquot). After 10 min of incubation at 37 °C, proteins were precipitated, separated on 10%–12% sodium dodecyl sulfate polyacrylamide gel electrophoresis (SDS-PAGE), and subjected to autoradiography. As illustrated in Fig. 2, treatment of monocytes with LPS results in changes of the phosphorylation state of a 36- and a 38-kDa (p36/38) cytosolic protein. This effect is shared by two other potent monocyte activators, the bacterial lipopeptide Pam$_3$ Cys-Ala-Gly and Bacillus Calmette-Guerin (BCG), indicating that phosphorylation of p36/38 seems to be a common event associated with activation (Heine et al. 1995). Increased phosphorylation was visible 30 min after incubation and after 24 h the labeled proteins were still detectable (Heine et al. 1995). Beside p36/38, other proteins have been described that change their phosphorylation state in response to LPS (Weinstein et al. 1991). The best characterized proteins belong to the MAPK family. These include MAP kinases p38/p42 and p44 (Han et al. 1994; Weinstein et al. 1992). MAP kinases are serine/threonine kinases that undergo rapid tyrosine phosphorylation (min) upon activation. This difference in kinetics and the failure of p36/38 to react with anti-MAPK antibodies clearly demonstrates that p36/38 are distinct from p38/p42 and p44 MAPK (Heine et al. 1995). Having shown that inhibitors of ADP-ribosylation prevent cytokine production, we tested whether these sub-

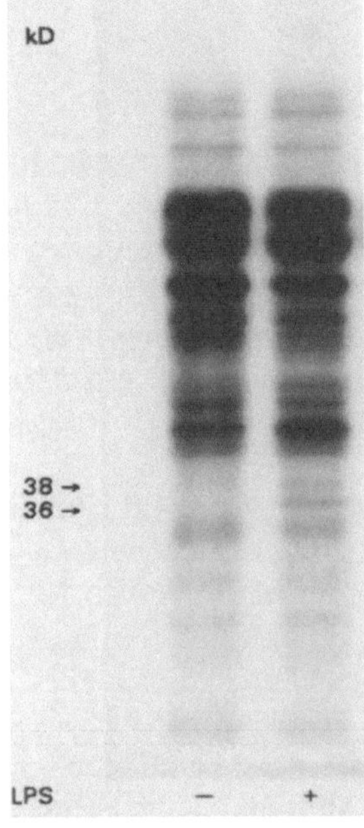

Fig. 2. Effect of lipopolysaccharide (*LPS*) on phosphorylation of cytosolic proteins. Monocytes (4×10^6/ml) were incubated in the presence and absence of LPS (10 ng/ml). After 4 h, cytosolic supernatants were prepared and incubated with [γ-^{32}P] adenosine triphosphate. Proteins were separated by sodium dodecyl sulfate polyacrylanide gel electrophoresis

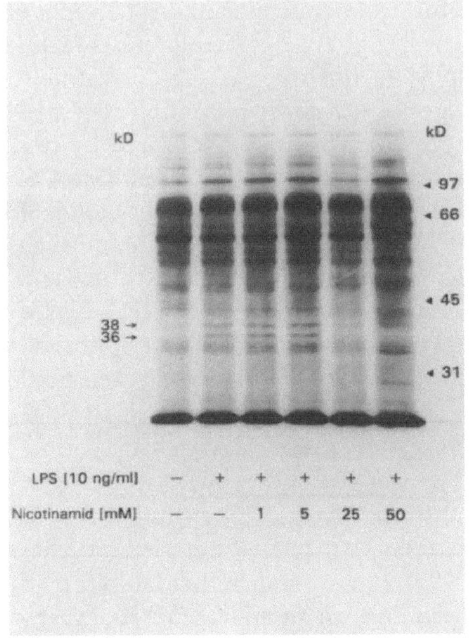

Fig. 3. Inhibition of lipopolysaccharide (*LPS*)-induced alteration in phosphate labeling of p36/38 by nicotinamide. Before stimulating monocytes (4×10^6/ml) with LPS (10 ng/ml) for 4 h, cells were preincubated with nicotinamide for 15 min. Cytosolic supernatants were prepared and incubated with [γ-^{32}P] adenosine triphosphate for 10 min. Proteins were separated on sodium dodecyl sulfate polyacrylamide gel electrophoresis (from Heine et al., 1995)

stances had any effect on LPS-induced protein phosphorylation. Monocytes (4×10^6/ml) were exposed to nicotinamide, MIBG, and novobiocin 15 min prior to incubation with LPS. After 4 h of incubation, the phosphorylation pattern of cytosolic proteins was analyzed. Increasing concentrations of all three inhibitors led to a diminished phosphorylation of p36/38. The effect of nicotinamide on the LPS-induced alteration in phosphorylation of cytosolic proteins is shown in Fig. 3. Nicotinamide inhibits both ADP-ribosyltransferase, as well as poly (ADP-ribose) synthetase activity (Rankin et al. 1989). Poly (ADP-ribose) synthetase which is localized in the nucleus catalyzes, in contrast to the ADP-ribosyltransferase, the covalent attachment of multiple residues of the ADP-ribose moiety of NAD to various proteins. Whereas low doses (µM) of nicotinamide are sufficient to inhibit poly (ADP-ribose) synthetase, higher concentrations (mM) are needed to block ADP-ribosyltransferase. The fact that phosphorylation of p36/38 is prevented by 25 mM nicotinamide implies the participation of mono-ADP-ribosylation in this process.

Identification of p36 as β/γ Actin

The close correlation between inhibition of p36/38 phosphorylation and inhibition of cytokine production points to a crucial role of the two proteins in LPS-initiated monocyte activation. To identify the nature of these proteins, we separated them by two-dimensional SDS-PAGE. P36 found in the cytosol of stimulated monocytes consisted of two spots (p36a and p36b), and p38 was hardly visible (Fig. 4). The p36b protein spot was excised and subjected to in-gel digestion with trypsin, followed by analysis by delayed extraction matrix-assisted laser desorption ionization (MALDI) mass spectrometry. P36b was identified as γ-actin and p36a as β/γ-actin (Hauschildt et al. 1997).

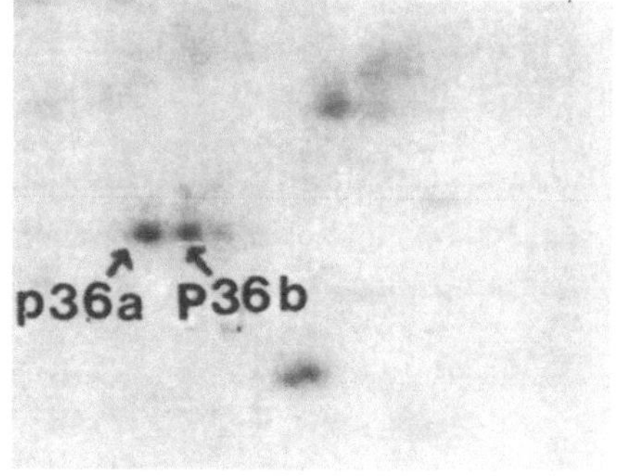

Fig. 4. Two-dimensional polyacrylamide gel electrophoresis of cytosolic proteins. Cytosolic supernatants from lipopolysaccharide-stimulated monocytes were incubated with [γ-^{32}P] adenosine triphosphate. Proteins were seperated by two-dimensional electrophoresis as described (Hauschildt et al. 1997)

Actins are highly conserved contractile proteins that are present in all eukaryotic cells. Of the three known actin isoforms, α, β, and γ, mammalian nonmuscle cells synthesize β- and γ-actin. Actins are the main components of microfilaments which, together with microtubuli, intermediate filaments, and associated proteins, form the cytoskeleton. The cytoskeleton pervades the entire cytoplasma and links the plasma membrane to the nucleus. It is reasonable to assume that such a system may transmit information from the cell surface to the nucleus and back again. Microfilaments are directly linked to the inner surface of the plasma membrane. They form a complex sub-membraneous network and give structural support to the cell. Due to their close vicinity to the cell membrane, they may be involved in regulating events occurring at the plasma membrane. It is therefore plausible to suggest that β/γ-actin, by changing its phosphorylation state, participates in the transmission of an LPS-induced signal from the outside into the interior of the cell. Upon exposure to a variety of stimuli, the cytoskeleton is reorganized, i.e., globular actin (G-actin) polymerizes to form filamentous actin (F-actin). To determine whether assembly of actin is involved in LPS-induced signal transduction, we preincubated monocytes (4×10^6/ml) for 15 min with cytochalasin D, an inhibitor of polymerization, before the addition of LPS. In the presence of 4 µM cytochalasin D, TNF-α concentrations decreased from 76 ng/ml to 41 ng/ml, suggesting a role of actin in LPS-induced cellular responses.

Is Uptake of LPS Required for Signaling?

To induce phosphorylation of β/γ-actin, as well as of other proteins, interactions of LPS with the plasma membrane are required. The membrane-bound glycosyl phosphatidyl-inositol-linked protein, membrane CD14 (m CD14), is the best characterized LPS-receptor molecule identified to date (Ulevitch and Tobias 1994). While the binding of LPS to CD14 is thought to be the first step in response to LPS, the succeeding steps are far less clear. It has been shown that LPS is internalized, but the relevance of this finding as to the ensuing signal transduction events is not known (Kang et al. 1990; Luchi and Munford 1993; Gallay et al. 1993). To examine the relation between LPS internalization and LPS responsiveness, we studied the uptake of the tetraacyl precursor Ia of lipid A (compound 406) in human monocytes. Compound 406 lacks the ability to induce cytokine production (Kovach et al. 1990). Monocytes were stimulated with 100 ng/ml compound 406, free lipid A, and LPS and, following varying incubation times, uptake was analyzed by confocal microscopy which allows the detection of internalized compounds.

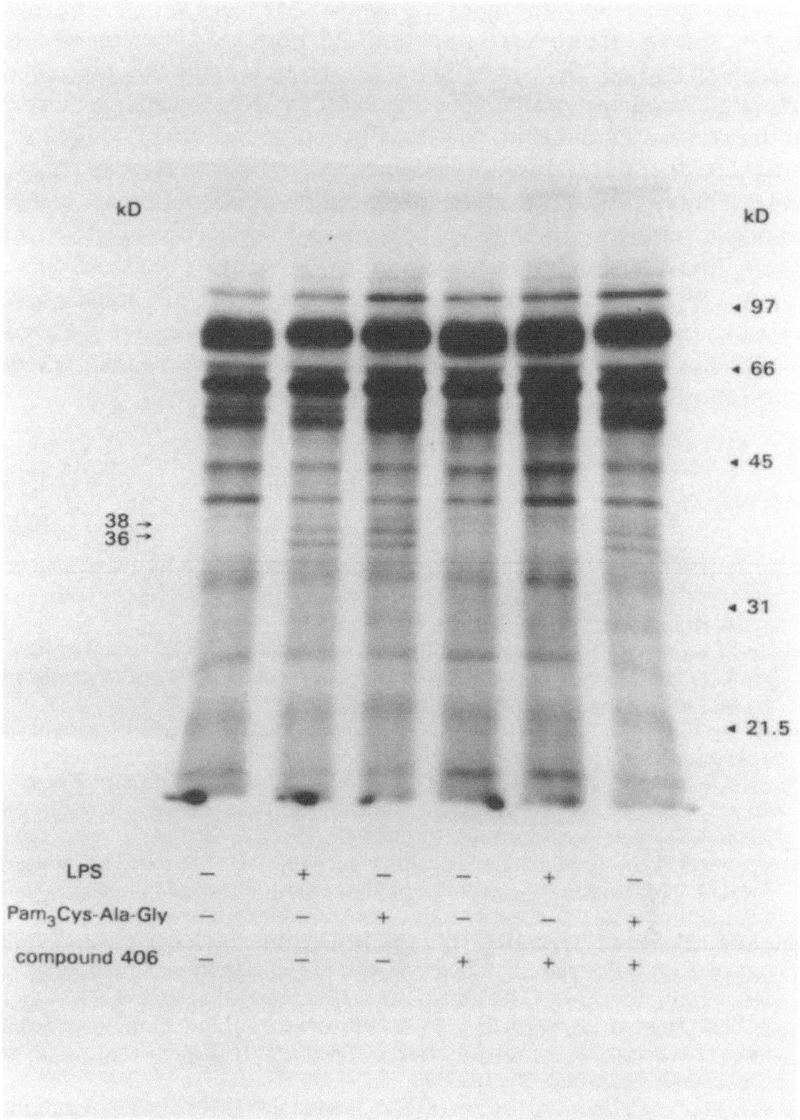

Fig. 5. Compound 406 inhibits lipopolysaccharide (*LPS*)-induced phosphorylation of p36/38. Monocytes (4×10^6/ml) were preincubated with compound 406 (10 µg/ml) before LPS (10 ng/ml) or Pam₃ Cys-Ala-Gly (10 ng/ml) was added. After 4 h, cytosolic supernatants were prepared and incubated with [γ-^{32}P] adenosine triphosphate. Proteins were separated by sodium dodecyl sulfate polyacrylamide gel electrophoresis (from Heine et al., 1995)

Similar to LPS and free lipid A, compound 406 was found to be internalized by human monocytes. Compound 406 inhibited LPS-induced cytokine release but had no effect on cytokine release induced by the monocyte activators BCG and bacterial lipopeptide Pam₃ Cys-Ala-Gly (Heine et al. 1995). In contrast to LPS and Pam₃ Cys-Ala-Gly, compound 406, although internalized, failed to induce phosphorylation of p36/38 (Fig. 5). However, it prevented LPS- but not Pam₃ Cys-Ala-Gly-induced phosphorylation of p36/38, suggesting a selective blockade of LPS-induced signal transduction mechanisms. These data and the observation that monocytes rendered unresponsive to LPS internalize LPS, clearly demonstrate that LPS uptake and LPS responsiveness are two distinct events and that internalization may occur in the absence of cellular responses. To what extent internalization is required for responsiveness remains to be established.

References

Dong Z, Qi X, Fidler IJ (1993) Tyrosine phosphorylation of mitogen activated protein kinases is necessary for activation of murine macrophages and synthetic bacterial products. J Exp Med 177:1071–1077

Gallay P, Jongeneel CV, Barras C, Burnier M, Baumgartner JD, Glauser MP, Heumann D (1993) Short time exposure to lipopolysaccharide is sufficient to activate human monocytes. J Immunol 150:5086–5093

Han J, Lee JD, Bibbs L, Ulevitch RJ (1994) A MAP kinase targeted by endotoxin and hyperosmolarity in mammalian cells. Science 265:808–811

Hauschildt S, Scheipers P, Bessler WG (1991) Inhibitors of poly (ADP-ribose) polymerase suppress lipopolysaccharide-induced nitrite formation in macrophages. Biochem Biophys Res Commun 179:865–871

Hauschildt S, Schwarz C, Heine H, Ulmer AJ, Flad HD, Rietschel ET, Jensen ON, Mann M (1997) Actin: a target of lipopolysaccharide-induced phosphorylation in human monocytes. Biochem Biophys Res Commun 241:670–674

Heine H, Ulmer AJ, Flad HD, Hauschildt S (1995) Lipopolysaccharide-induced change of phosphorylation of two cytosolic proteins in human monocytes is prevented by inhibitors of ADP-ribosylation. J Immunol 155:4899–4908

Kang YH, Dwivedi RS, Lee CH (1990) Ultrastructural and immunocytochemical study of the uptake and distribution of bacterial lipopolysaccharide in human monocytes. J Leuk Biol 43:316–332

Kovach NL, Yee E, Munford RS, Raetz CRH, Harlan JM (1990) Lipid IVA inhibits synthesis and release of tumor necrosis factor induced by lipopolysaccharide in human whole blood ex vivo. J Exp Med 172:77–84

Luchi M, Munford RS (1993) Binding, internalization, and deacylation of bacterial lipopolysaccharide by human neutrophils. J Immunol 151:959–969

Mc Manon KK, Piron KJ, Ha VT, Fullerton AT (1993) Developmental and biochemical characteristics of the cardiac membrane-bound arginine-specific mono ADP-ribosyltransferase. Biochem J 293:789–793

Novogrodsky A, Vanichkin A, Patya M, Gazit A, Osherov N, Levitzki A (1994) Prevention of lipopolysaccharide-induced lethal toxicity by tyrosine kinase inhibitors. Science 27:1319–1322

Rankin PW, Jacobson EL, Benjamin RC, Moss J, Jacobson MK (1989) Quantitative studies of inhibitors of ADP-ribosylation in vitro and in vivo. J Biol Chem 264: 4312–4317

Schuman EM, Meffert MK, Schulman H, Madison DV (1994) An ADP ribosyltransferase as a potential target for nitric oxide action in hippocampal long-term potential. Proc Natl Acad Sci USA 91:11958–11962

Sung S, Walters JA, Fu SM (1992) Stimulation of tumor necrosis factor alpha production in human monocytes by inhibitors of protein phosphatase 1 and 2A. J Exp Med 176:897–901

Tsuchiya M, Hara N, Yamada K, Osago H, Shimoyama M (1994) Cloning and expression of cDNA for arginine-specific ADP-ribosyltransferase from chicken bone marrow cells. J Biol Chem 269:27451–27457

Ulevitch RJ, Tobias PS (1994) Recognition of endotoxin by cells leading to transmembrane signaling. Curr Opin Immunol 6:125–130

Vedia ML, Mc Donald LB, Reep B, Brüne B, Di Silvio M, Billiar TR, Lapetina EG (1992) Nitric oxide induced S-nitrosylation of glyceraldehyde-3-phosphate dehydrogenase inhibits enzymatic activity and increases endogeneous ADP-ribosylation. J Biol Chem 267:24929–24932

Wang J, Nemoto E, Dennert G (1996) Regulation of CTL by ecto-nicotinamide adenine dinucleotide (NAD) involves ADP-ribosylation of a p56[lck]-associated protein. J Immunol 156:2819–2827

Weinstein SL, Gold MR, De Franco AL (1991) Bacterial lipopolysaccharide stimulates protein tyrosine phosphorylation in macrophages. Proc Natl Acad Sci USA 88: 4148–4152

Weinstein SL, Sanghera JS, Lemke K, DeFranco AL, Pelech SL (1992) Bacterial lipopolysaccharide induces tyrosine phosphorylation and activation of mitogen activated protein kinases in macrophages. J Biol Chem 267:14955–14962

Zolkiewska A, Moss J (1993) Integrin α7 as substrate for a glycosylphosphatidylinositol-anchored ADP-ribosyltransferase on the surface of skeletal muscle cells. J Biol Chem 268:25273–25276

Zolkiewska A, Nightingale MS, Moss J (1992) Molecular characterization of NAD: arginine ADP-ribosyltransferase from rabbit skeletal muscle. Proc Natl Acad Sci USA 89:11352–11356

Bacterial Lipopolysaccharides: Chemical Constitution, Endotoxic Activity, and Biological Neutralization

W. Brabetz, U. Mamat, C. Alexander, and E. Th. Rietschel

Introduction

In 1892, Richard Pfeiffer, a student of Robert Koch, was the first to describe bacterial endotoxins as heat-stable, cell-associated components of *Vibrio cholerae* which induced toxic reactions in guinea pigs [1]. He clearly distinguished these substances from the already known heat-labile exotoxins which are actively secreted by pathogenic bacteria [2]. Today we know that endotoxins structurally consist of a lipid and a carbohydrate component and, thus, constitute lipopolysaccharides (LPS). Therefore, both terms endotoxin and LPS are used as synonyms.

Endotoxins are characteristic components of the cell wall of most gram-negative bacteria (Fig. 1). This cell wall is characterized by an outer, asymmetrically constructed membrane, the inner layer of which contains phospholipids, whereas the outer layer, shaping the cell surface, consists of LPS. The unique composition of this outer membrane leads to specific biological characteristics which are often the result of the molecular structure of LPS. Thus, the lipid matrix of the outer membrane represents an efficient barrier for bile salts and hydrophobic antibiotics, and the LPS packing appears important for this function. The carbohydrate part of LPS is responsible for other functions such as shielding pathogenic bacteria from the attack by the immune system of the host organism. LPS have antigenic properties and can act as potent virulence factors. In addition, endotoxins are responsible for different immunomodulatory reactions when they are released into the bloodstream through lysis of bacteria during severe infectious diseases, in particular during the course of antibiotic therapy [3]. These released endotoxins can contribute locally and in small amounts to an enhanced killing of the microorganisms by causing stimulation of specific or non-specific defense mechanisms of the host. On the other hand, high quantities of circulating endotoxin may cause pathophysiological effects such as high fever, hypotension, leukopenia, tachycardia, tachypnoe, systemic intravascular coagulation and multi-organ failure – symptoms which are known as manifestations of bacterial sepsis. Thus, it appears that LPS play an important role in the mediaton of gram-negative sepsis. Severe sepsis and sep-

Symposium in Immunology VIII
Eibl/Huber/Peter/Wahn (Eds.)
© Springer Verlag Berlin Heidelberg 1999

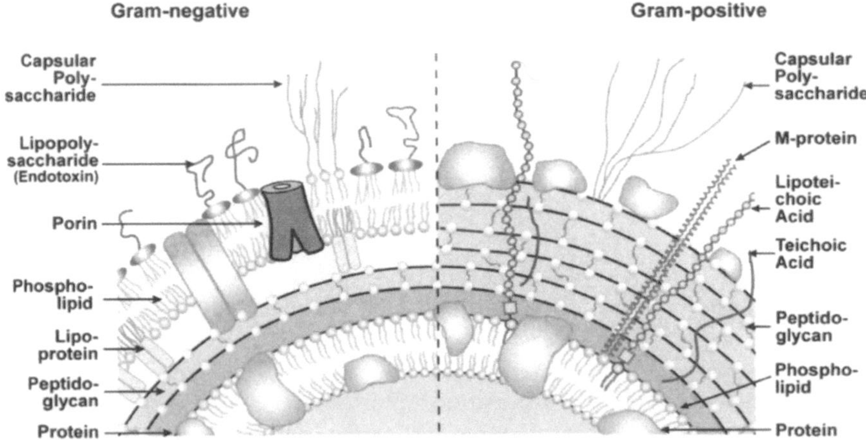

Fig. 1. The bacterial cell wall: The cellular compartment of bacteria is always surrounded by a cytoplasmic membrane consisting of a phospholipid bilayer and proteins. This membrane is outwardly followed by a covalent mesh work of peptidoglycan (murein) which, in the case of gram-negative bacteria, possesses only a few layers. As a peculiarity, this class of microorganisms has an outer membrane including a second cellular compartment (periplasmic space). Lipopolysaccharides form the outer leaf of the outer membrane. Porins (OmpF/C) mediate the selective uptake of hydrophilic nutrients, and structural proteins (OmpA, lipoprotein) contribute to the membrane's stability and its linkage with peptidoglycan. Capsular antigens are shown as examples of further glycosyl-based surface molecules. In contrast, gram-positive bacteria are surrounded by a thick murein multilayer. In addition, the cell wall of these microorganisms also consists of polysaccharides (lipoteichoic acid, teichoic acid, capsular polysaccharides) and/or proteins (partly also organized in complex surface layers)

Fig. 2. Effector mechanism of endotoxins. Bacterial endotoxins activate macrophages and monocytes to produce and release endogenous mediator molecules and antimicrobial factors. These can be classified into three different classes of substances. Reduced oxygen species and enzymes are efficient poisons for bacterial pathogens. Cytokines, especially tumor necrosis factor-α, are proteins which contribute to the enhancement of the inflammatory reaction, including the antimicrobial activity of phagocytes. Lipid mediators such as prostaglandin E_2 stemming from the metabolism of arachidonic acid partially inhibit an exuberant formation of mediators. Released in small quantities, an increased defense against infection is achieved by all these molecules. In the presence of large amounts of lipopolysaccharide, however, noxious overproduction of mediator molecules is induced which may lead to lethal shock through further reinforced cascade-like reactions. Interferon γ (*INF-γ*) stimulates macrophages also in the presence of low endotoxin concentrations to reacting in overproduction of mediator molecules and renders the host organism hyperreactive to endotoxin

tic shock are associated with a mortality rate of up to 50% and are responsible for approximately 150 000 cases of death annually in the USA alone [4–6].

The multitude and ambivalence of their effects suggest that endotoxins cannot be directly attributed to one single effector mechanism, as is known for many bacterial exotoxins [2]. Instead, LPS can be regarded as a bacterial mediator interacting specifically with different host cells and activating them

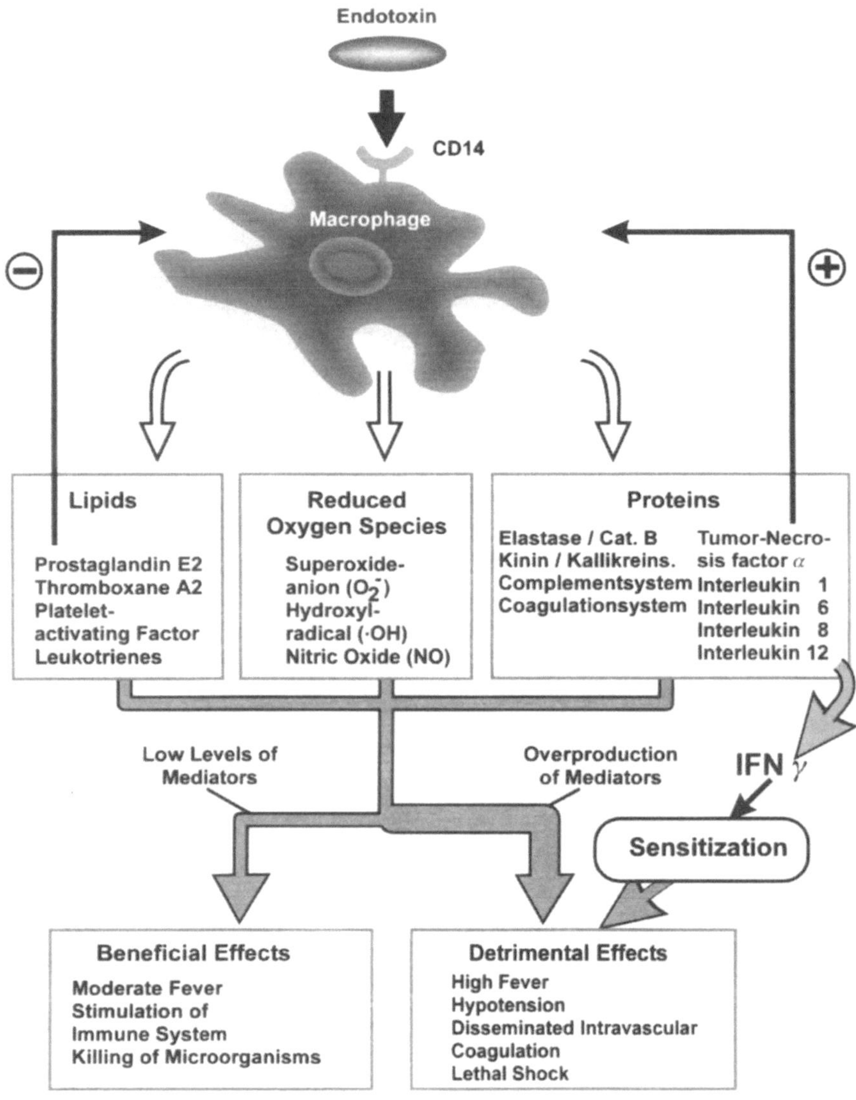

to synthesize and release various endogenous mediator and effector molecules. Among the cells in mice and humans known to be activated by endotoxins, macrophages and monocytes take a central position with their potential to produce proinflammatory cytokines [especially tumor necrosis factor-α (TNFα), interleukin 1 (IL-1), IL-6, IL-8, IL-12], eicosanoids, and reactive oxygen species (Fig. 2). High quantities of LPS lead to an overproduction of these endogenous mediators and, therefore, to pathophysiological consequences. Endotoxins are placed at the beginning of this chain reaction so that the elucidation of the molecular basis of their interaction with target cells is mandatory in order to develop effective strategies for prophylactic intervention and therapy of gram-negative sepsis.

Structure of Bacterial Endotoxins

The structure of endotoxins follows a general scheme which is shown in Fig. 3 for *Salmonella enterica*, as an example. Endotoxins are amphiphilic molecules consisting of a lipid component, termed lipid A, and a covalently bound polysaccharide. Because of genetic, biosynthetic, biological, and structural characteristics, the carbohydrate portion can be further divided into a lipid A-proximal core region and an O-specific side chain.

In general, O-specific chains are heteropolymers, made up of repeating oligosaccharide units (in enterobacteria up to 50) which consist of between two and eight monomers [9, 10]. Differing from this, a homopolymer of up to 75 molecules of legionaminic acid (5-acetamidino-7-acetamido-8-*O*-acetyl-3.5.7.9-tetradeoxy-D-*glycero*-L-*galacto*-non-2-ulosonic acid) has recently been described for *Legionella pneumophila* serotype 1 [11]. In nature, the great variety of the monomeric elements and the numerous possibilities of their linkage represent the basis for strain-specific O-chains. Therefore, LPS as O-antigens are of great diagnostic value and have been proven to be a reliable tool, for example, for serotyping of *Salmonella* according to the "Kaufmann-White scheme" [12]. It is further known for pathogenic enterobacteria that the O-chains of the LPS inhibit the phagocytosis of microorganisms by macrophages and may offer protection against the lytic effect of the complement system. O-specific chains are characteristic of so-called smooth LPS (S-form). This term was originally used to describe a corresponding colony morphology of wild-type bacteria and served as a differentiation to rough colonies of R-form mutants (Fig. 3) which could no longer express O-specific chains as a result of genetic defects. By creating these mutants it was shown that O-specific chains are not essential for growth of gram-negative bacteria. This is additionally proven by the fact that LPS structurally similar to that of R-forms are also found in pathogenic wild-

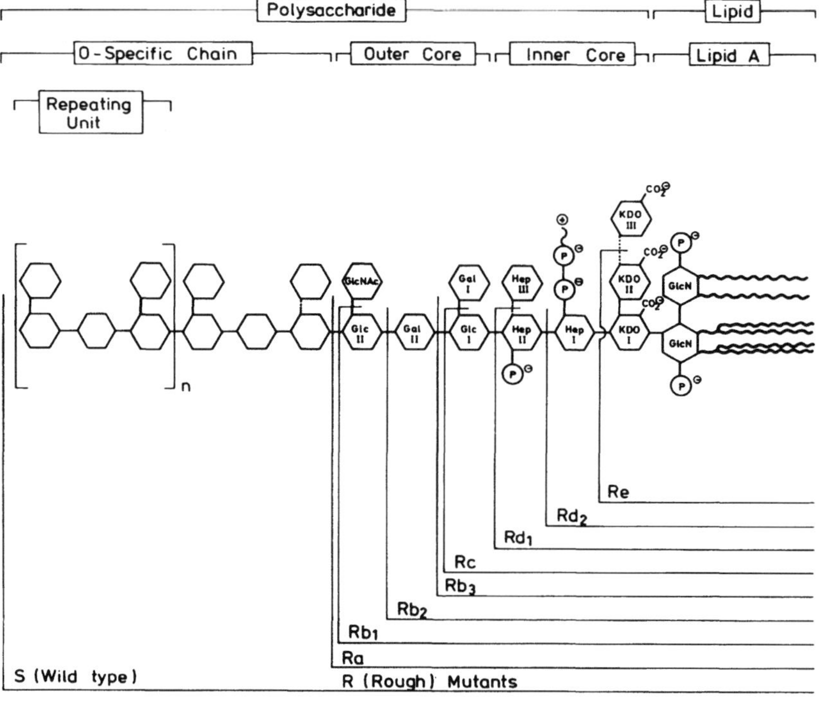

Fig. 3. Schematic representation of the structure of *Salmonella enterica*, wild type and rough mutant lipopolysaccharides (LPS). According to chemical, biosynthetic, biological and genetic criteria, LPS can be divided into three regions: O-specific chain, core oligosaccharide, and lipid A. The O-specific chain represents a polymer of repeating units characteristic of each bacterial strain. The terms Ra–Re refer to structures of LPS from rough mutants which, due to genetic defects, synthesize a truncated core oligosaccharide and, therefore, lack an O-specific chain. The smallest LPS structure which can be found in still viable *Salmonella enterica* strains consists of lipid A and two Kdo-residues (Re-mutant). Saccharide groups are depicted by *hexagons*, and *dotted lines* represent non-stoichiometric substitutions. *GlcN*, D-glucosamine; *Kdo*, 3-deoxy-D-*manno*-oct-2-ulosonic acid (2-Keto–3-deoxy-D-*manno*-octonic acid); *Hep*, L-glycero-D-*manno*-heptose; *Glc*, D-glucose; *Gal*, D-galactose; *GlcNAc*, N-acetyl-D-galactosamine; *P*, phosphate; *circle containing plus sign*, ethanolamine

type bacteria such as *Bordetella pertussis, Haemophilus influenzae, Neisseria meningitidis,* or of the genus *Chlamydia.*

The core region of LPS consists of a complex oligosaccharide and, as regards its structure, shows less variability in comparison to the O-specific chain [13]. In enterobacteria and some other families, one can differentiate between an outer core region with predominantly pyranosidic hexoses, such as D-glucose, D-galactose, 2-amino-2-deoxy-D-glucose or 2-amino-2-deoxy-D-galactose, and an inner core region. In all gram-negative bacteria, the latter contains 3-deoxy-D-*manno*-oct-2-ulosonic acid (2-keto–3-deoxy-D-*manno*-octonic acid, Kdo) and often LPS-specific L-*glycero*-D-*manno*-heptose (Hep). Defects in genes of the biosynthesis and the transfer of Kdo lead to a lethal phenotype, as shown for *Escherichia coli* and *S. enterica* [14, 15]. Furthermore, still viable mutants express an LPS consisting of lipid A and at least two Kdo-residues (*E. coli* Re mutant) [16, 17] or of a single but phosphorylated Kdo group (*H. influenzae* I-69) [18]. Therefore, a minimal structure of the core oligosaccharide with at least two negative charges seems to be important for the integrity of the outer membrane of gram-negative bacteria. In addition, other saccharides of the inner core region and non-stoichiometric substitutents such as phosphate, phosphoryl- and pyrophosphoryl-ethanolamine play an important role in the expression of the complete physiological capabilities of these microorganisms [7, 8].

Because of the essential character of the Kdo region in LPS, the biosynthetic enzymes are regarded as target molecules for the development of new antibiotics with a broad reactivity against all gram-negative bacteria [19, 20]. Core structures with one (*H. influenzae, B. pertussis, V. cholerae*) or two Kdo residues (enterobacteria, pseudomonas) have been identified up to now [13]. In addition, representatives of the genus *Chlamydia* have a unique, rough LPS consisting of a Kdo-trisaccharide of the structure αKdo-(2→8)-(αKdo-(2→4)-αKdo-(2→6) [21]. Remarkably, as shown for *H. influenzae* [22], *E. coli* [23], and *Chlamydia* [24–26], there is only one enzyme necessary for transfer of each Kdo residue, the transferase being therefore multifunctional.

Structurally, the lipid A component forms the most uniform part of LPS. It can be separated from the carbohydrate portion by mild acid hydrolysis leading to the cleavage of the glycosidic bond between Kdo I and lipid A (see Fig. 3) [27], and, hence, become accessible to a detailed structural elucidation [28]. Lipid A samples prepared from *E. coli* turned out to be as endotoxically active in vitro and in animal models as LPS [29], suggesting that lipid A represents the endotoxically active principle of LPS. This was unequivocally proven by chemical synthesis of lipid A from *E. coli* [30] and the demonstration of full biological activity of the synthetic product [29]. Because of the particular importance of this LPS component, a more detailed description of structural and functional aspects of the lipid A region and its interaction with host molecules will be given in the following sections.

Figure 4 shows the chemical structure of lipid A from four different gram-negative bacteria (*E. coli, H. influenzae, Chromobacterium violaceum,* and *N. meningitidis*) which express biologically highly active endotoxin [28]. In all cases, the core region is attached to the free hydroxyl group in position 6′ of the non-reducing glucosamine residue (GlcN II in Fig. 4). The molecules share a primary structure which is represented by a 1,4′ bisphosphorylated β-1,6-linked GlcN disaccharide acylated in positions 2, 3, 2′ and 3′ by four (*R*)-3-hydroxy fatty acids. These so-called primary fatty acids are character-

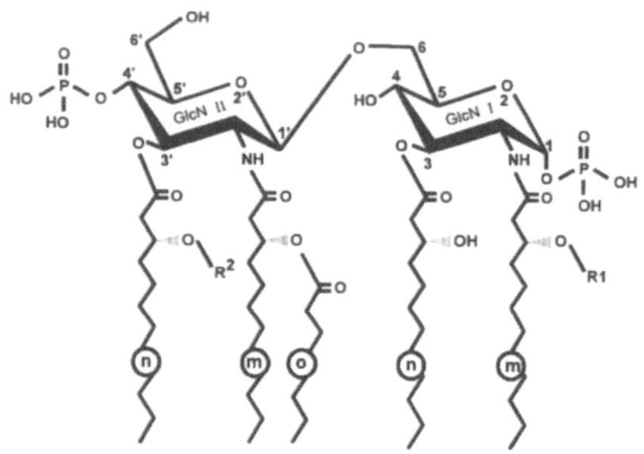

	Nature of		Number of carbon atoms		
	R^1	R^2	m	n	o
Escherichia coli	H	14:0	14	14	12
Haemophilus influenzae	H	14:0	14	14	14
Neisseria meningitidis	12:0	H	14	12	12
Chromobacterium violaceum	12:0	H	12	10	12

12:0, dodecanoic acid   14:0, tetradecanoic acid

Fig. 4. Primary structure of lipid A components of different gram-negative bacteria expressing endotoxically active lipopolysaccharide

istic of all LPS and represent the basis of a sensitive analytic system for endotoxins [31]. They can be acylated at their 3-hydroxyl groups by further secondary fatty acids. The structures have in common a fifth fatty acid which is ester linked to the 3-hydroxyl group of the C2'-bound primary fatty acid. However, there are differences in the linkage site of a sixth fatty acid, which may lead to a symmetric distribution of the acyl groups with respect to the saccharide backbone, as in the case of *N. meningitidis* and *C. violaceum* (R1 in Fig. 4; acylation type 3 + 3), or an asymmetric one in *E. coli* and *H. influenzae* (acylation type 4 + 2) where four fatty acids are bound to GlcN II (R2 in Fig. 4) and two to GlcN I. Additional differences concern the chain length of the fatty acids, which is larger on average in the case of asymmetrical acylation.

The described lipid A molecules exhibit a basic structural pattern which is realized in many gram-negative bacteria. But other LPS were isolated which showed a greater variability regarding their lipid A membrane anchor [review and literature in 28]. In *Campylobacter jejuni*, *Rhodopseudomonas viridis*, or *L. pneumophila*, GlcN is partly or totally replaced by 2,3-diamino-2,3-dideoxy-D-glucose (GlcN3N). These lipid A are also characterized by the presence of extremely long fatty acids (C22–C32). In addition, 3-oxo fatty acids, instead of the primary 3-hydroxyl fatty acids, were described in *Rhodobacter sphaeroides* and *Rb. capsulatus* (structure shown in Fig. 10). Remarkably, lipid A preparations from these bacteria are endotoxically inactive [32, 33]. Finally, the phosphate groups of lipid A can carry additional substituents or be missing, as shown for *Bacteroides fragilis* and *Rhizobium leguminosarum* biovar Phaseoli [34, 35]. Apart from these species- and strain-specific peculiarities, lipid A preparations exhibit a certain variability, especially regarding the quantitative distribution of the fatty acids, so that mature LPS always appears as a mixture of chemically slightly differing components [28].

LPS and Lipid A: Structure–Activity Relationships

The preparation and structural elucidation of lipid A from different bacteria, as well as the chemical synthesis of defined partial structures, made systematic examinations possible to determine the molecular parameters which are responsible for endotoxic activity. Among other parameters, the release of pro-inflammatory cytokines from murine macrophage cell lines and human peripheral monocytes was chosen as the biological analysis system to investigate this problem. The results of corresponding studies in the human system, which were carried out at the Research Center Borstel [36–38], are summarized in Fig. 5. It could be demonstrated that the structure of the hydrophilic saccharide backbone (β-1,6- linked GlcN- or GlcN3N-disaccharide) is a fundamental structural principle required for the expression of biological activity (Fig. 5a; cleavage of the glycosidic bond causes a decrease by a factor of 10^7) and that its phosphorylation has a decisive influence on endotoxicity (decrease by a factor of 10^2–10^4; Fig. 5a). Accordingly, the loss of secondary fatty acids dramatically reduces the molecule's activity ($>10^7$; Fig. 5b). Recently, these findings could be confirmed by using mutants of *E. coli* K-12 [39] and *H. influenzae* [40] in which the gene of an acyl transferase for secondary fatty acids had been inactivated. The strains are viable at 30 °C since the transfer of the Kdo residues and the further biosynthesis of the core

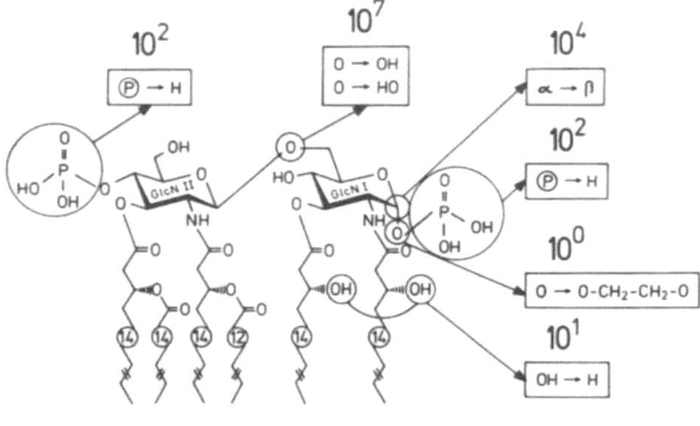

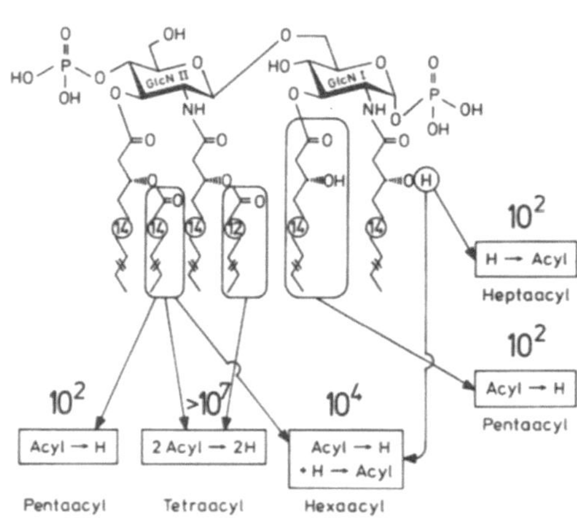

Fig. 5. The relationship between chemical structure and endotoxic activity of lipid A. Shown are chemical alterations of lipid A from *Escherichia coli* and the relative decrease of biological activity associated with them. **a** Modifications of the hydrophilic region (phosphorylated glucosamine disaccharide) of lipid A. **b** Modifications of the hydrophobic region (fatty acids) of lipid A

oligosaccharide can already occur at a lipid A precursor molecule with four fatty acids. As expected, these mutants express an LPS with a significantly reduced biological activity. In addition, lipid A preparations with an asymmetrical distribution of the secondary fatty acids show an increased endotoxicity compared to corresponding synthetic analogues with symmetrical acylation.

Lipid A and LPS are amphiphilic molecules forming supramolecular structures in an aqueous medium above their critical micellar concentrations (10^{-9}–10^{-7} M). These aggregate structures result from a peculiar con-

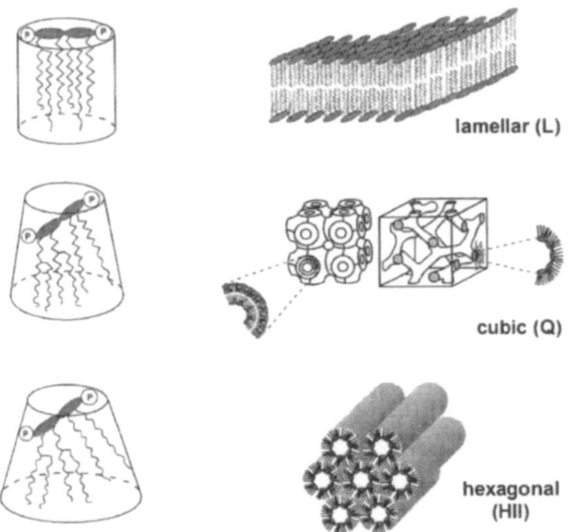

Fig. 6. Physical structure of endotoxically active and inactive lipid A. Endotoxically inactive lipid A possesses a cylindrical conformation and forms lamellar (*L*) supramolecular structures under approximately physiological conditions (for details see text). In contrast, biologically active lipid A molecules show a truncated conical shape which is enlarged in the hydrophobic region of the fatty acids and, therefore, leads to the formation of cubic (*Q*) or inverted hexagonal (H_{II}) supramolecular structures

formation of the monomers. The aggregation, however, is not only determined by the primary chemical structure of the molecules but also by environmental parameters such as temperature, water content, pH-value, and presence of divalent cations. By determining the physical structures of defined lipid A preparations under almost physiological conditions (37 °C, pH = 7, > 90% water content, presence of Mg^{2+}) [41–43], it could be demonstrated that endotoxically active molecules have a distinct tendency to form cubic (*S. enterica* serovar Minnesota) or inverted hexagonal (H_{II}, *Rb. gelatinosus*) supramolecular structures (Fig. 6). These physical structures correspond to monomers with a bigger volume of the hydrophobic fatty acid portion (conical shape) compared with the negatively charged saccharide backbone. In contrast, biologically inactive lipid A monomers, e.g., from *Rb. capsulatus*, are cylindrically shaped and associate to lamellar structures (Fig. 6).

It has been reported previously [44] that the biological effect of LPS in physiological solutions is mediated by larger aggregates. Newer findings [42, 45–48], however, show that there are rather small oligomeric units or monomers taking part in cell activation by endotoxins. The molecular shape of biologically active lipid A corresponds to a truncated cone-like conformation, which we call "endotoxic conformation" [49] and which, in turn, represents the specific and active counterpart for humoral and cell-bound receptor molecules of the host organism.

Interaction of LPS with Cells and Humoral Factors of the Host

LPS-dependent activation was described for many cell types from different higher organisms. Among these, cells of the immune system and of those, especially monocytes, macrophages, and granulocytes possess the greatest importance. Like phagocytes, these cell types are specialized in killing bacteria. They belong to the myeloid differentiation line of hematopoietic cells which evolutionarily represents the oldest component of the innate immune system. Therefore, it seems probable that, during evolution, LPS – as a widespread bacterial surface molecule – developed early into a host target structure as a result of the struggle of higher organisms with disease-causing bacteria.

Figure 7 shows the most important cell types known to be activated by LPS during infections with gram-negative bacteria. Each of the cell types react to endotoxin in a specific way, i.e., the production of mediator or effector molecules, phagocytosis, cell differentiation, and/or cell proliferation.

At the beginning of an infection, circulating monocytes and tissue-bound macrophages (see also Fig. 2) contribute to the formation of an inflammatory reaction. In addition, these cells play a key role in the development of sepsis. This could be proven experimentally by transfer of LPS-sensitive macro-

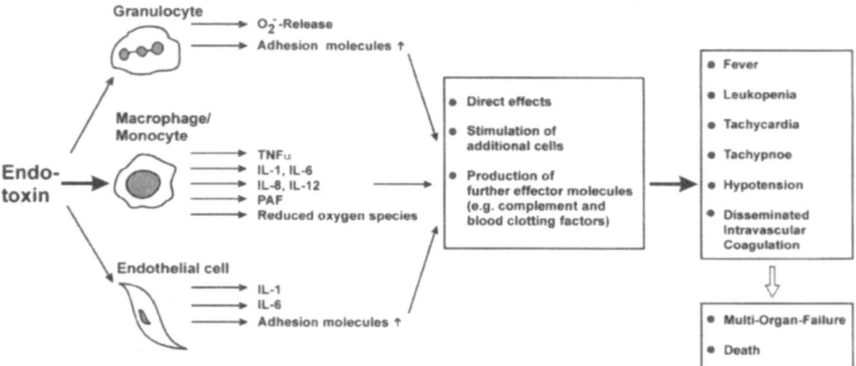

Fig. 7. Important target cells of endotoxins in humans. Endotoxins activate different cells to produce specific patterns of mediators and effectors. In the case of their overwhelming production, mediators in turn trigger successive reactions leading to the development of clinical manifestations of severe gram-negative sepsis. *TNF*, tumor necrosis factor; *IL*, interleukin; *PAF*, platelet-activating factor

phages into endotoxin-resistant C3H/HeJ mice [50]. In the presence of very low concentrations of LPS (< 1 ng/ml serum), macrophages and monocytes produce a great number of different mediators such as IL-1, IL-6, IL-8, IL-10, IL-12, the migration-inhibitory factor (MIF) [51], and especially TNFα [52]. These hormone-like molecules contribute to the accumulation and activation of further effector cells of the immune system at the site of infection [51, 53]. In addition, the general defense mechanism of the host organism is activated by moderate fever and the production of antimicrobial acute phase proteins from liver cells, contributing to antimicrobial host strategies. Thus, set free in small quantities, these mediators cause an effective limitation of the infection and elimination of the health-threatening microorganisms [53, 54]. However, if they are overproduced, e.g., in the course of severe sepsis, the host organism can no longer control the triggered inflammatory reaction, resulting in the damage of host cells and organs [55, 56]. Besides protein-like cytokines, monocytes and macrophages produce immuno-modulatory lipids such as products of the arachidonic acid metabolism (leukotrienes, prostaglandins) [51, 56–58], as well as derivatives of linoleic acid [59], in addition to platelet-activating factor (PAF) [60]. Finally, the phagocytic potency of the macrophages stimulated by endotoxins, as well as the production of reduced oxygen molecules (superoxide anion, hydrogen peroxide, hydroxyl racidals, nitric oxide; see also Fig. 2), essentially contribute to the killing of the bacteria or to the triggering of local or generalized inflammatory reactions.

Granulocytes (polymorphonuclear leukocytes; Fig. 7) also take up bacteria and their cell wall fragments, and their phagocytic activity is dramatically increased by endotoxins [59]. The activated cells augment the local inflammatory reaction in the early phase of an infection by sticking to the endothelial lining of blood capillaries and emigrating into the surrounding tissue by diapedesis. Thus, in the course of sepsis they cause damage to vessels and tissues. Granulocytes further contain enzymes (acyloxyacyl hydrolases) which degrade LPS into biologically inactive partial structures by specifically cleaving off the secondary fatty acids [61]. Activated by endotoxins and/or pro-inflammatory cytokines, granulocytes additionally release polycationic proteins from endosomal compartments which can specifically bind to LPS. Among these, the bactericidal/permeability increasing protein (BPI) is characterized best. It constitutes a 55-kDa membrane-associated protein of the primary granules of neutrophilic granulocytes which is cytotoxic for gram-negative bacteria and has an endotoxin neutralizing capacity [62–64]. BPI consists of two domains, an amino-terminal lipid A/LPS-binding site and a carboxy-terminal region with several membrane spanning domains [65, 66]. A recombinant 23-kDa fragment (rBPI$_{23}$) effectively inhibits the LPS-dependent release of TNFα, IL-1, IL-6, and IL-8 from human blood cells [66, 67] and also protects animal and human volunteers from phlogistic endotoxemia.

Apart from cells of the immune system, stimulation by LPS could also be shown for vascular cells (endothelial and smooth muscle cells). In these cases, stimulation by LPS yields the production of different cytokines such as IL-1, IL-6, and IL-8 [68–71], as well as of prostaglandins, nitric oxide, PAF, and growth factors for blood cells [72, 73]. In addition, following exposure to LPS as well as to IL-1 and TNFα [74–76], endothelial cells express adhesion molecules which, e.g., facilitate the attachment of blood platelets, granulocytes, and monocytes to the vessel wall and support their emigration to the subjacent tissue.

Because of the amphiphilic character of endotoxins, it was formerly suggested that their biological effect was due to a nonspecific intercalation into the membrane of host target cells. However, it is now recognized that different humoral and membrane-bound proteins interact specifically with LPS. Therefore, the concept of a receptor-mediated cell activation by endotoxins is generally accepted today.

The 53-kDa glycoprotein CD14 was identified as a LPS-binding molecule on the surface of monocytes, macrophages, and (in low concentration) neutrophilic granulocytes [77]. It is characteristic of all mature myeloid cells [77–80]. The protein has no membrane-spanning region but is integrated into the cell membrane via a glycosyl phosphatidyl inositol (GPI) anchor [80]. In addition to membrane-bound CD14 (mCD14; see Fig. 8), soluble isoforms of the protein (sCD14) with 55 kDa, 53 kDa or 48 kDa are found in serum (2–6 mg/ml in the circulation of healthy humans) [81, 82], which in CD14-positive cells are created by alternative protein modification or enzymatic cleavage of cell surface CD14 [83, 84]. The special role of mCD14 in LPS-mediated cell activation could be demonstrated in different experimental systems [77, 79, 85–87]. The endotoxin-dependent release of TNFα from monocytes, for example, can be inhibited by certain monoclonal antibodies against CD14 [77]. After transfection of the CD14-gene into LPS-resistant macrophage cell lines, a direct association between sensitivity to endotoxin and the expression of CD14 could be demonstrated [85]. Finally, CD14-deficient mice survive endotoxin doses of several orders of magnitude higher than the initial isogenic strain [87]. Nevertheless, sCD14 plays an important role in endotoxin activity in that it mediates the endotoxin-induced activation of CD14-negative endothelial cells [82, 88–91] (see Fig. 8). LPS binds to CD14 via the lipid A portion to a high affinity amino-terminal domain of the protein [92, 93]. Interestingly, CD14-dependent activation of monocytes could recently also be demonstrated for cell wall components of gram-positive bacteria such as peptidoglycan, arabinogalactan, and lipoarabinomannan [94–97]. Based on these findings, the concept was proposed that CD14 represented a pattern recognition receptor [96]. The structural prerequisites of these molecules for cell binding and the precise role of CD14 in these systems, however, are not yet known in detail.

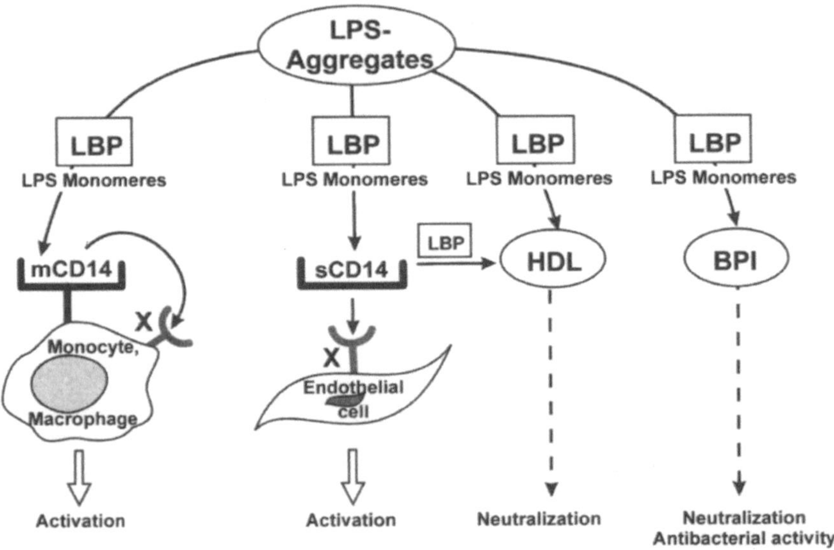

Fig. 8. Early stages of cell activation by endotoxins. The effect of lipopolysaccharide (*LPS*) is modulated by primary binding to serum proteins. In this process, LPS-binding protein (*LBP*) has an important function by liberating smaller oligomers and/or monomers from LPS aggregates and transmitting them to receptor molecules. Several mechanisms are discussed for the activation of target cells, where CD14 is of decisive importance in the case of low endotoxin concentrations ($<$ 10 ng/ml). A transmembrane, signal-transmitting receptor for LPS (here termed *X*) is not yet known. *HDL*, high density lipoprotein; *BPI*, bactericidal permeability-increasing protein; *mCD14*, membrane-bound CD14 molecule; *sCD14*, soluble (serum) CD14 molecule

The activation of cells by low concentrations of endotoxin is augmented about 1000-fold in the presence of serum [77, 89, 90]. This effect is due to the action of LPS binding protein (LBP) [98, 99]. LBP is a 58-kDa glycoprotein which is synthesized in hepatocytes and constantly released into the blood stream [100]. Its serum concentration of approximately 10–20 mg/ml can rise up to 200 mg/ml after infection during the host's acute phase response [100]. LBP shows 44% sequence similarity to BPI and, likewise, has a high affinity amino-terminal binding region for LPS or lipid A, respectively [98, 100]. The catalytic mechanism of LBP action has been examined intensively [48, 101, 102]. From today's point of view [46], LBP binds to LPS aggregates and resolves their supramolecular structure into LPS oligomers or monomers (Fig. 8). Subsequently, these are then transmitted as a complex with LBP to cell-bound and/or soluble CD14. Additionally, LBP catalyzes the transfer of LPS to BPI and to high-density lipoprotein (HDL) [48, 103–105], indicating that LBP also participates in the neutralization of endotoxins. It is, thus, conceivable that low amounts of LBP augment, whereas high doses inhibit LPS activity similar to sCD14 [145].

Although the importance of CD14 for specific binding of LPS and cell activation is indisputable, the first steps of the direct signal transduction into the cell has not been well defined to date. The CD14 protein possesses no domain spanning the cytoplasmic membrane [80] and can apparently – in a soluble form without GPI-anchor – also mediate an endotoxin-specific stimulation of endothelial cells [82, 88–91]. Therefore, the presence of another transmembrane protein for a CD14-dependent cell activation has been postulated which, as a receptor, has an LPS–CD14-binding and at the same time signal-transmitting function. It is known that macrophages and monocytes can also be stimulated by high endotoxin concentrations (>100 ng/ml) to release cytokines in a CD14-independent manner [106, 107]. This was also confirmed using macrophages from a CD14-negative mouse strain [108] and served as proof of an additional, CD14-independent pathway of cell activation by endotoxins. Recently, CD11c/CD18, a heterodimeric adhesion molecule of the integrin family, has been described as a functional transmembrane receptor mediating CD14-independent stimulation of macrophage-like cells in the presence of high LPS-concentrations [107]. It should be emphasized, however, that LPS-concentrations in these experiments are distinctly higher than corresponding serum values, e.g., during septic episodes.

In the search for a membrane signal transducer for a CD14-dependent way of cell activation in the presence of low amounts of endotoxin, a ligand binding test has recently been developed which permits the detection of lipid A binding to membrane proteins separated by gel electrophoresis and immobilized by transfer on to nitrocellulose membranes [109]. With the aid of this method, an 80-kDa protein from membranes of Mono-Mac–6-cells, a human monocyte cell line, could be demonstrated [109]. The protein binds lipid A only in the presence of serum or a mixture of purified sCD14 and LBP. It could further be shown to be present in cell membranes of human peripheral blood monocytes and endothelial cells. Whether this protein is involved in LPS-induced and LBP/CD14-dependent transduction remains to be elucidated.

Strategies for Treating Endotoxemia and Gram-Negative Septic Shock

Gram-negative sepsis represents a dramatic disease which is associated with high morbidity and mortality [4–6]. Despite considerable progress in the fields of modern antibiotic research and application, as well as intensive care medicine, the high sepsis lethality has not been successfully lowered over recent decades [110, 111]. Bacterial LPS constitutes a major factor responsible for pathological manifestations of gram-negative sepsis and its most dramatic manifestation – septic shock. LPS is released in higher amounts from bacteria, in particular, in the course of antibiotic therapies [3, 112] and the selective blockade of an overwhelming activation of different target cells caused by great quantities of circulating endotoxins represents an important approach to control this severe disease.

In principle, each step of the endotoxic activation cascade (see Figs. 2 and 7) could serve as a basis for the development of new therapy concepts [review in 112]. In our opinion, however, the early phases concerning the released bacterial toxin itself as the initial stimulus and its interaction with enhancing and inhibiting humoral factors (LBP, sCD14, BPI), as well as cell-bound receptors (mCD14), are of special interest. This concept is supported by the consideration that focussing on the early etiologic factors of the septic cascade would lead to an increased selectivity and, therefore, to less side effects regarding an antiseptic drug. In addition, an early therapeutic blockade, or even prophylactic medication, seem to be required from the clinician's point of view since, in practice, the development of septic shock is often difficult to predict [113]. In this chapter we will present only two concepts with promising clinical application, both followed on a basic research level at the Research Center Borstel.

Antagonists of Endotoxic Effects

During investigations characterizing in detail the nature of the interaction between lipid A and target cells, we determined the binding of radioactively- or fluorescently (fluorescein isothiocyanate)-labeled LPS to the murine macrophage cell line J774.1 or to human peripheral monocytes. For both systems, binding kinetics could be obtained which showed saturation [114]. This binding was completely inhibited by nanogram quantities of unlabeled R- or S-form LPS (Fig. 9). In further experiments, we examined defined partial structures of lipid A regarding its competitive effect in this binding test. After cleavage of the fatty acids from the hydrophilic saccharide backbone, no inhibition (which means no binding to the receptor) could be detected, comparable to the experiments regarding the release of cytokines. Therefore, the hydrophobic region of lipid A seemed to also be important for binding to target cells. However, a partial structure of lipid A could be identified – synthetic compound 406 – corresponding to a biosynthetic lipid A precursor molecule from *E. coli* with four fatty acids (lipid A precursor Ia or lipid IVa; for structure see Fig. 10a) which completely inhibited the binding of Re LPS (Fig. 9), but was not able to activate human, peripheral monocytes (see Fig. 5b). These results confirmed that initial specific binding of LPS to target cells takes place through the *hydrophilic* bisphosphorylated saccharide backbone

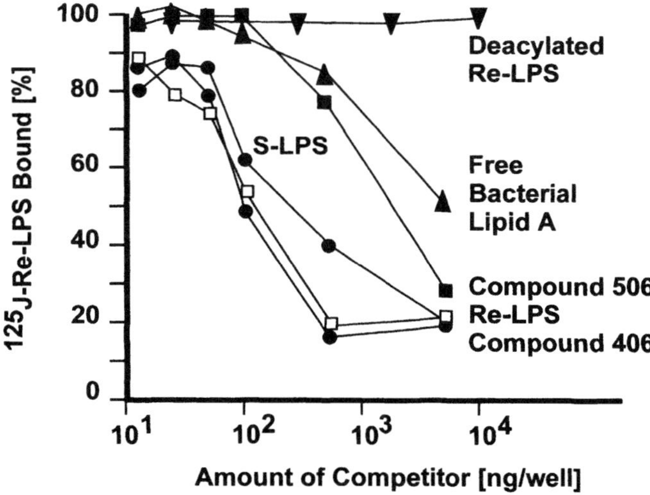

Fig. 9. Competitive inhibition of lipopolysaccharide (*LPS*) binding to the murine macrophage cell line J774.1. Binding of ^{125}J-labeled Re LPS was inhibited compared to control by increasing concentrations of LPS, free lipid A, or defined partial structures of Re LPS

(acyl groups also playing an important but non-specific role) before additional structural characteristics of the *hydrophobic* region of lipid A induce cell activation and release of cytokines.

This experimentally found separation of lipid A "binding" and lipid A-mediated "activation" suggested that endotoxically inactive LPS or partial structures may bind to target cells without activating them and, therefore, may probably represent inhibitors of endotoxic effects. This could be confirmed by our studies [36] and by others for the corresponding lipid A precursors from *E. coli* [36, 115, 116] and *S. enterica* serovar Typhimurium [117, 118]. The tetraacylated synthetic compound 406 inhibits specifically and in a dose-dependent manner the LPS-induced release of cytokines from human monocytes [36, 38, 115]. This inhibition takes place at a very early stage of cytokine production: Both the LPS-induced phosphorylation of proteins [119] and the specific synthesis of mRNA for IL-1 and TNFα [120] are suppressed. In addition, the LPS-induced expression of the intercellular adhesion molecule ICAM-1 [74] and the synthesis of IL-6 in the presence of serum [121] by endothelial cells could also be inhibited with this substance. Apart from the tetraacylated partial structure 406 of *E. coli*, non-toxic lipid A preparations from the phototrophic bacteria *Rb. sphaeroides* [33, 122] and *Rb. capsulatus* (Fig. 10b) [32, 121] also proved to be potent inhibitors of endotoxic effects. Recently, these observations resulted in the chemical synthesis of an antagonistic, pentaacylated analogue on the basis of lipid A from

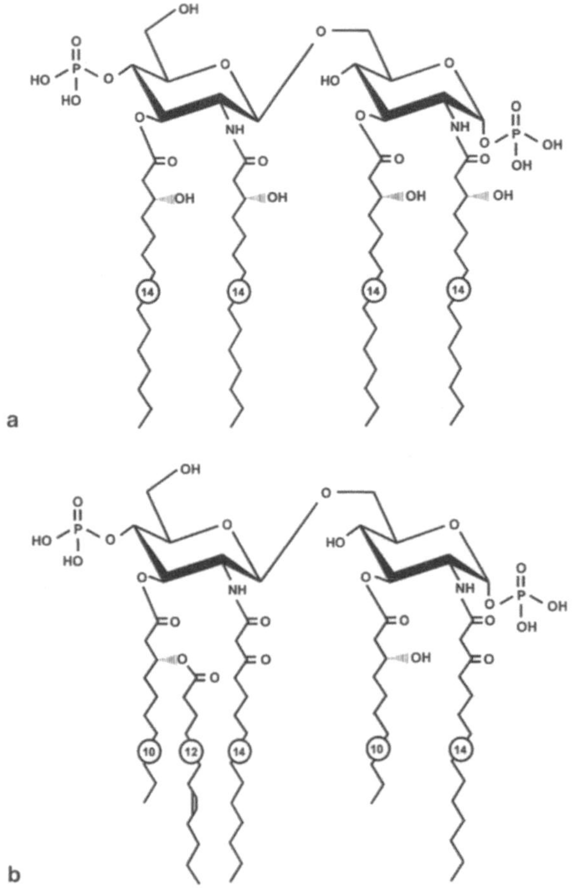

Fig. 10. Chemical structure of synthetic lipid A partial structure compound 406 (**a**) and non-toxic lipid A from *Rhodobacter capsulatus* (**b**)

Rb. capsulatus (substance E5531) [123]. This molecule reduces endotoxin-caused lethality in mice and, together with antibiotic medication, is able to protect the animals from *E. coli*-induced lethal peritonitis and a phase-1 clinical study with preparation E5531 shows its efficiency in inhibiting endotoxemic effects [123].

The mechanism of the inhibitory effect of lipid A partial structures such as compound 406 was intensively examined in different cell systems [36, 38, 114, 118, 124–127]. For cytokine induction of the murine macrophage cell line J774.1, as well as of peripheral human monocytes, we suppose a direct competition of these substances with active endotoxin for a surface-bound receptor. Our suggestion is supported by the fact that monokine production by other stimuli, such as phorbolester or lipopeptide, are not influenced by compound 406 [36, 38, 115]. In addition, the level of inhibition clearly depends on the competitor's dose and can be neutralized by an excess of LPS. Finally, an antagonistic effect could be proven by a quantitative evaluation of the binding using Lineweaver/Burk plots [126]. Because of these and further results not shown, we conclude that inhibitory preparations such as compound 406, lipid A from *Rb. sphaeroides*, or substance E5531 block an LPS-specific binding site on the target cells and so prevent binding and activation by endotoxins. CD14 could represent the decisive membrane protein for this inhibitory path since it is known that mCD14 can bind substance 406 and that the antagonistic effect of this lipid A partial structure is further neutralized by an antibody against CD14 [101]. This assumption, however, is not supported by other studies using the cell line THP-1 and suggesting a non-antagonistic mechanism for the preparation 406 [125].

Neutralizing Antibodies Against Endotoxin

Apart from antagonistic molecules which block the activity of endotoxins at the level of target cells, in particular those substances which can directly neutralize the activity of released endotoxins have recently been discussed for prophylaxis and therapy of gram-negative septic shock. Among these molecules, immunoglobulins represent classic therapeutic antitoxins which in many regards appear as a particularly suitable tool. Antibodies against endotoxins could interrupt the activation cascade of gram-negative sepsis at a very early stage. In addition, they are distinguished by a good host tolerance and long half-life in the patient's body because of their high specificity and low immunogenicity. Finally, antibodies in complexes with their specific antigen may activate the complement system or bind to Fc-receptors of phagocytes and, therefore, contribute to an accelerated non-inflammatory elimination of endotoxins. Due to these advantages, an immunological approach for the therapy of gram-negative sepsis has long been pursued.

In principle, all structural regions of the LPS molecule exhibit immunogenic and antigenic properties. Thus, polyclonal [128], as well as monoclonal [129, 130], antibodies against determinants of the O-specific chain turned out to be successfully protective in different endotoxin and infection models. However, the therapeutic benefit of these sera and antibodies are limited because of the high serotype variability of the O-specific chain, especially among the clinically relevant bacteria *E. coli*, *Klebsiella pneumoniae*, and *Pseudomonas aeruginosa*. The lipid A component of many pathogenic microorganisms proved instead to be an extraordinarily conserved region [28]. In addition, the center of endotoxic activity is localized in this LPS domain [28, 29], which therefore seemed to be predestined as a target structure for the production of neutralizing antibodies with a broad cross-reactivity with different pathogenic gram-negative bacteria. Interestingly, antibody specificities against free lipid A could hardly be detected in the serum of experimental animals which had been immunized with R- and S-form bacteria. Corresponding antisera [131] and monoclonal antibodies [132, 133] could, however, be generated with free lipid A as the immunogen and characterized with different lipid A preparations and partial structures regarding their specificity [134–136]. These antibodies showed cross-reactivity with different lipid A molecules which had been liberated from their polysaccharide portion [131, 134]. The epitopes of all investigated antibodies could be determined to be located in the hydrophilic saccharide backbone. However, no reactivity was found with lipid A still substituted with the saccharide portion of the core region [131]. The rationale for this seems to be that the primary hydroxyl group of the non-reducing GlcN residue (GlcNII in Fig. 4) serves as the epitope for lipid A-specific antibodies and, as such, substituted with Kdo, is not freely accessible in LPS. Thus, lipid A must be regarded as a neoantigen, and cross-reactivity between lipid A and LPS is unlikely [137]. Because of these circumstances, a protective effect of lipid A antibodies during a septic course is not to be expected. In fact, extensive clinical studies concluded with this result [138, 139].

The chemical analysis of core oligosaccharides of numerous LPS showed that this region within many strains and species of microorganisms contains conserved structural elements [13]. In particular, many clinically relevant isolates from the family of the *Enterobacteriaceae* have characteristics in common in the region of the inner core (Kdo and Hep) and its adjoining segments (Fig. 11; see also Fig. 3). By immunization of New Zealand black (NZB) mice with LPS from *E. coli* mutants with different core types (R1–R4) as immunogens, we have recently been able to produce monoclonal antibodies

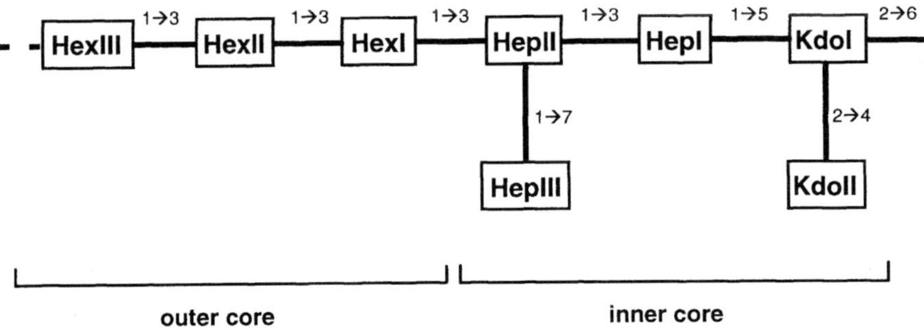

Fig. 11. Common structural characteristic of the core region of lipopolysaccharide from *Escherichia coli* and *Salmonella enterica*. All glycosyl bonds are α-pyranosidically configurated. *Hex*, D-glucose, D-galactose, or *N*-acetyl-D-glucosamine; *Hep*, L-*glycero*-D-*manno*-heptose; *Kdo*, 3-deoxy-D-*manno*-oct-2-ulosonic acid

which showed broad cross-reactivity with R- and S-form LPS from *E. coli*, *S. enterica*, and *Shigella* [140, 141]. In addition, these antibodies also exhibited anti-endotoxic qualities. One of these monoclonal antibodies, WN1 222-5 (IgG2a), was able to offer potent protection against the lethal effects of different endotoxins in mice (Table 1), as well as dramatically reduce the fever response of rabbits after LPS application [35]. In addition, a clear improvement in the survival rate was observed in infection experiments with mice (Table 2) [142]. For a conceivable application in patients, a human chimeric IgG1-isotype (SDZ 219-800) was finally created from WN1 222-5 [143] to achieve a better tolerance and half-life of the antibody. Figure 12 shows the

Table 1. Inhibition of LPS-induced lethality by monoclonal anti-LPS antibodies in mice

mAb (1 mg/mouse)	Surviving over treated animals after challenge with endotoxin derived from	
	S. enterica serovar Abortus equi (1 ng/mouse)	*E. coli* O16 (2 ng/mouse)
WN1 222–5	6/6	5/6
SDZ 219–800	6/6	5/6
HA-1A	0/6	1/6
Control	0/6	1/6

The monoclonal antibodies (mAB) were administered i.v. 2 h before i.v. application of LPS and i.p. administration of D-galactosamine (16 mg/mouse) in C57BL/6 mice

Table 2. Effects of anti-LPS antibodies on survival, blood bacterial counts, and TNFα levels in OF1 mice (outbred strain, IFFA credo) challenged i.v. with *E. coli* O111 (10^9 bacteria per mouse)

Treatment	Number of survivors/total	Blood bacterial counts (log CFU/ml) at [d]:		Blood TNFα levels (ng/ml) at 1.5 h [d]
		1.5 h	5 h	
Saline	0/8	7.3 ± 0.2	6.8 ± 0.3	38 ± 21
D6B3[a]	8/8	4.9 ± 0.2[c]	3.7 ± 0.3[c]	27 ± 17
WN1 222–5[b]	6/8	6.4 ± 0.3[c]	4.8 ± 0.4[c]	41 ± 12

[a] O-specific monoclonal antibody; 100 µg per mouse.
[b] 500 µg per mouse.
[c] $p < 0.001$ versus the saline group by Mann-Whitney test (two-tailed).
[d] Mean ± standard deviation.
TNFα, tumor necrosis factor-α.

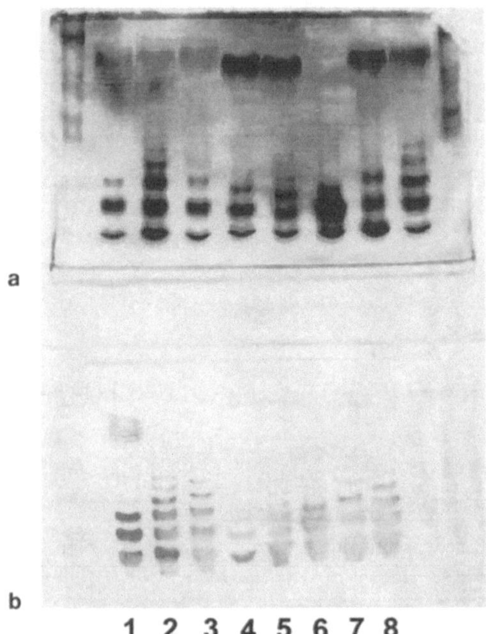

Fig. 12. Cross-reactivity of core oligosaccharide-specific, chimeric, monoclonal antibody SDZ 219-800 with clinically important *Escherichia coli* strains. **a** Sodium dodecyl sulfate polyacrylamide gel electrophoresis of lipopolysaccharide. Visualization was performed by silver nitrate staining after oxidation with periodic acid. **b** Immunoblot with monoclonal antibody SDZ 219-800. *1, Escherichia coli* O111; *2, E. coli* O86; *3, E. coli* O18; *4, E. coli* O16; *5, E. coli* O15; *6, E. coli* O12; *7, E. coli* O6; *8, E. coli* O4

cross-reactivity of this antibody with S-type LPS of a number of pathogenic *E. coli* strains in the form of an immunoblot. Further experiments proved also the binding to all clinical isolates from *E. coli, S. enterica* and some other *Enterobacteriaceae*. Apart from that, SDZ 219-800 could efficiently neutralize these endotoxins in different experimental systems in vitro and in vivo (Table 3) [140, 141].

The antibodies WN1 222-5 and SDZ 219-800 show no reactivity with free lipid A. The LPS-epitope which is accessible for the binding of these antibodies also in the presence of the O-specific chain, partially includes structural elements of the inner and outer core region (see Fig. 11). Therefore, no direct binding to the endotoxic center of LPS, i.e., lipid A, is necessary for the neutralizing effect of the antibodies. Steric effects of the bound antibody or a conformational change of LPS induced by the binding of the antibody could prevent the binding of endotoxins to LBP or CD14 [144]. In addition, an increased elimination of LPS/antibody complexes by Fc-receptors and/or the complement system is conceivable for the neutralizing effect in vivo.

Therefore, cross-reactive monoclonal antibodies against the core oligosaccharide of LPS can be regarded as potent neutralizing agents of endotoxin. In the near future, the further development and characterization of these antibodies may offer the chance for an immunotherapy of patients suffering from gram-negative sepsis. Present research projects at the Research Center

Table 3. Monoclonal anti-LPS core antibody SDZ 219-800 inhibits interleukin (IL)-6 secretion of mouse peritoneal macrophages induced by *E. coli* O111 LPS

Endotoxin from *E. coli* O111 (nM)	IL-6 secreted in culture supernatants in the absence or presence of mAb SDZ 219-800		
	Control	MAb SDZ 219-800	
		0.1 nM	1 nM
	ng/ml		
10	23.376	22.612	20.126
1	14.047	10.427	2.225
0.1	1.041	0.684	0.171
0.01	0.267	0.141	0.142
Control	0.125	0.128	0.224

IL-6 in culture supernatants was determined using the B13–29 hybridoma cell line. mAb, monoclonal antibody

Borstel include the extension of this concept to other clinically relevant bacteria including *Klebsiella* and *Pseudomonas* strains.

Final Remarks

As demonstrated in this short review, endotoxin represents a bacterial toxin which, in the case of overproduction, can trigger severe pathophysiological reactions in animals and humans. However, it is feasible that the overproduction and self-destructive overreaction of higher organisms only represent a rare exception. Perhaps LPS should actually be considered from another, but no less important, point of view which has to do with a more physiological role and the maintenance of human health. It is a well-known fact that endotoxin-free life does not exist. Each human organism carries about 10^{14} bacteria colonizing the digestive system, other mucosal areas, and the skin. Assuming that about 50% of these microorganisms belong to the class of gram-negative bacteria, our body is potentially confronted with 10–20 g endotoxin, of which 3–10 pg/ml LPS normally circulate in the blood. From the moment of birth on, our organism obviously has to struggle with gram-negative bacteria and their surface structures – and therefore above all also with LPS – and there are indications that this struggle is of decisive importance for the development of essential body systems such as the immune system. It can further be supposed that small LPS quantities are permanently resorbed from the intestinal flora and activate the immune system in a physiological manner and, so to speak, provide a particular tonus to it. Perhaps endotoxins represent vitamin-like substances produced by bacteria which are of great importance for the maintenance of the homeostasis of higher developed organisms such as humans. In this way it could be argued that in fact two million patients die of endotoxin-caused septic shock annually, but that on the other hand six billion people profit from its physiological effects of LPS [146]. Therefore, one of the most exciting problems of endotoxin research in the years to come will be the further characterization of the importance of endotoxin for the maintenance of human health.

Acknowledgments. The financial support of the DFG (Sonderforschungsbereich 367, projects B1 and B2, Sonderforschungsbereich 470, projects A1, B4, Graduiertenkolleg GRK 288, project A1), of the BMBF (grant 01KI/9471), and the Fonds der Chemischen Industrie (EThR) is gratefully appreciated. We thank Mrs. M. Kohlmorgen, and F. Richter for typing the manuscript, as well as I. Bouchain, M. Lohs, and G. Müller for the art and photographic work.

References

1. Pfeiffer R (1892) Untersuchungen über das Choleragift. Z Hyg 11:393–412
2. Bhakdi S, Grimminger F, Suttrop N, Walmrath D, Seeger W (1994) Proteinaceous bacterial toxins and pathogenesis of septic shock syndrome and septic shock: The unknown connection. Med Microbiol Immunol 183:119–144
3. Kirikae T, Nakano M, Morrison DC (1997) Antibiotic-induced endotoxin release from bacteria and its clinical significance. Micrbiol Immunol 41:285–294
4. Nogare D (1991) Southwestern internal medicine conference: Septic shock. Am J Med Sci 302:50–65
5. Bone RC (1993) Gram-negative sepsis: A dilemma of moderne medicine. Clin Micobiol Rev 6:57–68
6. Morrison DC, Danner RL, Dinarello CA, Munford RS, Natanson C, Pollack M, Spitzer JJ, Ulevitch RJ, Vogel SN, McSweegan E (1994) Bacterial endotoxins and pathogenesis of gram-negative infections: Current status and future direction. J Endotoxin Res 1:71–83
7. Schnaitman CA, Klena JD (1993) Genetics of lipopolysaccharide biosynthesis in enteric bacteria. Microbiol Rev 57:655–682
8. Whitfield C, Valvano MA (1993) Biosynthesis and expression of cell-surface polysaccharides in gram-negative bacteria. Adv Microb Physiol 35:135–246
9. Jann K, Jann B (1984) Structure and biosynthesis of O-antigens. In: Rietschel ET (ed) Handbook of Endotoxin, Vol. 1. Chemistry of Endotoxin. Elsevier Science Publisher, Amsterdam, pp 138–186
10. Knirel YA, Kochetkov NK (1994) The structure of lipopolysaccharides in gram-negative bacteria. III. The structure of O-antigens: A review. Biochem (Moscow) 59:1325–1383

11. Knirel YA, Rietschel ET, Marre R, Zähringer U (1994) The structure of the O-specific chain of *Legionella pneumophila* serotype 1 lipopolysaccharide. Eur J Biochem 221:239–245
12. Kaufmann F (1978) Das Fundament. Munksgaard, Copenhagen
13. Holst O, Brade H (1992) Chemical structure of the core region of lipopolysaccharides. In: Morrison DC, Ryan JL (eds) Bacterial endotoxic lipopolysaccharides, Vol. 1. CRC Press, Boca Raton, pp 135–170
14. Belunis CJ, Clementz T, Carty SM, Raetz CRH (1995) Inhibition of lipopolysaccharide biosynthesis and cell growth following inactivation of the *kdtA* gene in *Escherichia coli*. J Biol Chem 270:27646–27652
15. Rick PD, Osborn MJ (1977) Lipid A mutants of *Salmonella tyhimurium*. J Biol Chem 252:4895–4903
16. Zähringer U, Lindner B, Seydel U, Rietschel ET, Naoki H, Unger FM, Imoto M, Kusumoto S, Shiba T (1985) Structure of the de-O-acylated lipopolysaccharide from Escherichia coli Re mutant strain F515. Tetrahedron Lett 26:6321–6324
17. Brabetz W, Müller-Loennies S, Holst O, Brade H (1997) Deletion of the heptosyltransferase genes *rfaC* and *rfaF* in *Escherichia coli* K-12 results in an Re-type lipopolysaccharide with a high degree of 2-aminoethanol phosphate substitution. Eur J Biochem 247:716–724
18. Helander IM, Lindner B, Brade H, Altman K, Lindberg AA, Rietschel ET, Zähringer U (1988) Chemical structure of the lipopolysaccharide of *Haemophilus influenzae* strain I-69 Rd-/b+: Description of a new deep-rough phenotype. Eur J Biochem 177:483–492
19. Goldman RC, Kohlbrenner W, Lartey P, Pernet A (1987) Antimicrobial agents specifically inhibiting lipopolysaccharide biosynthesis. Nature 329:162–164
20. Hammond SM, Claesson A, Jansson AM, Larsson L-G, Pring BG, Town CM, Ekström B (1987) A new class of synthetic antibacterials acting on lipopolysaccharide. Nature 327:730–732
21. Brade H, Brabetz W, Brade L, Holst O, Lucakova M, Mamat U, Rozalski A, Zych K, Kosma P (1997) Chlamydial lipopolysaccharide. J Endotoxin Res 4:67–84
22. White KA, Kaltashov IA, Cotter RJ, Raetz CRH (1997) A mono-functional 3-deoxy-D-*manno*-octulosonic acid (Kdo) transferase and Kdo kinase in extracts of *Haemophilus influenzae*. J Biol Chem 272:16555–16563
23. Belunis CJ, Raetz CRH (1992) Biosynthesis of endotoxins. Purification and catalytic properities of 3-deoxy-D-*manno*-octulosonic acid transferase from *Escherichia coli*. J Biol Chem 267:9988–9997
24. Mamat U, Baumann M, Schmidt G, Brade H (1993) The genus-specific lipopolysaccharide epitope of *Chlamydia* is assembled in *C. psittaci* and *C. trachomatis* by glycosyltransferases of low homology. Mol Microbiol 10:391–399
25. Löbau S, Mamat U, Brabetz W, Brade H (1995) Molecular cloning, sequencing and functional characterization of the lipopolysaccharide biosynthetic gene kdtA encoding 3-deoxy-D-*manno*-octulosonic acid transferase of *Chlamydia pneumoniae* strain TW-183. Mol Microbiol 18:391–399
26. Belunis CJ, Mdluli KE, Raetz CRH, Nano FE (1992) A novel 3-deoxy-D-*manno*-octulosonic acid transferase from *Chlamydia trachomatis* required for expression of the genus-specific epitope. J Biol Chem 267:18702–18707
27. Westphal O, Lüderitz O (1954) Chemische Erforschung von Lipopolysacchariden Gram-negativer Bakterien. Angew Chem 66:407–417
28. Zähringer U, Lindner B, Rietschel ET (1994) Molecular structure of lipid A, the endotoxic center of bacterial lipopolysaccharides. Adv Carbohydr Chem Biochem 50:211–276

114 W. Brabetz et al.

29. Galanos C, Lüderitz O, Rietschel ET, Westphal O, Brade H, Brade L, Freudenberg MA, Schade FU, Imoto M, Yoshimura S, Kusumoto S, Shiba T (1985) Synthetic and natural *Escherichia coli* free lipid A express identical endotoxic activities. Eur J Biochem 148:1–5
30. Kusumoto S (1992) Chemical synthesis of lipid A. In: Morrison DC, Ryan JL (eds) Bacterial endotoxic lipopolysaccharides. Vol. 1. Molecular biochemistry and cellular biology. CRC Press, Boca Raton, pp 81–106
31. Maitra SK, Schotz MC, Yoshikawa TT, Guze LB (1978) Determination of lipid A and endotoxin in serum by mass spectroscopy. Proc Natl Acad Sci USA 75: 3993–3997
32. Loppnow H, Libby P, Freudenberg MA, Kraus JH, Weckesser J, Mayer H (1990) Cytokine induction by lipopolysaccharide (LPS) corresponds to the lethal toxicity and is inhibited by nontoxic *Rhodobacter capsulatus* LPS. Infect Immun 58:3743–3750
33. Quereshi N, Takayama K, Kurtz R (1991) Diphosphoryl lipid A obtained from the nontoxic lipopolysaccharide of *Rhodopseudomonas sphaeroides* is an endotoxin antagonist in mice. Infect Immun 59:441–444
34. Weintraub A, Zähringer U, Wollenweber H-W, Seydel U, Rietschel ET (1989) Structural characterization of the lipid A component of *Bacteroides fragilis* strain NCTC 9343 lipopolysaccharide. Eur J Biochem 183:425–431
35. Bhat NM, Forsberg LS, Carlson RW (1994) Structure of the lipid A component of *Rhizobium leguminosarum* hv. phaseoli lipopolysaccharide. J Biol Chem 269:14402–14410
36. Loppnow H, Brade H, Dürrbaum I, Dinarello CA, Kusumoto S, Rietschel ET, Flad H-D (1989) Interleukin 1 induction-capacity of defined lipopolysaccharide partial structures. J Immunol 142:3229–3238
37. Ulmer AJ, Feist W, Heine H, Kirikae T, Kirikae F, Kusumoto S, Kusama T, Brade H, Schade U, Rietschel ET, Flad H-D (1992) Modulation of endotoxin-induced monokine release in human monocytes by lipid A partial structures in hibiting the binding of ^{125}I-LPS. Infect Immun 60:5145–5152
38. Flad H-D, Loppnow H, Rietschel ET, Ulmer AJ (1993) Agonists and antagonists for lipopolysaccharide-induced cytokines. Immunbiology 187:303–316
39. Somerville JE Jr, Cassiano L, Bainbridge B, Cunningham MD, Darveau RP (1996) A novel *Escherichia coli* lipid A mutant that produces an antiinflammatory lipopolysaccharide. J Clin Invest 97:359–365
40. Nichols WA, Raetz CRH, Clementz T, Smith AL, Hanson JA, Ketterer MR, Sunshine M, Apicella MA (1997) htrB of *Haemophilus influenzae*. Determination of biochemical activity and effects on virulence and lipopolysaccharide toxicity. J Endotoxin Res 4:163–172
41. Seydel U, Labischinski H, Kastowsky M, Brandenburg K (1993) Phase behaviour, supramolecular structure, and molecular conformation of lipopolysaccharide. J Immunol 187:191–211
42. Brandenburg K, Mayer H, Koch MHJ, Weckesser J, Rietschel ET, Seydel U (1993) Influence of the supramolecular structure of free lipid A on its biological activity. Eur J Biochem 218:555–563
43. Brandenburg K, Seydel U, Schromm AB, Loppnow H, Koch MHJ, Rietschel ET (1996) Conformation of lipid A, the endotoxic center of bacterial lipopolysaccharide. J Endotoxin Res 3:173–178
44. Shnyra A, Hultenby K, Lindberg AA (1993) Role of the physical state of *Salmonella* lipopolysaccharide in expression of biological and endotoxic properties. Infect Immun 61:5351–5360

45. Takayama K, Mitchell DH, Din ZZ, Mukerjee P, Li C, Coleman DL (1994) Monomeric Re lipopolysaccharide from *Escherichia coli* is more active than the aggregated form in the *Limulus amoebocyte* lysate assay and in inducing Egr-1 mRNA in murine peritoneal macrophages. J Biol Chem 269:2241-2244

46. Schromm AB, Brandenburg K, Rietschel ET, Flad H-D, Carroll SF, Seydel U (1996) Lipopolysaccharide-binding protein mediates CD14-independent intercalation of lipopolysaccharide into phospholipid membranes. FEBS Letters 399:267-271

47. Schromm AB, Brandenburg K, Rietschel ET, Seydel U (1995) Do endotoxin aggregates intercalate into phospholipid membranes in a nonspecific, hydrophobic manner? J Endotoxin Res 2:313-323

48. Yu B, Wright SD (1996) Catalytic properies of lipopolysaccharide (LPS) binding protein. Transfer of LPS to soluble CD14. J Biol Chem 271:4100-4105

49. Rietschel ET, Brade H, Brade L, Brandenburg K, Schade U, Seydel U, Zähringer U, Galanos C, Lüderitz O, Westphal O, Labischinski H, Kusumoto S, Shiba T (1987) Lipid A, the endotoxic center of lipopolysaccharides: Relation of chemical structure to biological activity. Prog Clin Biol Res 231:25-53

50. Freudenberg MA, Keppler D, Galanos C (1986) Requirement for lipopolysaccharide responsive macrophages in galactosamin-induced sensitization to endotoxin. Infect Immun 51:891-895

51. Bernhagen J, Calandra T, Cerami A, Bucala R (1993) Macrophage migration inhibitory factor is a neuroendocrine mediator of endotoxaemia. Trends Microbiol 2:198-201

52. Nathan CF (1987) Secretory products of macrophages. J Clin Invest 79:319-323

53. Mastroeni P, Jannello D, Mastroeni PI (1993) TNFα as a modulator of the interaction between macrophages and intracellular parasites. Eur Bull Drug Res 2:163-174

54. Echternacher B, Falk W, Männel DN, Krammer PH (1990) Requirement of endogenous tumor necrosis factor cachectin for recovery from experimental peritonitis. J Immunol 145:3762-3766

55. Parillo JE (1993) Pathogenic mechanism of septic schock. N Engl J Med 328: 1471-1477

56. Vogel SN, Hogan MM (1990) The role of cytokines in endotoxin-mediated host response. In: Oppenheim JJ, Shevack EM (eds) Immunopharmacology – the role of cells and cytokines in immunity and inflammation. Oxford University Press, New York, pp 238-258

57. Schade FU, Burmeister I, Elekes E, Engel R, Wolter DT (1989) Mononuclear phagocytes and eicosanoids: Aspects of their synthesis and biological activities. Blut 59:475-485

58. Lüderitz T, Brandenburg K, Seydel U, Roth A, Galanos C, Rietschel ET (1989) Structural and physicochemical requirements of endotoxins for the activation of arachidonic acid metabolism in mouse peritoneal macrophages. Eur J Biochem 179:11-16

59. Schade FU, Burmeister I, Engel R (1987) Increased 1 3-hydroxyoctadecandienoic acid content in lipopolysaccharide-stimulated macrophages. Biochem Biophys Res Commun 147:695-700

60. Braquet P, Touqui L, Shen TY, Vargaftig BB (1987) Perspectives in platelet-activating factor research. Pharmacol Rev 39:97-112

61. Munford RS, Hall CL (1989) Purification of acyloxyacyl hydrolase, a leukocyte enzyme that removes secondary acyl chains from bacterial lipopolysaccharides. J Biol Chem 264:15613-15619

62. Mannion B, Kalatzis A, Weiss J, Elsbach P (1989) Preferential binding of the neutrophile cytoplasmic granule-derived bactericidal/permeability-increasing protein to target bacteria. Implications and use as a mean of purification. J Immunol 142:2807–2812

63. Marra MN, Wilde CG, Griffith JE, Snable JL, Scott RW (1990) Bactericidal/permeability-increasing protein has endotoxin-neutralizing activity. J Immunol 144:662–666

64. Marra MN, Wilde CG, Collins MS, Snable JL, Thornton MB, Scott RW (1992) The role of bactericidal/permeability-increasing protein as a natural inhibitor of bacterial endotoxin. J Immunol 148:532–537

65. Gray PW, Flaggs G, Leong SR, Gumina RJ, Weiss J, Ooi CE, Elsbach P (1989) Cloning of the cDNA of a human bactericidal protein. Structural and functional correlations. J Biol Chem 264:9505–9509

66. Meszaros K, Parent JB, Gazzano-Santoro H, Little R, Horwitz A, Parsons T, Theofan G, Grinna L, Weickmann J, Elsbach P, Weiss J, Conlon PJ (1993) A recombinant aminoterminal fragment of bactericidal/permeability increasing protein inhibits the induction of leucocyte response by LPS. J Leuk Biol 54:558–563

67. Weiss J, Elsbach P, Shu C, Castillo J, Horwitz A, Theofan G (1992) Human bactericidal/permeability-increasing protein and a recombinant NH_2-terminal fragment cause killing of serum-resistant gram-negative bacteria in whole blood and inhibit tumor necrosis factor release induced by the bacteria. J Clin Invest 90:1122–1130

68. Loppnow H, Libby P (1989) Adult human vascular endothelial cells express the IL-6 gene differently in response to LPS and IL-1. Cell Immunol 122:493–503

69. Loppnow H, Libby P (1990) Proliferating or IL-1 activated human vascular smooth muscle cells secrete copious IL-6. J Clin Invest 85:731–738

70. Loppnow H, Libby P (1992) Functional significance of human vascular smooth muscle cell-derived interleukin 1 in paracrine and autocrine regulation pathways. Exp Cell Res 198:283–290

71. Schönbeck U, Brandt E, Petersen F, Flad H-D, Loppnow H (1995) Interleukin 8 specifically binds to endothelial but not to smooth muscle cells. J Immunol 154:2375–2883

72. Mantovani A, Bussolino F (1991) Endothelium-derived modulators of leukocyte function. In: Gordon JL (ed) Vascular endothelium: Interaction with circulating cells. Elsevier, New York

73. Libby P, Loppnow H, Fleet JC, Palmer H, Li HM, Warner SJC, Salomon RN, Clinton SK (1991) Production of cytokines by vascular cells – an update and implications for artherogenesis. In: Gottlieb AI, Langille BL, Frederoff S (eds) Artheriosclerosis – cellular and molecular interactions in the artery wall. 1st Albsclul Symposium. Plenum, New York

74. Schönbeck U, Brandt E, Flad H-D, Rietschel ET, Loppnow H (1994) S-form lipopolysaccharide induces leukocyte adhesion to human vascular endothelial cells as potent as IL-1: Lipid A precursor Ia antagonizes induction of adhesion by LPS. J Endotoxin Res 1:4–13

75. Yu CL, Haskard DO, Cavender D, Ziff M (1986) Effects of bacterial lipopolysaccharides on the binding of lymphocytes to endothelial cell monolayers. J Immunol 136:569–573

76. Doherty DE, Zagarello L, Henson PM, Worthen GS (1989) Lipopolysaccharide stimulates monocyte adherence by effects on both the monocyte and endothelial cell. J Immunol 143:3673–3679

77. Wright SD, Ramos RA, Tobias PS, Ulevitch RJ, Mathison JC (1990) CD14, a receptor for complexes of lipopolysaccharide (LPS) and LPS binding protein. Science 249:1431–1433
78. Griffin JD, Ritz J, Nadler LM, Rossman SF (1981) Expression of myeloid differentiation antigens on normal and malignant myeloid cells. J Clin Invest 68: 932–941
79. Ziegler-Heitbrock H, Ulevitch RJ (1993) CD14: Cell surface receptor and differentiation marker. Immunol Today 14:121–125
80. Haziot A, Chen E, Ferrero E, Low MG, Siver R, Goyert SM (1988) The monocyte differentiation antigen, CD14, is anchored to the cell membrane by a phosphatidyinositol linkage. J Immunol 141:547–552
81. Bazil V, Baudys M, Hilgert I, Stefanova I, Low MG, Zbrozek J, Horejsi V (1989) Structural relationship between the soluble and membrane bound forms of human monocyte surface glycoprotein CD14. Mol Immunol 26:657–662
82. Frey EA, Miller DS, Jahr TG, Sundan A, Bazil V, Espevik T, Finlay BB, Wright SD (1992) Soluble CD14 participates in the response of cells to lipopolysaccharide. J Exp Med 176:1665–1671
83. Bazil V, Strominger JL (1991) Shedding as a mechanism of down-modulation on stimulated human monocytes. J Immunol 147:1567–1574
84. Derieux JJ, Vita N, Popescu O, Guette F, Calzadawack J, Munker R, Schmidt RE, Lupker J, Ferrara P, Ziegler-Heitbrock HWL, Labeta MO (1994) The two soluble forms of the lipopolysaccharide receptor, CD14: Characterization and release by normal human monocytes. Eur J Immunol 24:2006–2012
85. Lee JD, Dato K, Tobias PS, Kirkland TN, Ulevitch RJ (1992) Transfection of CD14 into 70Z/3 cells dramatically enhances the sensitivity to complexes of lipopolysaccharide (LPS) and LPS binding protein. J Exp Med 175:1697–1705
86. Haziot A, Tsuberi B, Goyert S (1993) Neutrophil CD14: Biochemical properties and role in secretion of tumor necrosis factor-α in response to lipopolysaccharide. J Immunol 150:5556–5565
87. Haziot A, Ferrero E, Kontgen F, Hijiya N, Yamamoto S, Silver J, Stewart CL, Goyert SM (1996) Resistance of CD14-deficient mice to endotoxin shock and reduced dissemination of gram-negative bacteria in CD14-deficient mice. Immunity 4:404–414
88. Pugin J, Schurer-Maly CC, Leturcq D, Moriarty A, Ulevitch RJ, Tobias PS (1993) Lipopolysaccharide activation of human endothelial and epithelial cells is mediated by lipopolysaccharide-binding protein and soluble CD14. Proc Nat Acad Sci USA 90:2744–2748
89. Haziot A, Rong G, Silver J, Goyert SM (1993) Recombinant soluble CD14 mediates the activation of endothelial cells by lipopolysaccharide. J Immunol 151: 1500–1507
90. Goldblum SF, Brann TW, Ding X, Pugin J, Tobias PS (1994) Lipopolysaccharide (LPS)-binding protein and soluble CD14 function as accessory molecules for LPS induced changes in endothelial barrier function in vitro. J Clin Invest 93:692–702
91. Arditi M, Zhou J, Dorio R, Rong GW, Goyert SM, Kim KS (1994) Endotoxin-mediated endothelial cell injury and activation: Role of soluble CD14. Infect Immun 61:3149–3156
92. Juan TS-C, Hailman E, Kelley MJ, Busse LA, Davy E, Empig CJM, Narhi LO, Wright SD, Lichenstein HS (1995) Identification of a lipopolysaccharide binding domain in CD14 between amino acids 57 and 64. J Biol Chem 270: 5219–5224

93. Viriyakosol S, Kirkland TN (1995) A region of human CD14 required for lipopolysaccharide binding. J Biol Chem 270:361–368

94. Weidemann B, Brade H, Rietschel ET, Dziarski R, Bazil V, Kusumoto S, Flad H-D, Ulmer AJ (1994) Soluble peptidoglykan-induced monokine production can be blocked by anti-CD14 monoclonal antibodies and by lipid A partial structures. Infect Immun 62:4709–4715

95. Weidemann B, Schletter J, Dziarski R, Kusumoto S, Stelter F, Rietschel ET, Flad H-D, Ulmer AJ (1997) Specific binding of soluble peptidoglycan and muramyl-dipeptide to CD14 on human monocytes. Infect Immun 65:858–864

96. Pugin J, Heumann D, Tomasz A, Kravchenko VV, Akamatsu Y, Nishijima M, Glauser MP, Tobias PS, Ulevitch RJ (1994) CD14 is a pattern recognition receptor. Immunity 1:509–516

97. Heumann D, Barras C, Severin A, Glauser MP, Tomasz A (1994) Gram-positive cell walls stimulate synthesis of tumor necrosis factor α and interleukin 6 by human monocytes. Infect Immun 62:2715–2721

98. Schumann RR, Leong SR, Flaggs GW, Gray PW, Wright SD, Mathison JC, Tobias PS, Ulevitch RJ (1990) Structure and function of lipopolysaccharide binding protein. Science 249:1431–1433

99. Schumann RR (1992) Function of lipopolysaccharide (LPS)-binding protein (LBP) and CD14, the receptor for LPS/LBP complexes: A short review. Res Immunol 170:11–15

100. Tobias PS, Ulevitch RJ (1993) Lipopolysaccharide binding protein and CD14 in LPS dependent macrophage activation. Immunbiology 187:227–232

101. Hailman E, Lichenstein HS, Wurfel MM, Miller DS, Johnson DA, Kelley M, Busse L, Zukowski MM, Wright SD (1994) Lipopolysaccharide (LPS)-binding protein accelerates the binding of LPS to CD14. J Exp Med 179:269–277

102. Tobias PS, Soldau K, Gegner JA, Mintz D, Ulevitch RJ (1995) Lipopolysaccharide binding protein-mediated complexation of lipopolysaccharide with soluble CD14. J Biol Chem 270:10482–10488

103. Wurfel MM, Kunitake ST, Lichenstein H, Kane JP, Wright SD (1994) Lipopolysaccharide (LPS)-binding protein is carried on lipoproteins and acts as a cofactor in the neutralization of LPS. J Exp Med 180:1025–1035

104. Horwitz AH, Williams RE, Nowakowski (1995) Human lipopolysaccharide-binding protein potentiates bactericidal activity of human bactericidal permeability-increasing protein. Infect Immun 63:522–527

105. Flegel WA, Baumstark MA, Weinstock C, Berg A, Northoff H (1993) Prevention of endotoxin-induced monokine release by human low- and high-density lipoproteins and by apolipoprotein A. Infect Immun 61:5140–5146

106. Lynn WA, Liu Y, Golenbock DT (1993) Neither CD14 nor serum is absolutely necessary for activation of mononuclear phagocytes by bacterial lipopolysaccharide. Infect Immun 61:4452–4461

107. Ingalls RR, Golenbock DT (1995) CD11c/CD18, a transmembrane signaling receptor for lipopolysaccharide. J Exp Med 181:1473–1479

108. Perera P-Y, Vogel SN, Detore GR, Haziot A, Goyert SM (1997) CD14-dependent and CD14-independent signaling pathways in murine macrophages from natural and CD14 knockout mice stimulated with lipopolysaccharide or taxol. J Immunol 158:4422–4429

109. Schletter J, Brade H, Brade L, Krüger C, Loppnow H, Kusumoto S, Rietschel ET, Flad H-D, Ulmer AJ (1995) Binding of lipopolysaccharide (LPS) to an 80-kDa membrane protein of human cells is mediated by soluble CD14 and LPS-binding protein. Infect Immun 63:2576–2580

110. Bone RC, Fisher CJ Jr, Clemmer TP, Slotman GJ, Metz CA, Balk RA, the Methylprednisolone Sepsis Study Group (1989) Sepsis syndrome: A valid clinical entity. Crit Care Med 17:389–393
111. Centers for Disease Control (1990) Increase in national hospital discharge survey cases for septicemia. MMWR 39:31–34
112. Levin J, Alving CR, Munford RS, Redl H (eds) (1995) Bacterial Endotoxins. Lipopolysaccharides from genes to therapy. Proceedings of the third conference of the international endotoxin society, Helsinki, Finland, 1994. Progress in Clinical and Biological Research, Vol. 392, Wiley-Liss, New York
113. Wenzel RP, Pinsky MR, Ulevitch RJ, Young L (1996) Current understandings of sepsis. Clin Infect Dis 22:407–413
114. Kirikae T, Schade FU, Kirikae F, Zähringer U, Brade H, Kusumoto S, Kusama T, Rietschel ET (1993) The significance of the hydrophilic backbone and the hydrophobic fatty acid regions of lipid A on macrophage binding and cytokine induction. FEMS Immunol Med Microbiol 8:13–26
115. Wang M-H, Flad H-D, Feist W, Brade H, Kusumoto S, Rietschel ET, Ulmer AJ (1991) Inhibition of endotoxin-induced interleukin 6 production by synthetic lipid A partial structures in human peripheral blood mononuclear cells. Infect Immun 59:4655–4664
116. Kovach NL, Lee E, Munford RS, Raetz CRH, Harlan JM (1990) Lipid IVa inhibits synthesis and release of tumor necrosis factor induced by lipopolysaccharide in human whole blood ex vivo. J Exp Med 172:77–84
117. Golenbock DT, Hampton RY, Qureshi N, Takayama K, Raetz CRH (1991) Lipid A-like molecules that antagonize the effects of endotoxins on human monocytes. J Biol Chem 266:19490–19498
118. Lynn WA, Golenbock DT (1992) Lipopolysaccharide antagonists. Immun Today 13:271–276
119. Heine H, Ulmer AJ, Flad H-D, Hauschildt S (1995) LPS-induced change of phosphorylation of two cytosolic proteins in human monocytes is prevented by inhibitors of ADP-ribosylation. J Immunol 155:4899–4908
120. Feist W, Ulmer AJ, Wang M-H, Musehold J, Schlüter C, Gerdes J, Herzbeck H, Brade H, Kusumoto S, Diamantstein T, Rietschel ET, Flad H-D (1992) Modulation of lipopolysaccharide-induced production of tumor necrosis factor, interleukin 1 and interleukin 6 by synthetic precursor Ia of lipid A. FEMS Micobiol Immunol 89:73–90
121. Loppnow H, Rietschel ET, Brade H, Feist W, Wang M-H, Heine H, Kirikae T, Schönbeck U, Dürrbaum-Landmann I, Grage-Griebenow E, Brandt E, Schade FU, Ulmer AJ, Campos-Portuguez S, Krauss J, Mayer H, Flad H-D (1993) Lipid A precursor Ia and Rhodobacter capsulatus LPS: Potent endotoxin antagonists. In: Levin E (ed) Endotoxin research series, Vol. 2. Excerpta Medica Elsevier, Amsterdam, pp 337–348
122. Takayama K, Quereshi N, Beutler B, Kirkland TN (1989) Diphosphoryl lipid A from *Rhodopseudomonas sphaeroides* ATCC 17023 blocks induction of cachectin in macrophages by lipopolysaccharide. Infect Immun 57:1336–1338
123. Christ WJ, Asano O, Robidoux ALC, Perez M, Wang Y, Dubuc GR, Gavin WE, Hawkins LD, McGuinness PD, Mullarkey MA, Lewis MD, Kishi Y, Kawata T, Bristol JR, Rose RR, Rossignol DP, Kobayashi S, Hishinuma I, Kimura A, Asakawa A, Katayama K, Yamatsu I (1995) E5531, a pure endotoxin antagonist of high potency. Science 268:80–83
124. Kitchens RL, Munford RS (1995) Enzymatically deacylated lipopolysaccharide (LPS) can antagonize LPS at multiple sites in the LPS recognition pathway. J Biol Chem 270:9904–9910

120   W. Brabetz et al.

125. Kitchens RL, Ulevitch RJ, Munford RS (1992) Lipopolysaccharide (LPS) partial structures inhibit responses to LPS in human macrophage cell line without inhibiting LPS uptake by a CD14-mediated pathway. J Exp Med 176:485–494

126. Heine H, Brade H, Kusumoto S, Kusama T, Rietschel ET, Flad H-D, Ulmer AJ (1994) Inhibition of LPS binding on human monoctes by phosphonooxyethyl analogs of lipid A. J Endotoxin Res 1:14–20

127. Kirikae T, Schade FU, Kirikae F, Qureshi N, Takayama K, Rietschel ET (1994) Diphosphoryl lipid A derived from the lipopolysaccharide (LPS) of *Rhodobacter sphaeroides* ATCC 17023 is a potent competitive inhibitor in murine macrophage-like J774.1 cells. FEMS Immunol Med Microbiol 9:237–244

128. Saxen H, Nurminen M, Kuusi N, Svenson SB, Mäkelä PH (1986) Evidence for the importance of O-antigen specific antibodies in mouse-protective *Salmonella* outer membrane protein (porin) antisera. Microbiol Pathog 1:433–441

129. Kirkland TN, Ziegler EJ (1984) An immunoprotective monoclonal antibody to lipopolysaccharide. J Immunol 132:2590–2592

130. Baumgartner JD, Heumann D, Gerain J, Weinbreck P, Grau GE, Glauser MP (1990) Association between protective efficacy of anti-lipopolysaccharide (LPS) antibodies and suppression of LPS induced tumor necrosis factor α and interleukin 6: Comparison of O-side chain specific antibodies with core LPS antibodies. J Exp Med 171:889–896

131. Galanos C, Freudenberg MA, Jay F, Nerkar D, Veleva K, Brade H, Schrittmatter W (1984) Immunogenic properities of lipid A. Rev Infect Dis 6:546–552

132. Dunn DI, Ewald DC, Chandan N, Cerra FB (1986) Immunotherapy of gram-negative bacterial sepsis. A single monoclonal antibody provides cross-genera protection. Arch Surg 121:58–62

133. Bogard WC Jr, Dunn DL, Albernethy K, Kilgariff C, Kung PC (1987) Isolation and characterization of murine monoclonal antibodies specific for gram-negative bacterial lipopolysaccharide: Association of cross-genus reactivity with lipid A specificity. Infect Immun 55:899–908

134. Brade H, Brade L, Rietschel ET (1988) Structure-activity relationships of bacterial lipopolysaccharides (endotoxins). Zentralbl Bakteriol Mikrobiol Hyg [A] 268:151–179

135. Kuhn H-M, Brade L, Appelmelk BJ, Kusumoto S, Rietschel ET, Brade H (1992) Characterization of the epitope specificity of murine monoclonal antibodies directed against lipid A. Infect Immun 60:2201–2210

136. Brade L, Holst O, Brade H (1993) An artificial glycoconjugate containing the bisphosphorylated glucosamine disaccharide backbone of lipid A binds lipid A monoclonal antibodies. Infect Immun 61:4514–4517

137. Brade L, Engel R, William JC, Rietschel ET (1997) A nonsubstituted primary hydroxyl group in the 6′ position of free lipid A is required for binding of lipid A monoclonal antibodies. Infect Immun 65:3961–3965

138. Baumgartner J-D, Glauser M-P (1993) Immunotherapy of endotoxemia and septicemia. Immunbiology 187:464–477

139. Wenzel R, Bone R, Fein A, Quenzero R, Schentag J, Gorelick KJ, Wedel NI, Perl T (1991) Results of a second double-blind, randomized, controlled trial of anti endotoxin antibody E5 in gram-negative sepsis (Abstract). Interscience Conference on Antimicrobial Agents and Chemotherapy, 294. ASM, Washington

140. Di Padova FE, Brade H, Barclay R, Poxton IR, Liehl E, Schuetze E, Kocker HP, Ramsay G, Schreier MH, McClelland DBL, Rietschel ET (1993) A broadly cross-protective monoclonal antibody binding to *Escherichia coli* and *Salmonella* lipopolysaccharids. Infect Immun 61:3863–3872

141. Di Padova FE, Gram H, Barclay R, Kreuser P, Liehl E, Rietschel ET (1993) New anticore LPS monoclonal antibodies with clinical potential. In: Levin J, Alving CR, Munford RS, Stuetz PL (eds) Bacterial endotoxin: Recognition and effector mechanisms. Elsevier, Amsterdam, pp 325–335
142. Bailat S, Neumann D, Le Roy D, Baumgartner JD, Rietschel ET, Glauser MP, Di Padova FE (1997) Similarities and disparities between core-specific and O-chain-specific antilipopolysaccharide monoclonal antibodies in models of endotoxemia and bacteremia in mice. Infect Immun 65:811–814
143. Di Padova FE, Mikol V, Barclay GR, Poxton IR, Rietschel ET (1994) Antilipopolysaccharide core antibodies. Prog Clin Biol Res 388:85–94
144. Pollack M, Ohl CA, Golenbock DT, Di Padova FE, Wahl LM, Koles NL, Guelde G, Monks BG (1997) Dual effects of LPS antibodies on cellular uptake of LPS and LPS-induced proinflammatory functions. J Immunol 159:3519–3530
145. Lamping N, Dettmer R, Schröder NWJ, Pfeil D, Hallatschek W, Burger R, Schuhmann RR (1988) LPS-binding protein (LBP) protects mice from septic shock caused by LPS or gram-negative bacteria. J Clin Invest (in press)
146. Bocci V (1992) The neglected organ: bacterial flora has a crucial immunostimulatory role. Perspect Biol Med 35:251–260

Membrane-Damaging Toxins and Inflammation

S. Bhakdi

Mechanism of Membrane Damage by Bacterial Protein Toxins

Transmembrane Pore Formation

The most widespread mechanism for membrane damage is the formation of transmembrane pores. This may be incurred by secreted proteins, or by surface-bound molecules that act when bacteria come into intimate contact with host target cells. Pore formation by secreted toxins follows a general pattern of events: (a) binding; (b) oligomerization); (c) insertion of amphipathic amino acid sequences into the bilayer. Thereby, oligomerization, i.e., formation of homotypic toxin aggregates, is a common but perhaps not obligatory feature.

Mechanisms underlying the binding of pore-forming toxins are poorly understood. In some cases, for example with staphylococcal α-toxin, specific binding sites are known to exist but they have not yet been identified (Bhakdi and Tranum-Jensen, 1991; Hildebrand et al., 1991). In other cases, e.g., for aerolysin, several binding molecules have been identified (Cowell et al., 1997; Nelson et al., 1997; Abrami et al., 1998). In no case is it known what happens to the toxin-receptor complexes after initial binding has occurred. Specifically, nothing is known regarding the direct involvement of any putative receptor in pore formation. Indeed, all pores isolated from target membranes have to date been found to consist solely of toxin molecules (Bhakdi and Tranum-Jensen, 1988; Bhakdi et al., 1996). This does not exclude the possibility that the participating receptor molecules have been removed from the complexes during the process of detergent solubilization and purification.

With most pore-forming toxins, binding is followed by oligomerization, which occurs when membrane-bound protomers diffuse laterally in the membrane plane and collide with each other. The ensuing oligomers may be homogeneous or heterogeneous. Most pore-forming toxins generate homogeneous oligomers with defined structure. Examples are the heptameric α-toxin (Gouaux et al., 1994; Song et al., 1996) and aerolysin pores (Moniatte et al., 1996), and the pores formed by *Vibrio cholerae* cytolysin (Zitzer et al.,

Symposium in Immunology VIII
Eibl/Huber/Peter/Wahn (Eds.)
© Springer Verlag Berlin Heidelberg 1999

1997). Such pores form fully circularized, cylindrical, or funnel-shaped complexes with channels of approximately 1-nm diameter running through their center. In all cases, it seems that assembly of the complete oligomer is a prerequisite of pore formation, i.e., no intermediates of smaller size have been detectable.

A different mode of pore formation underlies the action of streptolysin-O and related toxins. Here, protomers first bind reversibly to membrane cholesterol (Alouf, 1980; Palmer et al., 1995). Pore formation is probably initiated with the formation of dimers. It appears that this is caused by insertion of amphipathic sequences with the creation of small defects or "slits" in the bilayer, that are lined by the toxin on the one side and by lipid molecules on the other (Palmer et al., 1996, 1998a, 1998b). The toxin oligomers grow rapidly (within seconds and minutes) as further protomers associate with the nucleating complex, and this correlates to growth in pore size. Under optimal circumstances, lesions become completely circularized and are visible as large ring structures in the electron microscope (Bhakdi et al., 1985; Palmer et al., 1998b).

The mechanism of pore formation has been delineated for α-toxin. Here, it has been shown that immediately prior to pore formation, pre-pores assemble in which seven toxin molecules are aggregated, but have not yet inserted their pore-forming sequence into the bilayer (Walker et al., 1992, 1995; Valeva et al., 1997). Probably, energy released by the oligomerization step then drives the pore-forming amino acid sequences into the membrane. Thereby, seven amphipathic central domains encompassing amino acid residues 118–140 from each protomer form the walls of a water-filled channel in the form of a β-barrel, whose internal diameter is approximately 1 nm (Song et al., 1996; Valeva et al., 1996, 1997).

Enzymatic Attack

Phospholipases

Many pathogens elaborate phospholipases, the best known example being the phospholipase C of *Clostridium perfringens* (Titball, 1993). Cleavage of membrane phospholipids can directly lead to the breakdown of the permeability barrier and cause cellular dysfunction and death. Other potentially important phospholipases are the sphingomyelinases, elaborated for example by staphylococci, and phospholipase A2. Readers are referred to recent reviews for compilations on this subject (Roberts, 1996; Titball, 1993).

Proteases

Most pathogenic bacteria produce proteases, but their significance does not generally lie in their capacity to directly damage membranes. Readers are referred to recent reviews on this subject (Häse and Finkelstein, 1993; Iglewski and Nicas, 1985).

Pro-inflammatory Effects of Pore-Forming Toxins

Conventionally, pore-forming toxins have been thought to exert biological effects mainly through their cidal action on target cells. Many studies, however, have underlined the need to rectify this oversimplified concept. There is now much evidence to indicate that pore-forming toxins can provoke a plethora of inflammatory reactions via different pathways, the best studies of which are summarized here.

Pro-inflammatory Reactions Provoked by the Generation of Very Small Transmembrane Pores

Staphylococcal α-toxin is the best studied prototype of toxins in this category. When applied at low concentrations, α-toxin generates pores in mammalian cells that permit rapid diffusion of monovalent ions, but not Ca^{2+} or larger molecules (Walev et al., 1993). Therefore, the primary effect is a rapid loss of K^+ and influx of Na^+ and water. Cells typically swell within minutes and hours, but do not lyse. Adenosine triphosphate (ATP)-driven pumps strive to restore ionic homeostasis, and this leads to a reduction of ATP levels. Certain cells are able to repair the membrane lesions, apparently by closing the pores (Walev et al., 1994). In such cases, cells can fully recuperate from toxin attack. Other cells are not endowed with this capacity and will eventually die. In any event, cellular reactions occur that probably contribute to inflammation.

Activation of the calcium-independent phospholipase A_2 (iPLA$_2$) may be of primary importance. Recent evidence indicates that K^+ efflux is accompanied by enhanced activity of this phospholipase. This in turn is linked to important cellular events. K^+ depletion in monocytes by α-toxin (or by any other agent) thus causes rapid processing and release of biologically active interleukin (IL)-1β (Walev et al., 1995, and unpublished data).

Pro-inflammatory Effects Provoked by Ca²⁺-Permissive Pores

Many pathways are triggered by Ca^{2+} influx that will contribute to inflammation, and some well-defined reactions are summarized.

Stimulation of the Calcium-Dependent Phospholipase A₂ (cPLA₂)

This has been shown to occur in endothelial cells attacked by pore-forming toxins. The generation of arachadonic acid triggers subsets of reactions of the arachadonic cascade that will drive inflammation (Suttorp et al., 1985). Remarkable effects in whole organ systems, particularly in the isolated lung, have been observed. Here, the production of thromboxane leads to the development of pulmonary arterial hypertension and to leakage, which in turn underlie the development of pulmonary edema (Seeger et al., 1984, 1989).

Secretion

Secretory processes are generally stimulated by Ca^{2+}, so the finding that cells attacked by pore-forming toxins exocytose vesicular constituents is per se not surprising. When platelets are permeabilized, they rapidly secrete procoagulatory components and become foci for thrombus formation (Bhakdi et al., 1988). Permeabilized granulocytes release large amounts of their granular constituents; elastase is but one of the components whose inflammatory potential is obvious (Bhakdi et al., 1989).

Stimulation of cNOS

Ca^{2+} stimulates the constitutive form of nitric oxide synthase (cNOS), so the finding that toxin-permeabilized endothelial cells rapidly produce nitric oxide (NO) is readily explicable (Suttorp et al., 1993). NO production in turn will trigger a multitude of reactions that are relevant in the context of inflammation.

Cytoskeletal Dysfunction

Staphylococcal α-toxin and *Escherichia coli* hemolysin induce intercellular gap formation in cultured pulmonary artery endothelial cells, which results in the enhanced passage of fluid and macromolecules across the monolayer. This effect is probably due to contraction and rounding up of the adherent cells, because of Ca^{2+}-dependent rearrangement of the endothelial cytoskeleton (Suttorp et al., 1988, 1990).

Pro-inflammatory Processes of Unclarified Origin

Short-Circuiting of G-Protein-Dependent Signal Transduction Pathways

Certain pore-forming toxins short-circuit G-protein-regulated transduction pathways. This is exemplified by *E. coli* hemolysin and related toxins. How short-circuiting occurs is unknown and we are speculating that the toxins may gain immediate access to the G-proteins. As a result, these toxins are endowed with potent pseudo-chemokine effects that have been detected in polymorphonuclear granulocytes and monocytes. In granulocytes, *E. coli* hemolysin provokes massive production of diacylglycerol and IP3, which underlies triggering of the respiratory burst and secretion (Grimminger et al., 1991). These events are induced by very low concentrations of the toxin, and occur prior to the generation of transmembrane pores.

Activation of Shedding Metalloproteinases

Many membrane-associated, biologically important molecules can be released from cells by a proteolytic cleavage process called shedding. These include cytokines, receptors for cytokines and growth factors, and cellular adhesion proteins (Massagué and Pandiella, 1993; Bazil, 1995). Soluble receptors for cytokines and growth factors retain their ligand-binding capacity. In some cases, such soluble receptors can act as agonists. For example, soluble IL-6 receptor binds by specific interactions to receptorless bystander cells, rendering the latter sensitive to the action of the respective cytokines (Müllberg et al., 1993; Rose-John and Heinrich, 1994). An analogous phenomenon has been documented for the soluble lipopolysaccharide (LPS) receptor CD14, which binds to bystander cells and renders them susceptible to stimulation with LPS.

It has been found that cells dying from attack by pore-forming toxins activate their shedding membrane metalloproteinase via unknown mechanisms, and this leads to massive and rapid shedding of CD 14- and IL-6-receptor. The cleaved sIL-6-receptor is biologically active in transsignalling (Walev et al., 1996). These results have uncovered a novel mechanism by which pore-forming toxins can promote inflammatory processes.

Activation of the Immune System by "Planted" Bacterial Antigens

This effect has not been extensively studied, but its potential significance should be obvious. Binding of pore-forming toxins to cell surfaces is equatable with "planting" of potential antigens in the membranes. Because epitopes of the toxins always remain accessible at the surface, a straightforward mechanism for immune activation is via binding of antibodies and complement. Most pore-forming toxins are excellent immunogens and antibodies against these molecules are present in healthy individuals. The principle of auto-attack has been demonstrated for streptolysin-O after its binding to target human erythrocytes (Bhakdi et al. 1985). Complement activation was massive and the generation of anaphylatoxins can be expected to promote inflammation. Another pathway is triggered by pneumolysin, which contains a domain that directly activates complement independent of host antibody (Paton et al., 1993). Also in this case, proinflammatory reactions must be triggered at the site of toxin insertion into target cell membranes. In this context, the remarkable stability of oligomeric toxin pores is noteworthy. Toxin oligomers can usually not be destroyed at neutral pH by proteases, so they may be expected to represent long-lived foci of inflammation.

Synergisms Between Pore-Forming Toxins and Other Toxins

Pore-forming toxins can synergize with endotoxin. In a model study, priming of pulmonary cells in isolated lungs with endotoxin was found to potently enhance vascular abnormalities in response to subsequent application of α-toxin or *E. coli* hemolysin (Walmrath et al., 1994 a, b). Such synergisms are probably relevant to the pathogenesis of organ failure in systemic infections. In the future, it will be of interest to study possible synergisms between pore-forming toxins and superantigens.

Conclusions

The majority of important bacterial pathogens produce pore-forming toxins. Attack of these molecules on nucleated cells and platelets will evoke complex secondary reactions including secretion, stimulation of eicosanoid production, release of reactive oxygen species, and liberation of cytokines. These toxins, therefore, can influence homeostasis and trigger production and release of many potent mediators. Application of purified α-toxin or *E. coli* hemolysin in experimental animals has indeed been found to provoke acute symptoms of respiratory and circulatory failure and shock. Furthermore, administration of toxin producing *Staphylococcus aureus* or *E. coli* in isolated rabbit lungs produces severe lung vascular injury. It is of interest to note that pore-forming toxins need not necessarily be released in measurable quantities into body fluids or tissues to exert their action. Very few molecules are generally required to generate a membrane lesion, and attack on a susceptible cell may occur within a very small area when viable bacteria gain intimate contact with the target. This will probably suffice to evoke the various cytotoxic and proinflammatory effects discussed above. Overall, pore-forming toxins thus emerge as potent proinflammatory agents that are elaborated by medically important bacterial pathogens.

Acknowledgments. These studies have received the continued support of the Deutsche Forschungsgemeinschaft (SFB 311, grant D09; DFG Pa 539/1-1).

References

Abrami L, Fivac M, Glauser PE, Parton RG, van der Goot GF (1998) A pore-forming toxin interacts with a GPI-anchored protein and causes vacuolation of the endoplasmic reticulum. J Cell Biol 140:525–540

Alouf JE (1980) Streptococcal toxins (streptolysin O, streptolysin S, erythrogenic toxin). Pharmacol Ther 11:661–717

Bazil V (1995) Physiological enzymatic cleavage of leukocyte membrane molecules. Immunol Today 16:135–140

Bhakdi S, Tranum-Jensen J (1985) Complement activation and attack on autologous cell membranes induced by streptolysin-O. Infect Immun 48:713–719

Bhakdi S, Tranum-Jensen J (1988) Damage to cell membranes by pore-forming bacterial cytolysins. Prog Allergy 40:1–43

Bhakdi S, Tranum-Jensen J (1991) Alpha-toxin of Staphylococcus aureus. Microbiol Rev 55:733–751

Bhakdi S, Bayley H, Valeva A, Walev B, Walker B, Kehoe M, Palmer M (1996) Staphylococcal alpha-toxin, streptolysin-O, and *Escherichia coli* hemolysin: prototypes of pore-forming bacterial cytolysins. Arch Microbiol 165:73–79

Bhakdi S, Greulich S, Muhly M, Eberspächer F, Becker H, Thiele A, Hugo F (1989) Potent leukocidal action of *Escherichia coli* hemolysin mediated by permeabilization of target cell membranes. J Exp Med 169:737–754

Bhakdi S, Muhly M, Mannhardt U, Hugo F, Klapettek K, Mueller Eckhardt C, Roka L (1988) Staphylococcal alpha toxin promotes blood coagulation via attack on human platelets. J Exp Med 168:527–542

Bhakdi S, Tranum-Jensen J, Sziegoleit A (1985) Mechanism of membrane damage by streptolysin-O. Infect Immun 47:52–60

Cowell S, Aschauer W, Gruber HJ, Nelson KL, Buckley JT (1997) The erythrocyte receptor for the channel-forming toxin aerolysin is a novel glycoasylphosphatidylinositol-anchored protein. Mol Microbiol 25:343–350

Gouax JE, Braha O, Hobaugh MR, Song L, Cheley S, Shustak C, Bayley H (1994) Subunit stoichiometry of staphylococcal alpha-hemolysin in crystals and on membranes: a heptameric transmembrane pore. Proc Natl Acad Sci USA 91:12828–12831

Grimminger F, Sibelius U, Bhakdi S, Suttorp N, Seeger W (1991b) Escherichia coli hemolysin is a potent inductor of phosphoinositide hydrolysis and related metabolic responses in human neutrophils. J Clin Invest 88:1531–1539

Häse CC, Finkelstein RA (1993) Bacterial extracellular zinc-containing metalloproteases. Microbiol Rev 57:823–837

Hildebrand A, Pohl M, Bhakdi S (1991) *Staphylococcus aureus* a-toxin dual mechanisms of binding to target cells. J Biol Chem 266:17195–17200

Iglewski BH, Nicas TI (1985) Extracellular factors in the virulence of *Pseudomonas aeruginosa*. In: Roth JA (ed) Virulence mechanisms of bacterial pathogens. Springer, Berlin, p. 257–266

Massagué J, Pandiella A (1993) Membrane-anchored growth factors. Annu Rev Biochem 62:515–541

Moniatte M, van der Goot FG, Buckley JT, Pattus F, van Dorsselaer A (1996) Characterization of the heptameric pore-forming complex of the *Aeromonas* toxin aerolysin using MALDI-TOF mass spectrometry. FEBS Lett 384:269–272

Müllberg J, Schooltink H, Stoyan T, Günther M, Greave L, Buse G, Mackiewicz A, Heinrich PC, Rose-John S (1993) The soluble interleukin–6 receptor is generated by shedding. Eur J Immunol 23:473–480

Nelson KL, Raja SM, Buckely JT (1997) The GPI-anchored surface glycoprotein Thy-1 is a receptor for the channel-forming toxin aerolysin. J Biol Chem 272: 12170–12174

Palmer M, Harris JR, Freytag C, Tranum-Jensen J, Bhakdi S (1998a) Assembly mechanism of the oligomeric streptolysin O pore: the early membrane lesion is lined by a free edge of the lipid membrane and is extended gradually during oligomerization. EMBO J 17:1598–1605

Palmer M, Saweljew P, Vulicevic I, Valeva A, Kehoe M, Bhakdi S (1996) Membrane-penetrating domain of streptolysin-O identified by cysteine scanning mutagenesis. J Biol Chem 271:26664–26667

Palmer M, Valeva A, Kehoe M, Bhakdi S (1995) Kinetics of streptolysin-O self-assembly. Eur J Biochem 231:388–395

Palmer M, Vulicevic I, Saweljew P, Valeva A, Kehoe M, Bhakdi S (1998b) Streptolysin O: proposed model of allosteric interaction between a pore-forming protein and its target lipid bilayer. Biochemistry 37:2378–2383

Paton JC, Andrew PW, Boulnois GJ, Mitchell TJ (1993) Molecular analysis of the pathogenicity of *Streptococcus pneumoniae:* the role of pneumococcal proteins. Annu Rev Microbiol 47:89–115

Roberts MF (1996) Phospholipases: structural and functional motifs for working at an interface. FASEB J 10:1159–1172

Rose-John S, Heinrich PC (1994) Soluble receptors for cytokines and growth factors: generation and biological function. Biochem J 300:281–290

Seeger W, Bauer M, Bhakdi S (1984) Staphylococcal alpha-toxin elicits hypertension in isolated rabbit lungs. Evidence for thromboxane formation and the role of extracellular calcium. J Clin Invest 74:849–858

Seeger W, Walter H, Suttorp N, Bhakdi S (1989) Thromboxane-mediated hypertension and vascular leakage evoked by low doses of *Escherichia coli* hemolysin in rabbit lungs. J Clin Invest 84:220–227

Song L, Hobaugh MR, Shustak C, Cheley S, Bayley H, Gouaux JE (1996) Structure of a staphylococcal alpha-hemolysin, a heptameric transmembrane pore. Science 274:1859–1866

Suttorp N, Flöer B, Seeger W, Schnittler H, Bhakdi S (1990) Effects of *E. coli* hemolysin on endothelial cell function. Infect Immun 58:3796–3801

Suttorp N, Fuhrmann M, Tannert-Otto S, Grimminger F, Bhakdi S (1993) Pore-forming bacterial toxins potently induce release of nitric oxide in porcine endothelial cells. J Exp Med 178:337–341

Suttorp N, Hessz T, Seeger W, Wilke A, Koob R, Lutz F, Drenckhahn D (1988) Bacterial exotoxins and endothelial permeability for water and albumin. Am J Physiol 255:C369–C376

Suttorp N, Seeger W, Dewein E, Bhakdi S, Roka L (1985) Staphylococcal alpha-toxin-induced PG12 production in endothelial cells: role of calcium. Am J Physiol 248: C127-C135

Titball RW (1993) Bacterial phospholipase C. Microbiol Rev 57:347–366

Valeva A, Walev I, Pinkernell M, Walker B, Bayley H, Palmer M, Bhakdi S (1997) Transmembrane β-barrel of staphylococcal alpha-toxin forms in sensitive but not in resistant cells. Proc Natl Acad Sci USA 94:11607–11611

Valeva A, Weisser A, Walker B, Kehoe M, Bayley H, Bhakdi S, Palmer M (1996) Molecular architecture of a toxin pore: a 15-residue sequence lines the transmembrane channel of staphylococcal alpha-toxin. EMBO J 15:1857–1864

Walev I, Martin E, Jonas D, Mohamadzadeh M, Müller-Klieser W, Kunz L, Bhakdi S (1993) Staphylococcal alpha-toxin kills human keratinocytes by permeabilizing the plasma membrane for monovalent ions. Infect Immun 61:4972–4979

Walev I, Palmer M, Martin E, Jonas D, Weller U, Höhn-Bentz H, Husmann M, Bhakdi S (1994) Recovery of human fibroblasts from attack by the pore-forming alpha-toxin of *Staphylococcus aureus*. Microb Pathog 17:187–201

Walev, I, Reske K, Palmer M, Valeva A, Bhakdi S (1995) Potassium-inhibited processing of IL-1β in human monocytes. EMBO J 14:1607–1614

Walev I, Vollmer P, Palmer M, Bhakdi S, Rose-John S (1996) Pore-forming toxins trigger shedding of receptors for interleukin–6 and lipopolysaccharide. Proc Natl Acad Sci USA 93:7882–7887

Walker B, Krishnasastry M, Zorn L, Bayley H (1992) Assembly of the oligomeric membrane pore formed by staphylococcal alpha-hemolysin examined by truncation mutagenesis. J Biol Chem 267:21782–21786

Walker B, Braha O, Cheley S, Bayley H (1995) An intermediate in the assembly of a pore-forming protein trapped with a genetically engineered switch. Curr Biol 2: 99–105

Walmrath D, Ghofrani HA, Rosseau S, Schütte H, Cramer A, Kaddus W, Grimminger F, Bhakdi S, Seeger W (1994a) Endotoxin "priming" potentiates lung vascular abnormalities in response to *Escherichia coli* hemolysin: An example of synergism between endo- and exotoxin. J Exp Med 180:1437–1443

Walmrath D, Pilch J, Scharmann M, Grimminger F, Seeger W (1994) Severe ventilation-perfusion mismatch in perfused rabbit lungs evoked by sequential intravascular challenge with endotoxin and *E. coli* hemolysin. J Appl Physiol 74: 1972–1980

Zitzer A, Palmer M, Weller U, Wassenaar T, Biermann C, Tranum-Jensen J, Bhakdi S (1997) Mode of primary binding to target membranes and pore formation induced by *Vibrio cholerae* cytolysin (hemolysin). Eur J Biochem 247:209–216

Treatment Perspectives

The Interleukin-6 Family: Biological Function of the Soluble Receptors

S. ROSE-JOHN, P. VOLLMER, M. PETERS, P. MÄRZ, and J. MÜLLBERG

Introduction

The interleukin–6 (IL-6) family of cytokines comprises IL-6, IL-11, ciliary neurotrophic factor (CNTF), cardiotrophin-1 (CT-1), leukemia inhibitory factor (LIF) and oncostatin M (OSM) [79]. IL-6-type cytokines belong to a family of four helical cytokines with a unique protein fold [2, 74, 79]. Receptors for these cytokines are proteins with several immunoglobulin (Ig-) and fibronectin type-III domains. Two of these fibronectin type III domains form a cytokine-binding domain which is characterized by conserved cysteines and a tryptophane-serine-x-tryptophane-serine sequence motif [74].

IL-6-like cytokines act via receptor complexes which contain at least one subunit of the signal transducing protein gp130 [79]. IL-6, IL-11, CNTF and CT-1 first bind to specific receptors and these complexes associate with a homodimer of gp130 in the case of IL-6 and IL-11, or with a heterodimer of gp130 and the related protein LIF receptor (LIF-R) (Fig. 1). OSM and LIF first

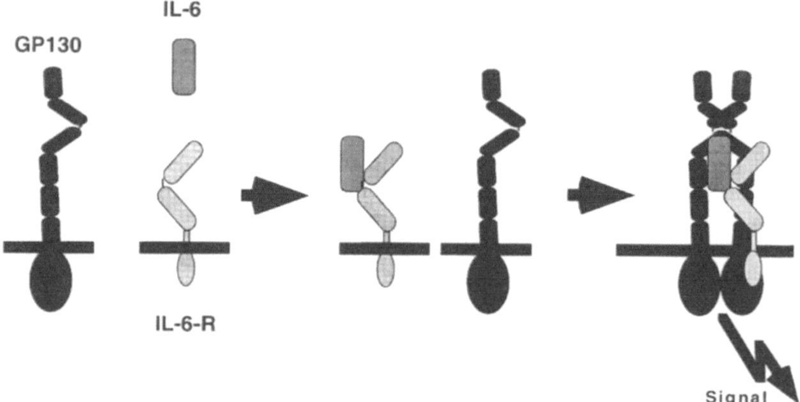

Fig. 1. Binding and signaling of interleukin-6 (*IL-6*) on the cell surface. IL-6 first binds to the IL-6 receptor (*IL-6R*). The IL-6/IL-6R complex associates with the signal transducing protein gp130 and induces dimerization of gp130. This assembled complex leads to triggering of IL-6-specific signaling

Symposium in Immunology VIII
Eibl/Huber/Peter/Wahn (Eds.)
© Springer Verlag Berlin Heidelberg 1999

bind directly to gp130 and LIF-R, respectively, and form heterodimers with LIF-R and gp130. Recently, a gp130-related protein was described which can heterodimerize with gp130 and form an alternative OSM receptor [48].

Structure function analysis of IL-6 [6, 7, 13, 30, 31, 37, 86], the IL-6 receptor (IL-6R) [26, 97] and gp130 [23] have clarified the understanding of the molecular contacts between the three proteins [17, 93]. One site was identified as the contact region (site 1) between IL-6 and the IL-6R [13, 30, 31], whereas two distinct sites turned out to establish the contact between IL-6 and two gp130 proteins [13, 72, 73].

Cytokines of the IL-6 family have been implicated with inflammatory reactions, as well as with various steps of hematopoiesis [24, 47, 58]. Recent review articles have concentrated on soluble cytokine receptors in general [19], the mechanisms of generation of soluble receptors [22, 69] and on various aspects of the IL-6 cytokine family [29, 79]. This article will focus mainly on the biological activity of the IL-6-type cytokines complexed with their soluble receptors on various target cell types, including hematopoietic and neuronal cells.

Generation and Occurence of Soluble Receptors

Many, if not all, transmembrane proteins also occur in a soluble form which usually consists of the entire extracellular domain. This phenomenon has been observed for type-I and type-II transmembrane proteins [22, 69]. Two independent mechanisms lead to the generation of such soluble proteins.

Transmembrane proteins can be cleaved by a transmembrane metallo-proteinase which is most likely a protease other than a matrix-type metallo-proteinase (MMP) to yield the soluble extracellular domain of the proteins. This mechanism has been studied in detail for the human IL-6R [51–55]. Cleavage is controlled by protein kinase C and occurs at a distinct site which is not strictly sequence-specific [53]. The generation of the soluble IL-6R (sIL-6R) can be prevented by hydroxamic acid compounds [52] which have been previously shown to inhibit the processing of the membrane form of tumor necrosis factor (TNF) [44, 46]. A TNF-processing metalloproteinase has recently been cloned [4, 49] and shown to belong to the large family of disintegrin domains containing metalloproteinases (ADAMs) [94]. It is unclear whether different family members of the ADAMs are highly substrate-specific or whether one protease is able to cleave more than one protein.

Alternatively, the generation of soluble counterparts of transmembrane proteins has been shown to occur via translation from alternatively spliced mRNAs [69]. In particular, a soluble form of the IL-6R can be synthesized by various cells from a spliced mRNA, yielding a protein which differs at its COOH-terminus by 14 amino acid residues [35, 36], indicating that for one given transmembrane protein both mechanisms of generation, shedding and alternative splicing may exist.

sIL–6R protein has been shown to occur in the blood of normal individuals at concentrations of 50–80 ng/ml [21]. Increased concentrations have been detected after infections and during malignant disorders [15, 21, 33]. Interestingly, bacterial proteins have been shown to massively induce the shedding of several membrane proteins via the activation of metalloproteinases [90]. Moreover, metalloproteases secreted by several bacteria have been shown to cleave membrane proteins and thereby generate biologically active soluble receptors [88]. This might represent a novel pathogenic mechanism of microbial metalloproteinases [88].

IL-6-Type Cytokines Transsignaling via Soluble Receptors

Soluble receptor proteins have been shown to bind their ligands with similar affinities as the cognate transmembrane receptors [69]. Most soluble receptors for cytokines and growth factors compete with their membrane-bound counterparts for the binding of the ligand and are therefore antagonists [69]. In contrast, the soluble receptors of the IL-6 cytokine family, when complexed with their ligands, exhibit agonistic biological activities. These complexes can directly recruit and activate homodimers of gp130 (in the case of IL-6 and IL-11) or heterodimers of gp130 and LIF-R (in the case of CNTF and CT-1) [1, 11, 38, 62, 78]. Cells which do not express specific receptors for IL-6, IL-11, CNTF or CT-1 are not able to respond to these cytokines. The presence of soluble receptors leads to responsiveness of these cells (Fig. 2). This process has been named transsignaling [69]. Of note, soluble forms of gp130 and LIF-R exist in vivo and have been demonstrated to possess antagonistic biological activity [34, 57].

Biological Properties of sIL–6R

With the help of co-immunoprecipitation techniques, it was demonstrated that sIL–6R in the presence of IL-6 associates with gp130 [77]. Consequently, release of a sIL–6R by human peripheral blood mononuclear cells (PBMC) was demonstrated and it was shown that sIL–6R, together with IL-6, suppressed the proliferative responses of PBMC [21]. The in vivo biological activity of sIL–6R has been demonstrated using a murine tumor rejection

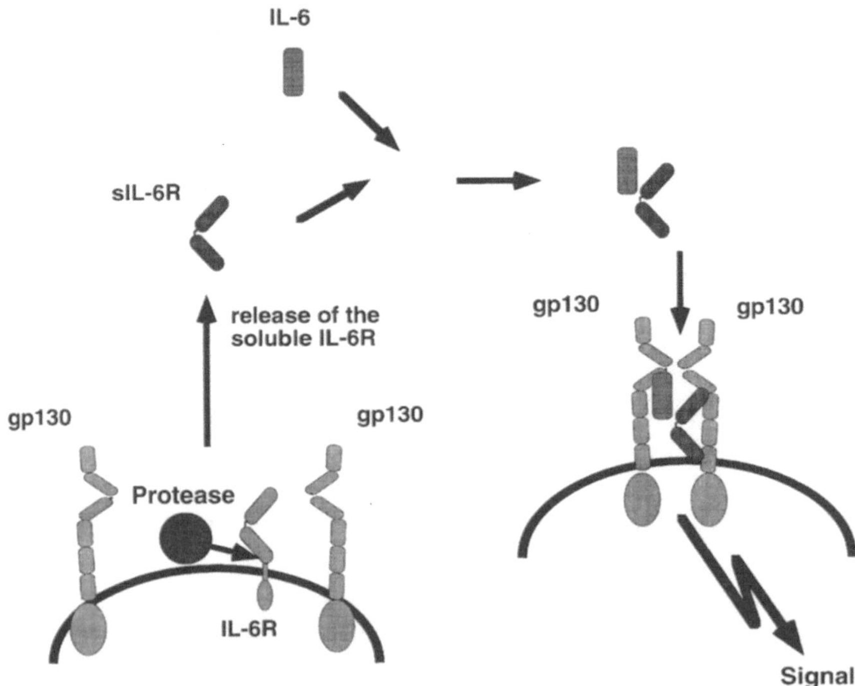

Fig. 2. Transsignaling of soluble receptors of the interleukin-6 (*IL-6*) cytokine family. An IL-6 receptor (*IL-6R*)-expressing cell (*left*) releases a soluble receptor (*sIL-6R*) by shedding or alternative splicing. This soluble receptor binds IL-6 and induces homodimerization of gp130 on a target cell (*right*) which expresses gp130 but no IL-6R. The target cell in the absence of soluble IL-6R would not be responsive to IL-6

model [39]. In this assay, highly tumorigenic murine melanoma cells (B78) were used. B78 cells injected into syngeneic mice caused the formation of tumors and metastases, whereas cells transfected with a cDNA coding for IL-6 protected the animals. Surprisingly, transfection of B78 cells with a cDNA coding for the murine sIL–6R resulted in an even more effective protection of the animals, indicating that the sIL-6R interacted with the endogenous murine IL-6 [39].

In order to study the in vivo function of sIL–6R, we have constructed transgenic mice which express a human IL-6R cDNA into which a translational stop codon had been introduced upstream of the transmembrane region. Expression of this soluble receptor was under the transcriptional control of the liver-specific phosphoenolpyruvate carboxykinase (PEPCK) promoter [63]. Human IL-6 stimulates human and murine cells, whereas murine IL-6 only stimulates murine cells [87]. Due to this species-specificity of IL-6, the transgenic human sIL–6R did not bind the endogenous murine

IL-6 and consequently the transgenic animals showed no transgene-specific phenotype. Upon injection of human IL-6 into transgenic and nontransgenic control mice, the IL-6-specific induction of hepatic genes was analysed [63]. It turned out that the sIL-6R sensitized hepatocytes towards IL-6 (Fig. 3a) and prolonged the IL-6-induced expression of hepatic haptoglobin mRNA by prolonging the plasma half-life of IL-6 (Fig. 3b).

It was recently shown that human IL-6-dependent myeloma were unable to grow in the presence of low IL-6 concentrations when the medium was

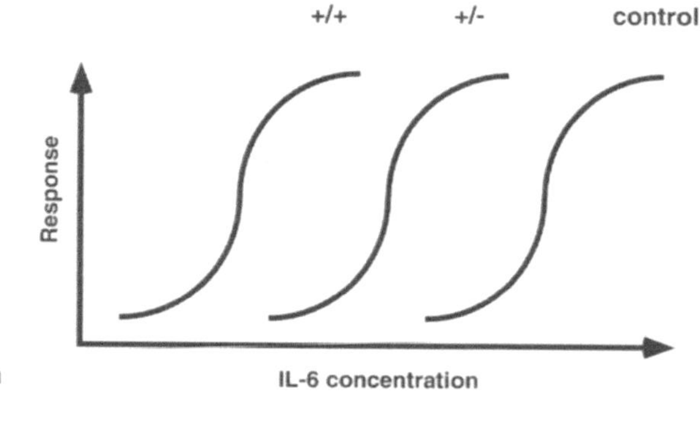

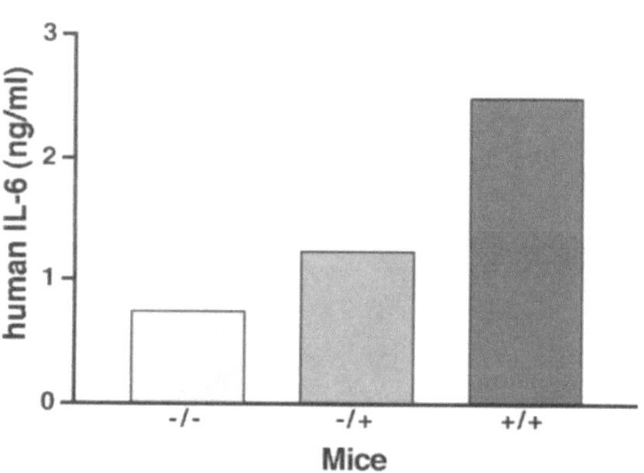

Fig. 3. Sensitization of target cells and increase of the plasma half-life of interleukin-6 (*IL-6*) in mice transgenic for the human soluble IL-6 receptor (*IL-6R*). **a** Mice expressing the human soluble IL-6R are more sensitive to human IL-6 than non-transgenic control mice. Liver haptoglobin was measured in the different mouse strains. **b** Serum levels of human IL-6 after being injected into control mice, heterozygous (–/+) or homozygous (+/+) transgenic mice expressing the human soluble IL-6R was measured 4 h after injection by a human IL-6-specific enzyme-linked immunosorbent assay

depleted of sIL-6R produced by these cells. These data indicated that in the two human myeloma cell lines used, the membrane-bound IL-6R was not sufficient to mediate the growth-stimulating signal of IL-6 and might point to a more general importance of the IL-6/sIL-6R complex for gp130-mediated signaling [16].

Definition of New Target Cells of the IL-6/sIL–6R Complex

The function of the sIL-6R can be deduced from a situation depicted in Fig. 4a. Cells which express gp130 and the specific IL-6R can be stimulated with human IL-6 or human IL-6 together with the human IL-6R. Figure 4b schematically shows a hypothetical target cell which would only be responsive to the complex of IL-6 and sIL-6R. To address the question of whether such target cells existed in vivo, we compared the phenotype of mice transgenic for IL-6 alone with one of the mice transgenic for both, human IL-6 and human sIL-6R [64, 65].

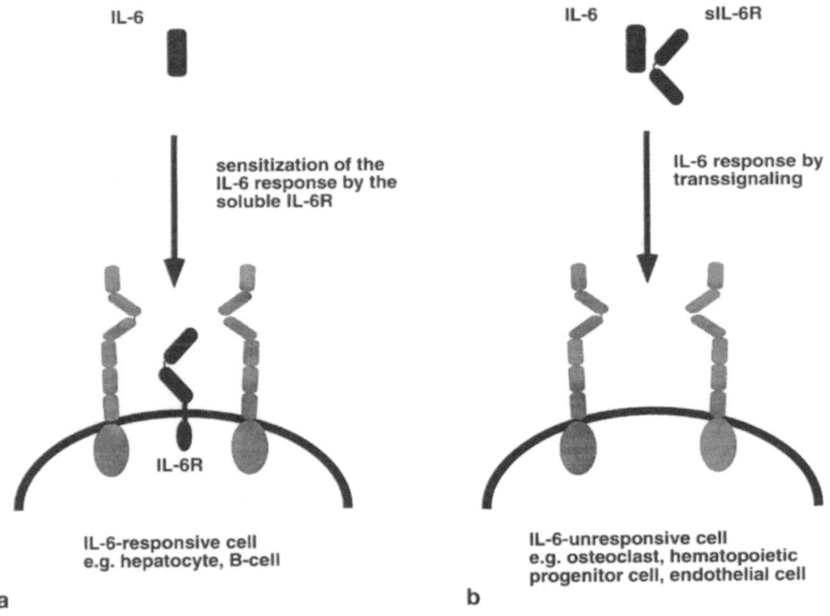

Fig. 4. Target cells of interleukin-6 (*IL-6*) and the IL-6/soluble IL-6R (*sIL-6R*) complex. **a** Cells which express gp130 (*gray*) and membrane bound IL-6R (*black*) are responsive to IL-6 and are sensitized by the presence of sIL-6R. **b** Cells which only express gp130 but no membrane-bound IL-6R are unresponsive to IL-6, but can be stimulated by the complex of IL-6 and sIL-6R

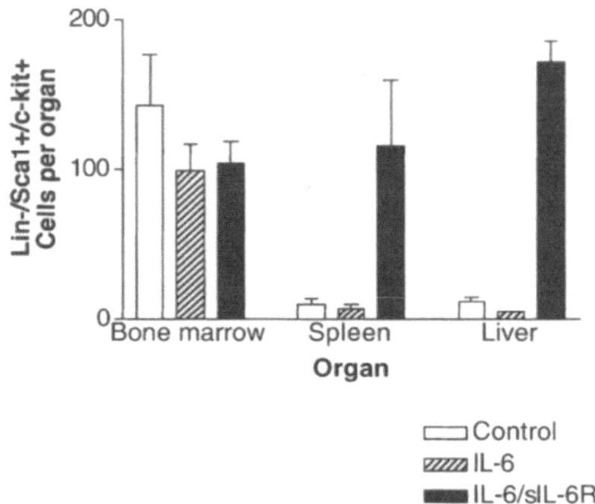

Fig. 5. Early hematopoietic progenitor cells in control, interleukin-6 (*IL-6*) or IL-6/ soluble IL-6R (*sIL-6R*) transgenic mice. The presence of Lin$^-$/Sca1$^+$/c-kit$^+$ cells present in bone marrow, spleen and liver of control mice, IL-6 transgenic mice and IL-6/sIL-6R double-transgenic mice was analyzed by fluorescence-activated cell sorter and expressed as total cells per organ

It turned out that the main difference between single- and double-transgenic mice was a massive extramedullary hematopoiesis in liver and spleen of the adult animals [65]. As shown in Fig. 5, the livers and spleens of IL-6/sIL–6R double-transgenic mice contain a highly elevated number of Lin-/Sca1$^+$/c-kit$^+$ cells, which have been demonstrated to contain a very high percentage of hematopoietic stem cells [60, 61] (M. Peters and A. Müller, manuscript in preparation). Moreover, spleen and liver contain highly elevated numbers of granulocytes, macrophages, Sca1$^+$ hematopoietic progenitor cells and B cells. The presence of hematopoietic progenitor cells in liver and spleen resulted in a time-dependent massive increase of peripheral blood cell numbers in IL-6/sIL–6R double-transgenic mice. These effects were completely absent in single-transgenic IL-6 mice.

In murine embryogenesis, the first hematopoietic cells are generated in the yolk sac at day 7.5 (E 7.5) of gestation. The first intraembryonic tissue with multilineage and long-term repopulating activity is the splanchnopleural mesoderm/AGM (aorta, genital ridge, mesonephros) region between E 8.5–11 of gestation [12]. Later, hematopoietic progenitor and stem cells can be found in the fetal liver and around birth in the spleen and bone marrow. The presence of multipotent hematopoietic progenitor cells and cells with a stem cell phenotype in double-transgenic adult animals might point to the fact that the adult liver retains a hematopoietic microenvironment and hematopoietic stem cells from the fetal developmental stage independent of other hematopoietic tissues, such as spleen and bone marrow. Bone marrow hematopoiesis in double-transgenic mice is unaffected by the presence of IL-6 and IL-6R [65]. This suggests that both tissues are affected in a different manner by IL-6 and sIL-6R.

Several studies have described functional changes in the hematopoietic system during development (reviewed in [5]). It was reported that human fetal liver cells have a higher proliferation and self-renewal rate compared to cord blood cells, and that cord blood cells have a higher proliferative and self-renewal capacity than adult bone marrow cells [32, 89]. There is now growing evidence that the functional difference of stem cells isolated from different developmental stages is reflected by a developmental-specific cytokine/growth factor receptor expression pattern on the surface of hematopoietic cells. Several lines of evidence support this notion: While cells isolated from bone marrow are optimally expanded with a combination of Flt-3 ligand, stem cell factor (SCF) and IL-3 [66, 100], cord blood cells require Flt-3 ligand, IL-6 and the sIL-6R for efficient expansion [100]. A further example of developmental-specific growth factor activity of a member of the IL-6 family of cytokines is OSM. Mukouyama et al. report that stimulation by OSM leads to the expansion of AGM-derived multipotent hematopoietic progenitors, but no stimulation of colony formation was detected with bone marrow-derived cells [50].

Taken together, the data from the single- and double-transgenic mice indicate that expansion of early extramedullary hematopoietic progenitor cells could only be stimulated by IL-6 in the presence of sIL-6R. This finding is strongly supported by recent data from Tajima et al. who found that CD34[+] cells can be subdivided into IL-6R-expressing and -nonexpressing cells. Both cell populations express gp130. It was demonstrated that IL-6R-expressing cells can be stimulated to form granulocyte-macrophage colonies, whereas IL-6R-negative cells, upon stimulation with IL-6 and sIL-6R, form various types of colonies including erythroid bursts, granulocyte-macrophage colonies, megacaryocytes and mixed colonies [80]. These findings are further supported by data from McKinstry et al. who demonstrate that the number of IL-6R on hematopoietic progenitor cells increases significantly with maturation of these cells [45]. These results indicate that the CD34[+] subpopulation which does not express IL-6R includes most of the erythroid, megacaryocytic and primitive human hematopoietic progenitors. Such cells are target cells for IL-6/sIL-6R, but not for IL-6 alone.

Endothelial Cells as Targets for the IL-6/sIL–6R Complex

It was recently noted that IL-6 -/- mice, after application of a local inflammatory stimulus, showed an impaired leukocyte accumulation in subcutaneous air pouches [68]. This defective leukocyte accumulation was not due to defective migratory capacity of IL-6 -/- leukocytes, but rather was associated with a reduced in situ production of chemokines. Analysis of IL-6 stimulation of endothelial cells in vitro demonstrated that these cells express only the gp130 signal transducing chain, but not the subunit-specific IL-6R. Therefore, endothelial cells are unresponsive to IL-6. IL-6 responsiveness, however, can be completely restored by the addition of recombinant sIL-6 R. In vivo and in vitro, evidence supports the concept that the IL-6 system plays an important role in local inflammatory reactions. The immune reaction seems to be completely dependent on the presence of both IL-6 and sIL-6R [68]. This might represent an important in vivo example of a reaction which, in the presence of IL-6, completely depends on the presence of sIL-6R. In this respect, it will be interesting to examine the responsiveness of smooth muscle cells with regard to IL-6 alone or the combination of IL-6 and sIL-6R.

Neuronal Cells are Stimulated by the IL-6/sIL-6R Complex

Rat pheochromocytoma cells (PC12) have been shown to undergo neuronal differentiation under the influence of IL-6 [71]. These results, however, seem to be only reproducible with subclones of the PC12 cell line [95]. We recently demonstrated that neurite outgrowth of PC12 cells can efficiently be stimulated by the combination of IL-6 and sIL-6R, but not with IL-6 [43]. Survival of rat primary sympathetic neurons is triggered by nerve growth factor (NGF). Treatment of these cells with IL-6 alone did not result in a survival response. When the primary sympathetic neurons were incubated with IL-6 in the presence of sIL-6R, cells survived to a similar extent as when treated with NGF [41]. Similar results have recently been obtained with dorsal root ganglions [82].

Many neuronal cells synthesize and secrete bioactive IL-6, but fail to be stimulated by this cytokine. Addition of recombinant sIL-6R resulted in a survival response of primary sympathetic neurons [41]. These data indicate that sIL-6R can be generated by one cell and acts in a paracrine fashion on a separate cell which secretes IL-6. This view is supported by the recent finding that cerebrospinal fluid contains levels of sIL-6R of several orders of magnitude higher than IL-6 [42]. The expanded spectrum of target cells by the transsignaling mechanism might shed new light on the intercellular communication network in the nervous system.

Osteoclasts Are Stimulated by IL-6 in the Presence of sIL-6R

IL-6 alone is not sufficient for the induction of osteoclast formation in cocultures of mouse bone marrow cells and osteoblastic cells. The addition of sIL-6R to such cocultures, however, strongly triggered osteoclast formation [81]. Treatment of cells with glucocorticoids triggered IL-6R mRNA and protein expression [70]. As described above, sIL-6R can be generated from membrane IL-6R protein or from IL-6R mRNA [69]. After addition of the synthetic glucocorticoid dexamethasone to cocultures of bone marrow cells and osteoblastic cells, IL-6 could stimulate osteoclast formation without the addition of sIL-6R [85]. This effect was due to a massive upregulation of IL-6R mRNA by dexamethasone. Osteoblastic cells from transgenic mice constitutively expressing human IL-6R could support osteoclast development in the presence of human IL-6 alone in cocultures with normal spleen cells. In contrast, osteoclast progenitors in spleen cells from transgenic mice overexpressing human IL-6R were not able to differentiate into osteoclasts in response to IL-6 in cocultures with normal osteoblastic cells. These results clearly indicate that the ability of IL-6 to induce osteoclast differentiation depends on signal transduction mediated by IL-6R expressed on osteoblastic cells but not on osteoclast progenitors [85].

Stimulation of Hematopoietic Progenitor Cells with the IL-6/sIL-6R Complex in vitro

Experimental strategies to expand hematopoietic cells often used cytokines of the IL-6 family [24, 47, 58]. Sui et al. were the first to demonstrate that stimulation of gp130 by IL-6 and sIL-6R resulted in superior ex vivo expansion of human primitive hematopoietic progenitor cells compared with IL-6 alone [76]. In this study, human cord blood CD34$^+$ cells were stimulated by SCF combined with IL-6 and sIL-6R (Fig. 6). These studies were extended by

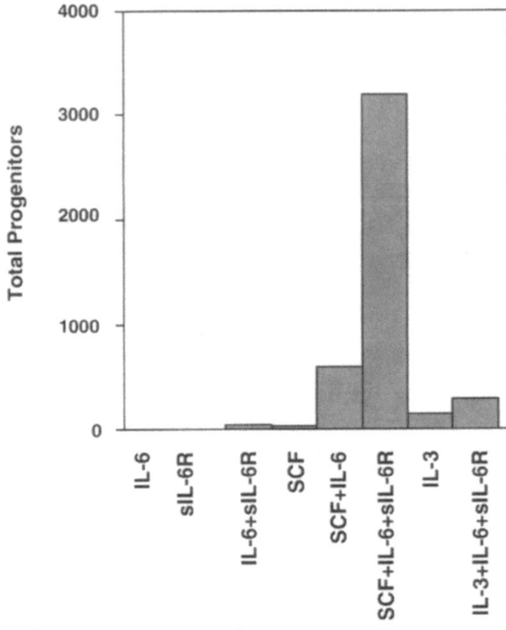

Fig. 6. Expansion of CD34$^+$ cells from human cord blood in the presence of interleukin-6 (*IL-6*) or IL-6/soluble IL-6R (*sIL-6R*). Generation of total progenitors from 2000 CD34$^+$ cord blood cells containing 684 progenitors in serum containing suspension culture supplemented with the factors indicated. *SCF*, stem cell factor. Adapted from [76]

the same group [28, 80] and have meanwhile been confirmed by several laboratories [8, 14, 100]. The most interesting aspect of these studies is that direct stimulation of gp130 seems not to be a proliferative stimulus by itself but, in combination with SCF and IL-3, seems rather to attenuate differentiation of hematopoietic cells [14, 76, 100].

A Designer Cytokine Which Directly Stimulates gp130

The effective concentration of IL-6 (50 ng/ml) and sIL-6R (>1000 ng/ml) [76] necessary for the stimulation of human hematopoietic progenitor cells is high considering a dissociation constant (K_d) of around 1 nM [70, 96]. It has recently been reported that the ligand/receptor interaction is mainly determined by the off-rate [92], suggesting that the average half-life of the IL-6/sIL-6R complex might be shorter than the time needed to assemble the

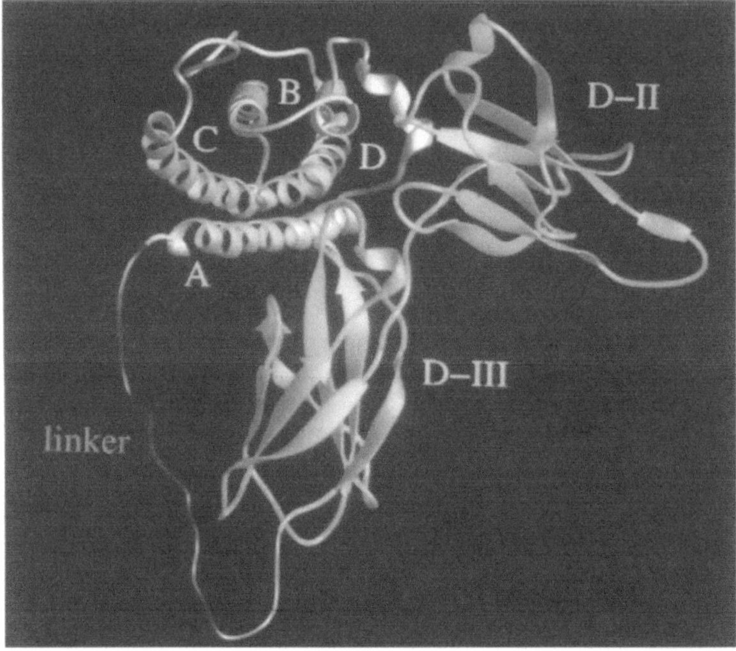

Fig. 7. Hyper-interleukin-6 (*IL-6*): a highly active designer cytokine consisting of IL-6 and soluble IL-6 receptor (*sIL-6R*). Molecular model of the fusion protein of IL-6 and sIL-6R (Hyper-IL-6) consisting of IL-6 and sIL-6R fused by a flexible peptide linker. *A–D* denote the four helices of IL-6; *D-II* and *D-III* are the two cytokine-binding receptor domains of sIL-6R used for the construction of the fusion protein

IL-6/sIL-6R/gp130 complex. Accordingly, to lower the effective dose needed for IL-6 bioactivity, IL-6 muteins with a lower off-rate have been selected to render the complexes with IL-6R more stable [83]. As a novel approach we postulated that the formation of the IL-6/sIL-6R complex could be enhanced by converting it into single protein by using a flexible polypeptide as a linker (Fig. 7). The distance between the C-terminus of IL-6R and the N-terminus of IL-6 was calculated from our three-dimensional model of the complex to be in the order of 40 Å [17]. Consequently, we used the 16 N-terminal non-helical, and presumably flexible, amino acid residues of IL-6, together with a 13-residue sequence rich in glycine and serine, to connect IL-6 and sIL-6R [14]. The fusion protein was called Hyper-IL-6.

On gp130-expressing cells the fusion protein turned out to be fully active at 100–1000-fold lower concentrations than the combination of unlinked IL-6 and IL-6R. The fusion protein was therefore tested for its ability to stimulate expansion of hematopoietic progenitor cells in vitro. It turned out that stimulation with Hyper-IL-6 was at least as effective as IL-6/sIL-6R at 100 times lower concentrations than those used for unlinked IL-6 and IL-6R [8, 14].

gp130 Stimulation in Hematopoiesis

Hematopoiesis is arranged in a descending hierachy: Clonogenic hematopoietic stem cells pass through several stages of differentiation and finally produce functionally mature blood cells, including erythrocytes, megakaryocytes, granulocytes, monocytes, macrophages, mast cells and the different classes of lymphocytes [84]. The ability of a cell to generate and sustain the production of both mature myeloid and lymphoid cells for many weeks after being transplanted into a hematologically compromised host has now been widely accepted as a useful functional definition for its assignment to the stem cell compartment [9, 59].

In the double-transgenic IL-6/sIL-6R mice, hematopoietic progenitor cells in liver and spleen have been detected [65]. At present, it can not be decided whether these hematopoietic progenitor cells were resident in liver or spleen or whether they immigrated via the circulation. It is clear, however, that these cells must have been expanded and that during several weeks of hepatic and spleenic hematopoiesis, renewal of hematopoietic progenitor cells must have occurred. In this respect, it is noteworthy that in double-transgenic IL-6/sIL-6R mice, but not in single-transgenic IL-6 mice, we find a massive upregulation of SCF mRNA and cell surface protein expression in the liver, which might contribute to stimulation and homing of hematopoietic progenitor cells (M. Peters, unpublished results).

So far it is not clear whether gp130 stimulation contributes to hematopoiesis in vivo. From our transgenic-mice data, together with the data from Zandstra et al., it is likely that gp130 stimulation is more important during fetal liver than during adult medullary hematopoiesis [65, 100]. Accordingly, gp130-deficient mice die perinatally between day 12.5 and term. The mutant embryos have reduced numbers of pluripotential and committed hematopoietic progenitors in the liver and differentiated lineages such as T cells in the thymus [99]. In contrast, mice which lack LIF-R have normal hematologic compartments [91]. These data argue against an important role of cytokines interacting with LIF-R during fetal hematopoiesis (CNTF, CT-1, LIF).

The case of OSM is somewhat more complicated since human OSM can interact with both gp130/LIF-R and gp130/OSM-R complexes [48]. Also, murine OSM seems only to interact with the gp130/OSM-R complex [25]. In transgenic mice which overexpressed OSM, however, no hematological abnormalities have been reported [40]. However, it was recently reported that OSM is expressed in the AGM region and that it stimulated expansion of multipotential hematopoietic progenitor cells in vitro [50].

We conclude that gp130 is required for normal fetal liver hematopoiesis and that among the cytokines of the IL-6 family, only IL-6 and IL-11, which use gp130 homodimers for signaling, may play a role in hematopoiesis in vivo. IL-11 has been demonstrated to possess thrombopoietic potential and can induce serial repopulating ability of murine hematopoietic stem cells [18]. IL-11R-deficient mice, however, do not show hematological abnormalities [56]. IL-6 is involved in the regulation of stem cells and committed progenitors in vivo, but hematopoiesis still occurs in IL-6-deficient mice [3]. A likely explanation for these findings is that IL-6 and IL-11, and possibly OSM, can compensate for one another. It cannot be excluded that other, as yet unidentified, gp130-stimulating cytokines which possess hematopoietic activities exist.

The second question which arises from the reviewed data is whether soluble receptors (e.g. sIL-6R or sIL-11R) are involved in gp130 stimulation during hematopoiesis. Since several reports indicate that hematopoietic progenitor cells do not express IL-6R [45, 65, 80], gp130 stimulation on these cells might involve soluble receptors or intercellular stimulation as depicted in Fig. 8. It is, however, hard to discriminate between the two models. The only way to ultimately clarify the biological role of sIL-6R will be to generate mice unable to produce a sIL-6R. The generation of such an animal model, however, is a complex undertaking, since the generation of sIL-6R by shedding and splicing would have to be blocked. Therefore, a mouse lacking the exon used for the alternatively spliced sIL-6R [35] would have to be constructed. This mutation would then have to be combined with a mutation resulting in the deletion of the shedding sites of the IL-6R [53, 88, 90], or alternatively, with a mutation resulting in the deletion of the shedding protease. Problems

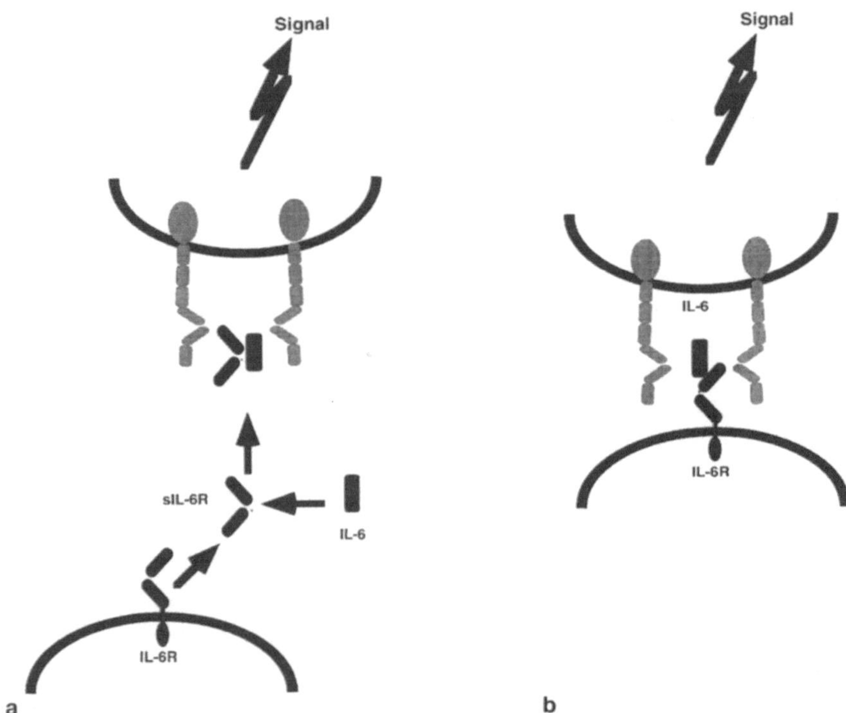

Fig. 8. gp130 Stimulation via soluble or membrane-bound interleukin-6 receptor (*IL-6R*). **a** A donor cell (*bottom*) releases the soluble IL-6R (*sIL-6R*) which, in the presence of IL-6, stimulates the target cell (*top*) to dimerize gp130 (*gray*) and initiate signal transduction. **b** The contact between donor cell (*bottom*) and target cell (*top*) is mediated by the membrane-bound IL-6R of the donor cell, IL-6 and the two gp130 molecules of the target cell, leading to gp130 dimerization and signaling. For reasons of simplicity, on donor cells, gp130 has been omitted

in this respect might arise from our finding that at least three different cleavage sites can be used by the shedding protease [53, 88, 90] and that the IL-6R shedding protease has not yet been molecularly defined.

gp130 Stimulation During Development

The receptor subunit gp130 is ubiquitously expressed [20]. To investigate the physiological roles of gp130 and to examine pathological consequences of a lack of gp130, mice deficient in gp130 have been prepared [99]. Embryos homozygous for the gp130 mutation progressively died between 12.5 days postcoitum and term. On 16.5 days postcoitum and later, they showed hypo-plastic ventricular myocardium without septal and trabecular defect. The subcellular ultrastructures in gp130-/-cardiomyocytes appeared normal. Re-markably, the mutant embryos have greatly reduced numbers of pluripoten-tial and committed hematopoietic progenitors in the liver. Moreover, differ-entiated lineages, such as T cells in the thymus, were greatly reduced. Some gp130-/-embryos showed anemia reflecting impaired development of eryth-roid lineage cells. The reduction of hematopoietic progenitor cells in the liver was consistent with a crucial role of gp130 stimulation during hepatic hematopoiesis [65]. Interestingly, in gp130-deficient mice the number of osteoclasts was about twice as high as that in wild-type animals. The volume of mineralized trabecular bones was also decreased at mandibulae, accom-panied by an increased number of osteoclasts in gp130-deficient mice com-pared with wild-type and heterozygous mice. These results suggest that the formation of osteoclasts is not solely dependent on gp130 signaling, at least during fetal development. The osteoclastic bone resorption in gp130-defi-cient mice might be caused by the functional redundancy of bone-resorbing hormones and cytokines other than those of the IL-6 family [27].

Cellular Responsiveness Depends on the Ratio Between gp130 and IL-6R

The tissue expression of gp130 is believed to be ubiquitous and the cellular expression seems not to be the subject of major transcriptional regulation [20, 79]. The IL-6R, however, is only expressed on some cell types [79, 96], including hepatocytes and B cells. While the number of gp130 signal trans-ducers is believed to be relatively constant on all cells of the body, the num-ber of IL-6R molecules expressed on the surface of target cells may vary from one cell type to another (Fig. 9). Cells that express no, or very little, IL-6R on their surface can be stimulated only by the IL-6/sIL-6R complex and are insensitive to IL-6 alone (Fig. 9a). Examples of such cells are hematopoietic progenitor cells [65], endothelial cells [68], osteoclasts [81] and many neuro-nal cells [41, 43]. Cells that express fewer IL-6R molecules on their surface than gp130 signal transducers respond to IL-6 alone, and this response can be enhanced by the presence of sIL-6R (Fig. 9b). Examples of such cells are hepatocytes and plasmacytoma cells. Cells that express IL-6R and gp130 with equal numbers on their surface respond to IL-6, and this response is not altered by sIL-6R (Fig. 9c). Theoretically, on cells that express more IL-6R molecules than gp130 proteins, low IL-6 concentrations might not induce a response, whereas high IL-6 concentrations might even antagonize the IL-6 response, since the formation of inactive complexes containing only one

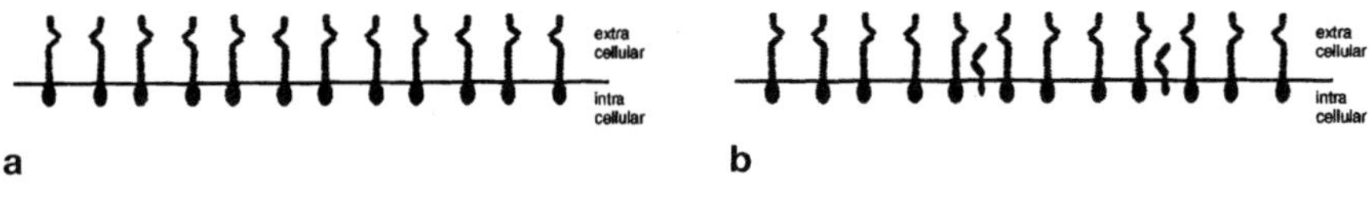

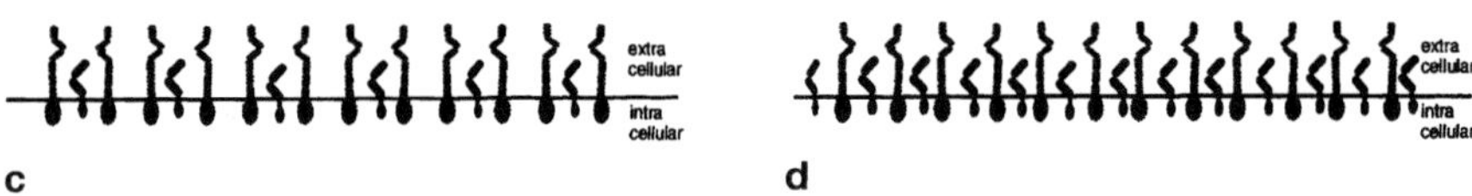

Fig. 9. Cellular responsiveness to interleukin-6 (*IL-6*) or IL-6/soluble IL-6R receptor (*sIL-6R*) is determined by the expression levels of IL-6R and gp130. The number of the ubiquitously expressed gp130 proteins (*gray*) is believed to be constant on all cells of the organism. The number of IL-6R molecules (*black*) varies on different cell types. **a** Cells that express no, or very little, IL-6R on their surface can be stimulated only by the IL-6/sIL-6R complex and are insensitive to IL-6 alone. **b** Cells that express fewer IL-6R molecules on their surface than gp130 signal transducers respond to IL-6 alone, and this response can be enhanced by the presence of sIL-6R. **c** Cells that express IL-6R and gp130 in equal numbers on their surface respond to IL-6, and this response is not altered by sIL-6R. **d** On cells that express more IL-6R molecules than gp130 proteins, low IL-6 concentrations might not induce a response, whereas high IL-6 concentrations might even antagonize the IL-6 response, since the formation of inactive complexes containing only one gp130 molecule is favored

gp130 molecule could be favored (Fig. 9d). Using transfected cells, such a situation has recently been mimicked using the IL-11 receptor system [10].

gp130 Stimulation and Inhibition of Differentiation

As outlined above, the stimulation of gp130 on hematopoietic progenitor cells might result in a differentiation-inhibiting activity. This is reminiscent of the activity of LIF on embryonic stem cells which are now widely used to generate chimeric animals in the process of establishing knock-out animals [75]. Interestingly, LIF can also be replaced by other cytokines of the IL-6 family which interact with the gp130/LIR heterodimer like OSM and CNTF [67]. Embryonic stem cell differentiation is also completely prevented when cells are treated with the combination of IL-6 and sIL-6R [98]. It is therefore tempting to speculate that the consequence of gp130 stimulation on early hematopoietic progenitor cells and on neuronal cells might be an inhibition of differentiation related to that seen in embryonic stem cells. Further experiments are needed to support such a provocative hypothesis.

Conclusions

The reviewed data indicate that gp130 stimulation is of importance for hematopoiesis and neuropoiesis in vivo. Cytokines which directly stimulate gp130 will be of use for in vitro expansion of hematopoietic progenitor cells and should replace IL-6, which is commonly used in such cytokine cocktails. A therapeutic application of gp130-stimulating cytokines on hematopoietic progenitor cells and neuronal cells can be anticipated.

References

1. Baumann H, Wang Y, Morella KK, Lai CF, Dams H, Hilton DJ, Hawley RG, Mackiewicz A (1996) Complex of the soluble IL-11 receptor and IL-11 acts as IL-6-type cytokine in hepatic and nonhepatic cells. J Immunol 157:284–290
2. Bazan JF (1990) Haemopoietic receptors and helical cytokines. Immunol Today 11:350–354
3. Bernad A, Kopf M, Kulbacki R, Weich N, Koehler G, Gutierrez Ramos JC (1994) Interleukin-6 is required in vivo for the regulation of stem cells and committed progenitors of the hematopoietic system. Immunity 1:725–731
4. Black RA, Rauch CT, Kozlosky CJ, Peschon JJ, Slack JL, Wolfson MF, Castner BJ, Stocking KL, Reddy P, Srinivasan S, Nelson N, Boiani N, Schooley KA Gerhart M, Davis R, Fitzner JN, Johnson RS, Paxton RJ, March CJ, Cerretti DP (1997) A metalloproteinase disintegrin that releases tumour-necrosis factor-alpha from cells. Nature 385:729–733
5. Bonifer C, Faust N, Geiger H, Müller AM (1998) Developmental changes in the differentiation capacity of haematopoietic stem cells. Immunol Today, in press
6. Brakenhoff JP, Hart M, Aarden LA (1989) Analysis of human IL-6 mutants expressed in Escherichia coli. Biologic activities are not affected by deletion of amino acids 1–28. J Immunol 143:1175–1182
7. Brakenhoff JP, Hart M, De Groot ER, Di Padova F, Aarden LA (1990) Structure-function analysis of human IL-6. Epitope mapping of neutralizing monoclonal antibodies with amino- and carboxyl-terminal deletion mutants. J Immunol 145:561–568
8. Chebath J, Fischer D, Kumar A, Oh JW, Kolett O, Lapidot T, Fischer M, Rose-John S, Nagler A, Slavin S, Revel M (1997) Interleukin-6 receptor-interleukin-6 fusion proteins with enhanced interleukin-6 type pleiotropic activities. Eur Cytokine Netw 8:359–365
9. Conneally E, Cashman J, Petzer A, Eaves CJ (1997) Expansion in vitro of transplantable human cord blood stem cells demonstrated using a quantitative assay of their lympho-myeloid repopulating activity in NOD/SCID mice. Proc Natl Acad Sci USA 94:9836–9841
10. Curtis DJ, Hilton DJ, Roberts B, Murray L, Nicola N, Begley CG (1997) Recombinant soluble interleukin-11 (IL-11) receptor alpha-chain can act as an IL-11 antagonist. Blood 90:4403–4412

11. Davis S, Aldrich TH, Ip NY, Stahl N, Scherer S, Farruggella T, DiStefano PS, Curtis R, Panayotatos N, Gascan H, Chevalier S, Yancopulos GD (1993) Released form of CNTF receptor alpha component as a soluble mediator of CNTF responses. Science 259:1736–1739

12. Dzierzak E, Medvinsky A (1995) Mouse embryonic hematopoiesis. Trends in Genetics 11:359–365

13. Ehlers M, Grötzinger J, deHon FD, Müllberg J, Brakenhoff JP, Liu J, Wollmer A, Rose-John S (1994) Identification of two novel regions of human IL-6 responsible for receptor binding and signal transduction. J Immunol 153:1744–1753

14. Fischer M, Goldschmitt J, Peschel C, Kallen KJ, Brakenhoff JPJ, Wollmer A, Grötzinger J, Rose-John S (1997) A designer cytokine with high activity on human hematopoietic progenitor cells. Nature Biotech 15:142–145

15. Frieling JTM, van Deuren M, Wijdenes J, van der Meer JWM, Clement C, van der Linden CJ, Sauerwein RW (1995) Circulating interleukin-6 receptor in patients with sepsis syndrome. J Infect Dis 171:469–472

16. Gaillard J-P, Liautard J, Klein B, Brochier J (1997) Major role of the soluble interleukin-6/interleukin-6 receptor complex for the proliferation of interleukin-6-dependent human myeloma cell lines. Eur J Immunol 27:3332–3340

17. Grötzinger J, Kurapkat G, Wollmer A, Kalai M, Rose-John S (1997) The family of the IL-6-type cytokines: Specificity and promiscuity of the receptor complexes. Proteins 27:96–109

18. Hawley RG, Hawley TS, Fong AZ, Quinto C, Collins M, Leonard JP, Goldman SJ (1996) Thrombopoietic potential and serial repopulating ability of murine hematopoietic stem cells constitutively expressing interleukin 11. Proc Natl Acad Sci USA 93:10297–10302

19. Heaney ML, Golde DW (1996) Soluble cytokine receptors. Blood 87:847–857

20. Hibi M, Murakami M, Saito M, Hirano T, Taga T, Kishimoto T (1990) Molecular cloning and expression of an IL-6 signal transducer, gp130. Cell 63:1149–1157

21. Honda M, Yamamoto S, Cheng M, Yasukawa K, Suzuki H, Saito T, Osugi Y, Tokunaga T, Kishimoto T (1992) Human soluble IL-6 receptor: its detection and enhanced release by HIV infection. J Immunol 148:2175–2180

22. Hooper NM, Karran EH, Turner AJ (1997) Membrane protein secretases. Biochem J 321:265–279

23. Horsten U, Schmitz-Van de Leur H, Müllberg J, Heinrich PC, Rose-John S (1995) The membrane distal half of gp130 is responsible for the formation of a ternary complex with IL-6 and the IL-6 receptor. FEBS Lett 360:43–46

24. Ikebuchi K, Wong GG, Clark SC, Ihle JM, Hirai Y, Ogawa M (1987) Interleukin 6 enhancement of interleukin 3-dependent proliferation of multipotential hematopoietic progenitors. Proc Natl Acad Sci USA 84:9035–9039

25. Ishihara M, Hara T, Kim H, Murate T, Miyajima A (1997) Oncostatin M and leukemia inhibitory factor do not use the same functional receptor in mice. Blood 90:165–173

26. Kalai M, Montero-Julian FA, Grötzinger J, Wollmer A, Morelle D, Brochier J, Rose-John S, Heinrich PC, Brailly H, Content J (1996) Participation of two Ser-Ser-Phe-Tyr repeats in interleukin-6 (IL-6)-binding sites of the human IL-6 receptor. Eur J Biochem 238:714–723

27. Kawasaki K, Gao YH, Yokose S, Kaji Y, Nakamura T, Suda T, Yoshida K, Taga T, Kishimoto T, Kataoka H, Yuasa T, Norimatsu H, Yamaguchi A (1997) Osteoclasts are present in gp130-deficient mice. Endocrinology 138:4959–4965

28. Kimura T, Sakabe H, Tanimukai S, Abe T, Urata Y, Yasukawa K, Okano A, Taga T, Sugiyama H, Kishimoto T, Sonoda Y (1997) Simultaneous activation of signals through gp130, c-kit, and interleukin-3 receptor promotes a trilineage blood cell production in the absence of terminally acting lineage specific factors. Blood 90:4767–4778
29. Kishimoto T, Akira S, Narazaki M, Taga T (1995) Interleukin-6 family of cytokines and gp130. Blood 86:1243–1254
30. Krüttgen A, Rose-John S, Dufhues G, Bender S, Lütticken C, Freyer P, Heinrich PC (1990) The three carboxy-terminal amino acids of human interleukin-6 are essential for its biological activity. FEBS Lett 273:95–98
31. Krüttgen A, Rose-John S Moller C, Wroblowski B, Wollmer A, Müllberg J, Hirano T, Kishimoto T, Heinrich PC (1990) Structure-function analysis of human interleukin-6. Evidence for the involvement of the carboxy-terminus in function. FEBS Lett 262:323–326
32. Lansdorp PM, Dragowska W, Mayani H (1993) Ontogeny-related changes in proliferative potential of human hematopoietic cells. J Exp Med 178:787–791
33. Lavabre Bertrand T, Exbrayat C, Liautard J, Gaillard JP, Baskevitch PP, Poujol N, Duperray C, Bourquard P, Brochier J (1995) Detection of membrane and soluble interleukin-6 receptor in lymphoid malignancies. Br J Haematol 91: 871–877
34. Layton MJ, Cross BA, Metcalf D, Ward LD, Simpson RJ, Nicola NA (1992) A major binding protein for leukemia inhibitory factor in normal mouse serum: identification as a soluble form of the cellular receptor. Proc Natl Acad Sci USA 89:8616–8620
35. Lust JA, Donovan KA, Kline MP, Greipp PR, Kyle RA, Maihle NJ (1992) Isolation of an mRNA encoding a soluble form of the human interleukin-6 receptor. Cytokine 4:96–100
36. Lust JA, Jelinek DF, Donovan KA, Frederick LA, Huntley BK, Braaten JK, Maihle NJ (1995) Sequence, expression and function of an mRNA encoding a soluble form of the human interleukin-6 receptor (sIL-6R). Curr Top Microbiol Immunol 194:199–206
37. Lütticken C, Krüttgen A, Moller C, Heinrich PC, Rose-John S (1991) Evidence for the importance of a positive charge and an alpha-helical structure of the C-terminus for biological activity of human IL-6. FEBS Lett 282:265–267
38. Mackiewicz A, Schooltink H, Heinrich PC, Rose-John S (1992) Complex of soluble human IL-6-receptor/IL-6 up-regulates expression of acute-phase proteins. J Immunol 149:2021–2027
39. Mackiewicz A, Wiznerowicz M, Roeb E, Karczewska A, Nowak J, Heinrich PC, Rose-John S (1995) Soluble interleukin 6 receptor is biologically active in vivo. Cytokine 7:142–149
40. Malik N, Haugen HS, Modrell B, Shoyab M, Clegg CH (1995) Developmental abnormalities in mice transgenic for oncostatin M. Mol Cell Biol 15:2349–2358
41. März P, Cheng J-C, Gadient RA, Patterson P, Stoyan T, Otten U, Rose-John S (1998) Sympathetic neurons can produce and respond to interleukin-6. Proc Natl Acad Sci USA 95:3251–3256
42. März P, Heese K, Hock C, Golombowski S, Müller-Spahn F, Rose-John S, Otten U (1997) Interleukin-6 (IL-6) and soluble forms of IL-6 receptors are not altered in cerebrospinal fluid of Alzheimer's disease patients. Neurosci Lett 239:29–32
43. März P, Herget T, Lang E, Otten U, Rose-John S (1997) Activation of gp130 by IL-6/soluble IL-6 receptor induces neuronal differentiation. Eur J Neurosci 9: 2765–2773

154 S. Rose-John et al.

44. McGeehan GM, Becherer JD, Bast RC Jr, Boyer CM, Champion B, Connolly KM, Conway JG, Furdon P, Karp S, Kidao S, McElroy AB, Nichols J, Pryzwanszky M, Schoenen F, Sedut L, Truesdale A, Verghese M, Warner J, Ways JP (1994) Regulation of tumour necrosis factor-alpha processing by a metalloproteinase inhibitor. Nature 370:558–561

45. McKinstry WJ, Li CL, Rasko JE, Nicola NA, Johnson GR, Metcalf D (1997) Cytokine receptor expression on hematopoietic stem and progenitor cells. Blood 89:65–71

46. Mohler KM, Sleath PR, Fitzner JN, Cerretti DP, Alderson M, Kerwar SS, Torrance DS, Otten Evans C, Greenstreet T, Weerawarna K, Kronheim SR, Petersen M, Gerhart M, Kozlosky CJ, March CJ, Black RA (1994) Protection against a lethal dose of endotoxin by an inhibitor of tumour necrosis factor processing. Nature 370:218–220

47. Morrison SJ, Uchida N, Weissman IL (1995) The biology of hematopoietic stem cells. Ann Rev Cell Dev Biol 11:35–71

48. Mosley B, De Imus C, Friend D, Boiani N, Thoma B, Park LS, Cosman D (1996) Dual oncostatin M (OSM) receptors. Cloning and characterization of an alternative signaling subunit conferring OSM-specific receptor activation. J Biol Chem 271:32635–32643

49. Moss ML, Jin SL, Milla ME, Bickett DM, Burkhart W, Carter HL, Chen WJ, Clay WC, Didsbury JR, Hassler D, Hoffman CR, Kost TA, Lambert MH, Leesnitzer MA, McCauley P, McGeehan G, Mitchell J, Moyer M, Pahel G, Rocque W, Overton LK, Schoenen F, Seaton T, Su JL, Warner J, Willard D, Becherer JD (1997) Cloning of a disintegrin metalloproteinase that processes precursor tumour-necrosis factor-alpha. Nature 385:733–736

50. Mukouyama Y-S, Hara T, Xu M-J, Tamura K, Donovan PJ, Kim H-J, Kogo H, Tsuji K, Nakahata T, Miyajima A (1998) In vitro expansion of murine multipotential hematopoietic progenitors from the embryonic aorta-gonad-mesonephros region. Immunity 8:105–114

51. Müllberg J, Dittrich E, Graeve L, Gerhartz C, Yasukawa K, Taga T, Kishimoto T, Heinrich PC, Rose-John S (1993) Differential shedding of the two subunits of the interleukin-6 receptor. FEBS Lett 332:174–178

52. Müllberg J, Durie FH, Otten Evans C, Alderson MR, Rose-John S, Cosman D, Black RA, Mohler KM (1995) A metalloprotease inhibitor blocks shedding of the IL-6 receptor and the p60 TNF receptor. J Immunol 155:5198–5205

53. Müllberg J, Oberthur W, Lottspeich F, Mehl E, Dittrich E, Graeve L, Heinrich PC, Rose-John S (1994) The soluble human IL-6 receptor. Mutational characterization of the proteolytic cleavage site. J Immunol 152:4958–4968

54. Müllberg J, Schooltink H, Stoyan T, Gunther M, Graeve L, Buse G, Mackiewicz A, Heinrich PC, Rose-John S (1993) The soluble interleukin-6 receptor is generated by shedding. Eur J Immunol 23:473–480

55. Müllberg J, Schooltink H, Stoyan T, Heinrich PC, Rose-John S (1992) Protein kinase C activity is rate limiting for shedding of the interleukin-6 receptor. Biochem Biophys Res Commun 189:794–800

56. Nandurkar HH, Robb L, Tarlinton D, Barnett L, Kontgen F, Begley CG (1997) Adult mice with targeted mutation of the interleukin-11 receptor (IL-11Ra) display normal hematopoiesis. Blood 90:2148–2159

57. Narazaki M, Yasukawa K, Saito T, Ohsugi Y, Fukui H, Koishihara Y, Yancopoulos GD, Taga T, Kishimoto T (1993) Soluble forms of the interleukin-6 signal-transducing receptor component gp130 in human serum possessing a potential to inhibit signals through membrane-anchored gp130. Blood 82:1120–1126

58. Ogawa M (1993) Differentiation and proliferation of heamtopoietic stem cells. Blood 81:2844–2853
59. Orkin SH (1995) Transcription factors and hematopoietic development. J Biol Chem 270:4955–4958
60. Osawa M, Hanada K, Hamada H, Nakauchi H (1996) Long-term lymphohematopoietic reconstitution by a single CD34-low/negative hematopoietic stem cell. Science 273:242–245
61. Osawa M, Nakamura K, Nishi N, Takahasi N, Tokuomoto Y, Inoue H, Nakauchi H (1996) In vivo self-renewal of c-Kit+ Sca-1+ Lin(low/-) hemopoietic stem cells. J Immunol 156:3207–3214
62. Pennica D, Arce V, Swanson TA, Vejsada R, Pollock RA, Armanini M, Dudley K, Phillips HS, Rosenthal A, Kato AC, Henderson CE (1996) Cardiotrophin-1, a cytokine present in embryonic muscle, supports long-term survival of spinal motoneurons. Neuron 17:63–74
63. Peters M, Jacobs S, Ehlers M, Vollmer P, Müllberg J, Wolf E, Brem G, Meyer zum Büschenfelde KH, Rose-John S (1996) The function of the soluble interleukin 6 (IL-6) receptor in vivo: sensitization of human soluble IL-6 receptor transgenic mice towards IL-6 and prolongation of the plasma half-life of IL-6. J Exp Med 183:1399–1406
64. Peters M, Odenthal M, Schirmacher P, Blessing M, Fattori E, Ciliberto G, Meyer zum Büschenfelde KH, Rose-John S (1997) Soluble IL-6 receptor leads to a paracrine modulation of the IL-6-induced hepatic acute phase response in double transgenic mice. J Immunol 159:1474–1481
65. Peters M, Schirmacher P, Goldschmitt J, Odenthal M, Peschel C, Dienes HP, Fattori E, Ciliberto G, Meyer zum Büschenfelde KH, Rose-John S (1997) Extramedullary expansion of hematopoietic progenitor cells in IL 6/sIL-6R double transgenic mice. J Exp Med 185:755–766
66. Petzer AL, Zandstra PW, Piret JM, Eaves CJ (1996) Differential cytokine effects on primitive (CD34+CD38-) human hematopoietic cells: novel responses to Flt3-ligand and thrombopoietin. J Exp Med 183:2551–2558
67. Piquet-Pellorce C, Grey L, Mereau A, Heath JK (1994) Are LIF and related cytokines functionally equivalent? Exp Cell Res 213:340–347
68. Romano M, Sironi M, Toniatti C, Polentarutti N, Fruscella P, Ghezzi P, Faggioni R, Luini W, van Hinsbergh V, Sozzani S, Bussolino F, Poli V, Ciliberto G, Mantovani A (1997) Role of IL-6 and its soluble receptor in induction of chemokines and leukocyte recruitment. Immunity 6:315–325
69. Rose-John S, Heinrich PC (1994) Soluble receptors for cytokines and growth factors: generation and biological function. Biochem J 300:281–290
70. Rose-John S, Schooltink H, Lenz D, Hipp E, Dufhues G, Schmitz H, Schiel X, Hirano T, Kishimoto T, Heinrich PC (1990) Studies on the structure and regulation of the human hepatic interleukin-6 receptor. Eur J Biochem 190:79–83
71. Satoh T, Nakamura S, Taga T, Matsuda T, Hirano T, Kishimoto T, Kaziro Y (1988) Induction of neuronal differentiation in PC12 cells by B-cell stimulatory factor 2/interleukin-6. Mol Cell Biol 8:3546–3549
72. Savino R, Ciapponi L, Lahm A, Demartis A, Cabibbo A, Toniatti C, Delmastro P, Altamura S, Ciliberto G (1994) Rational design of a receptor super-antagonist of human interleukin-6. EMBO J 13:5863–5870
73. Savino R, Lahm A, Salvati AL, Ciapponi L, Sporeno E, Altamura S, Paonessa G, Toniatti C, Ciliberto G (1994) Generation of interleukin-6 receptor antagonists by molecular-modeling guided mutagenesis of residues important for gp130 activation. EMBO J 13:1357–1367

74. Sprang SR, Bazan JF (1993) Cytokine structural taxonomy and mechanism of receptor engagement. Curr Opin Struct Biol 3:815–827
75. Stewart CL (1994) Leukaemia inhibitory factor and the regulation of pre-implantation development of the mammalian embryo. Mol Reprod Dev 39: 233–238
76. Sui X, Tsuji K, Tanaka R, Tajima S, Muraoka K, Ebihara Y, Ikebuchi K, Yasukawa K, Taga T, Kishimoto T, Nakahata T (1995) gp130 and c-Kit signalings synergize for ex vivo expansion of human primitive hemopoietic progenitor cells. Proc Natl Acad Sci U S A 92:2859–2863
77. Taga T, Hibi M, Hirata Y, Yamasaki K, Yasukawa K, Matsuda T, Hirano T, Kishimoto T (1989) Interleukin-6 triggers the association of its receptor with a possible signal transducer, gp130. Cell 58:573–581
78. Taga T, Kishimoto T (1990) Immune and hematopoietic cell regulation: cytokines and their receptors. Curr Opin Cell Biol 2:174–180
79. Taga T, Kishimoto T (1997) gp130 and the interleukin-6 family of cytokines. Annu Rev Immunol 15:797–819
80. Tajima S, Tsuji K, Ebihara Y, Sui X, Tanaka R, Muraoka K, Yoshida M, Yamada K, Yasukawa K, Taga T, Kishimoto T, Nakahata T (1996) Analysis of interleukin-6 receptor and gp130 expressions and proliferative capability of human CD34 + cells. J Exp Med 184:1357–1364
81. Tamura T, Udagawa N, Takahashi N, Miyaura C, Tanaka S, Yamada Y, Koishihara Y, Ohsugi Y, Kumaki K, Taga T, Kishimoto T, Suda T (1993) Soluble interleukin-6 receptor triggers osteoclast formation by interleukin 6. Proc Natl Acad Sci U S A 90:11924–11928
82. Thier M, März P, Otten U, Weis J, Rose-John S (1998) Interleukin-6 (IL-6) supports survival of sensory neurons: Autocrine trophic effects of IL-6 and soluble IL-6 receptor and enhanced activity of an IL-6 designer cytokine. J Neurosci Res, submitted
83. Toniatti C, Cabibbo A, Sporena E, Salvati AL, Cerretani M, Serafini S, Lahm A, Cortese R, Ciliberto G (1996) Engineering human interleukin-6 to obtain variants with strongly enhanced bioactivity. EMBO J 15:2726–2737
84. Uchida N, Fleming WH, Alpern EJ, Weissman IL (1993) Heterogeneity of hematopoietic stem cells. Curr Opin Immunol 5:177–184
85. Udagawa N, Takahashi N, Katagiri T, Tamura T, Wada S, Findlay DM, Martin TJ, Hirota H, Taga T, Kishimoto T, Suda T (1995) Interleukin (IL)-6 induction of osteoclast differentiation depends on IL-6 receptors expressed on osteoblastic cells but not on osteoclast progenitors. J Exp Med 182:1461–1468
86. van Dam M, Müllberg J, Schooltink H, Stoyan T, Brakenhoff JP, Graeve L, Heinrich PC, Rose-John S (1993) Structure-function analysis of interleukin-6 utilizing human/murine chimeric molecules. Involvement of two separate domains in receptor binding. J Biol Chem 268:15285–15290
87. van Snick J (1990) Interleukin-6: an overview. Annu Rev Immunol 8:253–279
88. Vollmer P, Walev I, Rose-John S, Bhakdi S (1996) Novel pathogenic mechanism of microbial metalloproteinases: liberation of membrane anchored molecules in biologically active form exemplified by studies with the human interleukin-6 receptor. Infect Immun 64:3646–3651
89. Vormoor J, Lapidot T, Pflumio F, Risdon G, Patterson B, Broxmeyer HE, Dick JE (1994) Immature human cord blood progenitors engraft and proliferate to high levels in severe combined immunodeficient mice. Blood 83:2489–2497
90. Walev I, Vollmer P, Palmer M, Bhakdi S, Rose-John S (1996) Pore-forming toxins trigger shedding of receptors for interleukin 6 and lipopolysaccharide. Proc Natl Acad Sci U S A 93:7882–7887

91. Ware CB, Horowitz MC, Renshaw BR, Hunt JS, Liggitt D, Koblar SA, Gliniak BC, McKenna HJ, Papayannopoulou T, Thoma B, Cheng L, Donovan PJ, Peschon JJ, Bartlett PF, Willis CR, Wright BD, Carpenter MK, Davison BL, Gearing DP (1995) Targeted disruption of the low-affinity leukemia inhibitory factor receptor gene causes placental, skeletal, neural and metabolic defects and results in perinatal death. Development 121:1283–1299

92. Wells JA (1996) Binding in the growth hormone receptor complex. Proc Natl Acad Sci USA 93:1–6

93. Wells JA (1996) Hematopoietic receptor complexes. Annu Rev Biochem 65: 609–634

94. Wolfsberg TG, White JM (1996) ADAMs in fertilization and development. Dev Biol 180:389–401

95. Wu YY, Bradshaw RA (1996) Induction of neurite outgrowth by interleukin-6 is accompanied by activation of Stat3 signaling pathway in a variant PC12 cell (E2) line. J Biol Chem 271:13023–13032

96. Yamasaki K, Taga T, Hirata Y, Yawata H, Kawanishi Y, Seed B, Taniguchi T, Hirano T, Kishimoto T (1988) Cloning and expression of the human interleukin-6 (BSF-2/IFN beta 2) receptor. Science 241:825–828

97. Yawata H, Yasukawa K, Natsuka S, Murakami M, Yamasaki K, Hibi M, Taga T, Kishimoto T (1993) Structure-function analysis of human IL-6 receptor: dissociation of amino acid residues required for IL-6-binding and for IL-6 signal transduction through gp130. EMBO J 12:1705–1712

98. Yoshida K, Chambers I, Nichols J, Smith A, Saito M, Yasukawa K, Shoyab M, Taga T, Kishimoto T (1994) Maintenance of the pluripotential phenotype of embryonic stem cells through direct activation of gp130 signaling pathways. Mech Dev 45:163–171

99. Yoshida K, Taga T, Saito M, Suematsu S, Kumanogoh A, Tanaka T, Fujiwara H, Hirata M, Yamagami T, Nakahata T, Hirabayashi T, Yoneda Y, Tanaka K, Wang WZ, Mori C, Shiota K, Yoshida N, Kishimoto T (1996) Targeted disruption of gp130, a common signal transducer for the interleukin 6 family of cytokines, leads to myocardial and hematological disorders. Proc Natl Acad Sci USA 93: 407–411

100. Zandstra PW, Conneally E, Piret JM, Eaves CJ (1998) Ontogeny-determined changes in the cytokine responses of primitive human hematopoietic cells. Brit J Haematol 101:770–778

IgE-Mediated Allergen Presentation via FcεRI$\alpha\gamma$ Complexes on Dendritic Antigen-Presenting Cells

D. Maurer and G. Stingl

Introduction

The syndrome of atopy consists of three major symptoms, i.e., allergic rhinoconjunctivitis, allergic asthma, and atopic dermatitis [1], and is usually associated with elevated serum immunoglobulin E (IgE). Whereas the pathogenetic role of allergen-specific IgE is clearly established in the case of allergic rhinoconjunctivitis and allergic asthma, the manifestation of atopic dermatitis cannot be easily explained by the occurrence of type I allergic immune reactions. In fact, the clinical and histopathological picture, as well as the emergence kinetics of atopic eczema, roughly follow the criteria of delayed-type (type IV) immune reactions.

IgE-Binding Structures on Dendritic Cells

First evidence for a possibly causative role of IgE in the pathogenesis of atopic dermatitis (AD) was derived from studies showing that skin from atopic dermatitis patients harbors large numbers of IgE$^+$ dendritic cells (DC) in the epidermis (Langerhans cells, LC) as well as in the dermis (dermal dendritic cells, DDC) [2, 3]. While the epidermis of healthy individuals is devoid of IgE$^+$ DC, the detection of these cells can be regarded as an almost diagnostic finding in AD. Initial attempts to characterize the critical IgE-binding structure on LC suggested that these cells express the low affinity IgE receptor, FcεRII/CD23, in situ [4], and that this receptor is upregulated following exposure of LC to certain cytokines [5]. However, (a) the failure of specific anti-CD23 monoclonal antibodies (mAbs) to entirely block IgE binding to LC [4], (b) the obvious high affinity of this IgE-binding structure, and (c) the fact that LC of both normal and atopic skin are capable of binding IgE [2, 6], prompted the search for IgE-binding moieties other than CD23. Recently, this issue was clarified by the demonstration that epidermal LC and DDC of even healthy persons bind monomeric IgE via the high affinity IgE receptor FcεRI (6–9), previously thought to be exclusively expressed on mast cells and baso-

Symposium in Immunology VIII
Eibl/Huber/Peter/Wahn (Eds.)
© Springer Verlag Berlin Heidelberg 1999

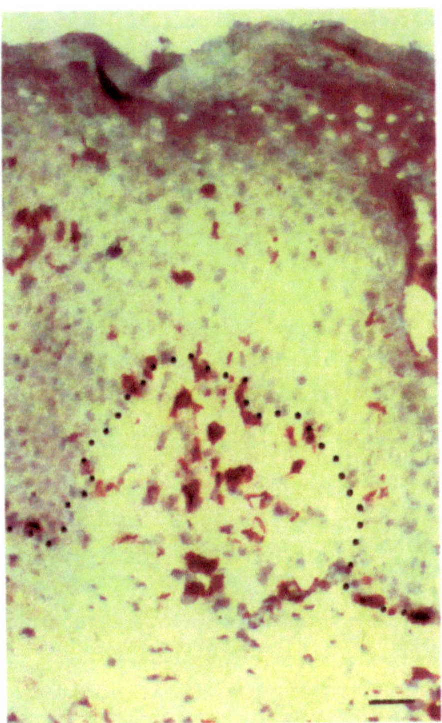

Fig. 1. Anti-FcεRI labeling of dendritic cells in lesional atopic dermatitis skin. The tissue section was incubated with the anti-FcεRIα monoclonal antibody 15-1 and bound antibody revealed using an indirect immunoperoxidase procedure. *Black dots* delineate the dermal–epidermal junction. Scale bar, 30 μm

phils. Our group has now shown that the high affinity IgE receptor FcεRI expressed by epidermal LC and DDC in diseased atopic skin (Fig. 1) is biologically the most relevant cellular IgE-binding structure in this inflammatory atopic tissue reaction [10]. Recent investigations demonstrate that, in addition to basophils, there exists a minor peripheral blood mononuclear cell population capable of binding monomeric IgE via FcεRIb [11]. Further experiments revealed that these FcεRI-expressing cells are peripheral blood DC (PB-DC) based on their immunophenotype [human leukocyte antigen (HLA)-DR^{high}, HLA-DQ^{high}; cluster of differentiation (CD)4$^+$, CD11a$^+$, CD32$^+$, CD33$^+$, B7/2 (CD86)$^+$; CD11b^{low}, CD14^{low}, CD40^{low}, CD54^{low}, CD64^{low}], typical cell morphology, and the capacity to induce primary alloreactive T cell responses [11].

IgE–Binding Structures on Monocytes/Macrophages

Until recently, it was generally believed that monocytes/macrophages express only low affinity IgE binding sites, i.e., the inducible form of the low affinity IgE receptor CD23 [12] and the IgE-binding protein εBP [13]. This led to the assumption that these cell types preferentially bind preformed IgE complexes rather than monomeric IgE. We have recently found that monocytes of atopic individuals and, to a lesser extent, healthy subjects can bind monomeric IgE and that this binding occurs via FcεRI [14]. Pronounced monocyte FcεRI expression was detected in most atopic dermatitis patients (70%–80%) and in a proportion of allergic rhinoconjunctivitis patients (~ 50%). However, this demonstration of FcεRI on monocyte surfaces does not exclude the possibility that, under in vivo conditions, the binding of polyclonal serum IgE to monocytes occurs predominantly via FcεRII or εBP. We have experimentally addressed this issue and found that freshly isolated monocytes of atopics, but not of non-atopics, carry cell surface-bound IgE in vivo and that the majority of IgE-binding sites are occupied by (elevated) serum IgE [15]. The further observation that lactic-acid but not lactose treatment of the cells almost completely removed in vivo-bound IgE molecules argued against a possible role of εBP in this process, but did not exclude an important role for CD23 as a relevant IgE-binding molecule in vivo. For this purpose, we exposed lactic acid-treated monocytes to sera from birch pollen-sensitized individuals, either in the presence or absence of inhibiting mAbs to FcεRI or CD23, and visualized the binding of birch pollen-specific serum IgE by a subsequent incubation step with biotinylated recombinant Bet *v* I, the major birch pollen allergen. Selectively, the mAb to FcεRI abolished the binding of polyclonal serum IgE to monocyte surfaces [15]. These results indicate that, in analogy to LC, monocytes of allergic individuals carry FcεRI-bound, allergen-specific IgE in vivo and that the interaction with polyvalent allergen is followed by the triggering of FcεRI rather than CD23.

Structural Analysis of FcεRI on APC

On basophils and mast cells, FcεRI is expressed as a tetrameric holoreceptor composed of one α-chain, one β-chain and one γ-chain homodimer [16]. Molecular and biochemical studies revealed that DC [11] and monocytes of atopic persons [14] co-express the IgE-binding FcεRIα and the signal transducing FcεRIγ chains both at the mRNA and protein level and that FcεRIα and FcεRIγ chains expressed by these cells are physically associated and thereby form functional FcεRIαγ$_2$ complexes [11]. In fact, transfection experiments have shown that this chain composition suffices for functional cell surface expression of the human but not of the murine receptor [19, 20]). The COOH-terminal intracytoplasmic portion of the β-chain has been found to contain a conserved protein sequence motif (immunoreceptor tyrosine-based activation motif, ITAM) [19] which allows the physical associa-

Table 1. Structure and cellular distribution of FcεRI in humans and genetically modified mice. (Adapted from Dombrowicz et al. [22])

	Mice	Humans	FcεRIαβγ$_2$ mice	FcεRIαγ$_2$ mice
Mast cells	αβγ$_2$	αβγ$_2$	αβγ$_2$	αγ$_2$
Basophils	αβγ$_2$	αβγ$_2$	αβγ$_2$	αγ$_2$
Dendritic cells	–	αγ$_2$	αγ$_2$	αγ$_2$
Monocytes	–	αγ$_2$	αγ$_2$	αγ$_2$

tion with members of the src protein tyrosine kinase (PTK) family. Recent findings re-emphasize the functional importance of the β subunit by showing that the constitutively β-associated PTK lyn is crucial for phosphorylation and activation of the FcεRIγ subunit. FcεRIγ thus modified can then activate the PTK syk and initiate further downstream signaling events, i.e., the phosphorylation and activation of phospholipase $C_{\gamma 1}$, the breakdown of phosphoinositols, and the elevation of the cytosolic calcium concentration [20]. Despite the apparent lack of β, FcεRI on APC is capable of mediating PTK activation [21] and calcium mobilization [14, 21], indicative of competent signaling via this receptor. Thus, it is tempting to speculate about the presence of a putative β-like structure that functionally substitutes for the "classical" FcεRIβ chain in APC.

That DC can express FcεRIαγ$_2$ rather than FcεRIαβγ$_2$ complexes has been convincingly reproduced in transgenic/knock-out mouse models [22]. While DC from wild-type and FcεRIβ$^{-/-}$ mice fail to express endogenous FcεRI on their surface, DC from mice transgenic for human (hu) FcεRIα under control of the huFcεRIα promoter and bred onto either a murine (mu) FcεRIα$^{-/-}$FcεRIβ$^{+/+}$ or a muFcεRIα$^{-/-}$FcεRIβ$^{-/-}$ background express FcεRI and display this receptor in the αγ$_2$ but not αβγ$_2$ configuration. As to be expected, mast cells from huFcεRIα transgenic, muFcεRIα$^{-/-}$FcεRIβ$^{+/+}$ animals express FcεRI as an αβγ$_2$ complex (Table 1). Furthermore, these findings indicate that the promoter region of the huFcεRIα gene, but not of the muFcεRIα gene, contains sequences necessary for FcεRIα transcription in DC.

Biological Consequences of Allergen-IgE Binding to FcεRI on APC

The binding of allergen-specific IgE to FcεRI on mast cells and basophils, followed by bridging of the membrane-bound IgE molecules by soluble, multivalent allergens results in cellular degranulation and, consequently, in the release of proinflammatory substances such as histamine, serotonin, prostaglandins, and leukotrienes, as well as in the synthesis and secretion of cyto-kines such as interleukin (IL)-3, IL-4, IL-5, IL-6, granulocyte-macrophage colony-stimulating factor (GM-CSF), and interferon-γ (IFN-γ) [23]. The fact that FcεRI on APC constitutes a functional cell-surface receptor and that APC are potent producers of cytokines [24–28] and eicosanoids [29, 30] makes it likely that FcεRI-induced release of biological effector molecules by APC occurs and, moreover, critically modulates, or even initiates, allergic inflammatory responses in allergen-exposed tissues.

We recently found that, besides its putative cytokine-inducing properties, FcεRI on professional APC functions as an allergen-focusing receptor struc-ture. Using sera from grass- or birch pollen-sensitized donors and recombi-nant birch (rBet *v* 1) and grass pollen (rPhl *p* 2) allergens, as well as hapten (hydroxy-nitrophenacetyl, NP)-specific, monomeric IgE (cIgE) and NP-con-jugated allergens, we observed that the presence of cell surface-bound IgE

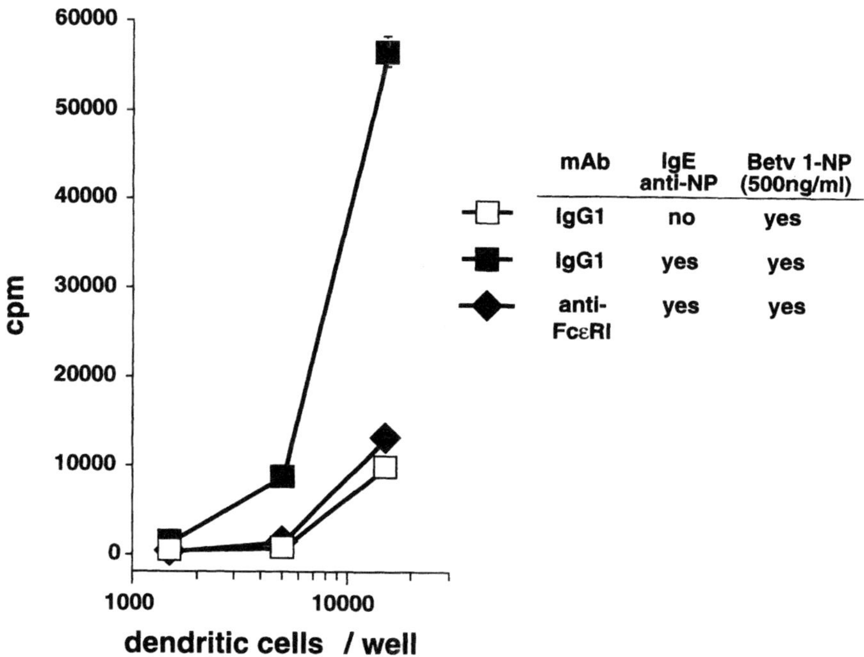

Fig. 2. Dendritic cells (DC) use FcεRI to present allergen to major histocompatibility complex (MHC) class II-restricted T cells in an immunoglobulin (Ig)E-dependent manner. Indicated numbers of peripheral blood DC were reacted with IgG1 (*open squares*), IgG1 plus hydroxy-nitrophenacetyl (*NP*)-specific monomeric IgE (*cIgE*) (*closed squares*), or monoclonal antibody 15-1 (anti-FcεRIα) plus NP-specific cIgE (*diamonds*) followed by the addition of 500 ng/ml NP-conjugated rBet *v* 1. T cells of T cell clone WD24 were added as responders and (³H)-thymidine uptake was meas-ured (*cpm*, ordinate)

results in efficient allergen binding to APC of atopics [15]. MAb-blocking experiments revealed that FcεRI, rather than FcεRII, is the pivotal moiety that mediates this event. Even more importantly, cIgE-mediated allergen binding to APC of atopic persons resulted in a 100–1000-fold amplification of rBet *v* 1 or rPhl *p* 2 presentation to autologous T cell clones (TCCs) with peptide specificities for Bet *v* 1 or Phl *p* 2 [11, 15]. The addition of the anti-FcεRIα-chain mAb, but not of an anti-CD23 mAb, reduced this cIgE-enhanced, allergen-specific TCC response to levels seen in the absence of cIgE (Fig. 2). This demonstrates that FcεRI, but not FcεRII, mediates IgE-dependent allergen uptake, processing, and presentation by professional APC from atopics.

Antigen Targeting by FcεRI on DC

Selective antigen targeting may profoundly affect the occurrence, quantity, and perhaps also the quality of antigen-specific T-cell responses. Antigen-uptake receptors known so far include lectin receptors, e.g., the macrophage mannose receptor and DEC-205, as well as members of the Ig supergene family, i.e., the B-cell receptor, FcγRI, FcγRII, ILT3, and FcεRI [31]. Recently, we demonstrated that FcεRI-bound IgE, after polyvalent but not monovalent ligation, is efficiently internalized into acidic, proteolytic compartments, degraded, and delivered into organelles containing major histocompatibility complex (MHC) class II, HLA-DM, and lysosomal proteins [peptide loading compartments termed MIICs (MHC class II compartments)] [32] (Fig. 3a,b). To follow the fate of the fragmented ligand, we sought to interfere with invariant chain (li) degradation, a process critical for peptide loading of nascent MHC class II molecules. We found DC to express cathepsin (Cat) S, a cysteine protease involved in li processing by B cells. Exposure of DC to a specific, active-site inhibitor of Cat S resulted in the loss of anti-Cat S immunoreactivity, led to the appearance of a N-terminal li remnant, and decreased the export of newly synthesized MHC class II to the DC surface. Furthermore, inactivation of Cat S, as well as blockade of protein neo-synthesis by cyclocloheximide, strongly reduced IgE/FcεRI-mediated antigen presentation by DC. Thus, multimeric ligands of FcεRI, instead of being delivered into a recycling MHC class II pathway, are efficiently channeled into lysosomal, MIIC-like compartments of DC where Cat S-dependent li processing and peptide loading of newly synthesized MHC class II molecules occurs. This IgE/FcεRI-dependent signaling pathway in DC may be a particularly effective route for immunization and a promising target for interfering with the early steps of allergen presentation.

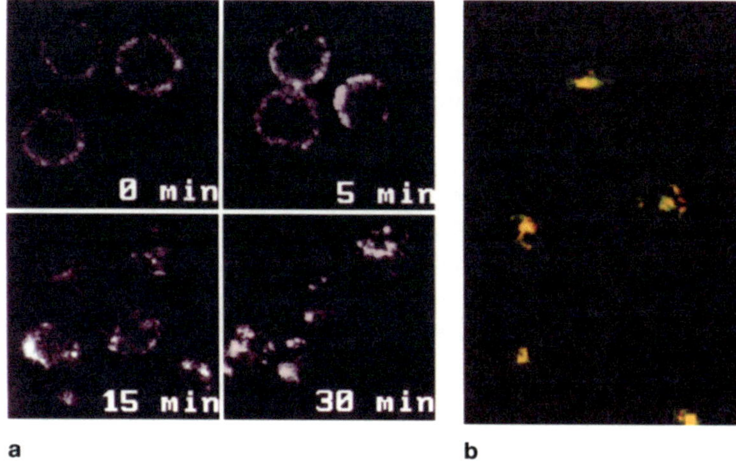

Fig. 3a. Immunoglobulin (Ig) E-FcεRI complexes are efficiently internalized and progressively accumulate in distinctive cytosolic dendritic cell (DC) compartments. Purified DC were mounted onto slides and subjected to IgE-tetramethylrhodamine isothiocyanate (TRITC)-labeling and FcεRI crosslinking. Cells were either fixed immediately after the labeling procedure or incubated at 37 °C for the indicated periods prior to fixation and analysis by confocal laser scanning microscopy. IgE-FcεRI complexes display pronounced patching, capping, and partial internalization at 5 min and, thereafter, are transported to certain distinctive cytosolic DC organelles which occur in a perinuclear location, as well as adjacent to the cell membrane. Little or no fluorescent material remained on the cell surface. **b** FcεRI delivers ligands into major histocompatibility complex class II compartment (MIIC)-like vesicles of DC. Purified DC were mounted onto glass slides and FcεRI-bound IgE was crosslinked with TRITC-labeled secondary antibodies. After 40 min at 37 °C, DC were permeabilized and exposed to fluorescein isothiocyanate (FITC)-labeled monoclonal antibodies recognizing human leukocyte antigen class II β-chain. To demonstrate the relative positional distribution of the material internalized via FcεRI (TRITC, *red*)- and of FITC (*green*)-labeled major histocompatibility complex (MHC) class II, the images collected in the two channels were merged. The (sub)cellular areas where the TRITC and the FITC fluorescence is co-localized appear in *yellow*. As visualized, the intracellular vesicles which are accessible for IgE-/FcεRI complexes stain for MHC class II antigens (**b**) and are HLA-DM- and lysosome-associated membrane protein (LAMP)-2-positive (not shown)

In vivo Relevance of Allergen-IgE Binding to FcεRI on APC

With regard to IgE-mediated cutaneous allergy, these findings may be of pathogenetic significance for delayed-type atopic inflammation occurring in the skin and, perhaps, also in other tissues. If repeated allergenic exposure of skin and/or mucosal tissue results in the production of allergen-specific IgE, the interaction of allergen with IgE bound to FcεRI on skin APC may result in: (a) IgE-facilitated allergen presentation to T cells in lymphoid and non-lymphoid organs and, furthermore, in (b) allergen/IgE-dependent activation and cytokine secretion by FcεRI-expressing cells within the tissue.

This may not only be true for exogenous allergens. Very recently, Valenta et al. [33] showed that atopic individuals, particularly those suffering from severe atopic dermatitis, frequently exhibit IgE responses to human proteins expressed in histogenetically different cell types. It is quite conceivable that presentation of these IgE-reactive human proteins by FcεRI$^+$ APC will result in a continuously growing and widening autoallergenic immune response. In fact, it is tempting to speculate that this autoallergic sensitization may account for the chronicity of the atopic tissue reaction, even in the absence of exogenous allergen.

In particular, monocytic cells secrete IL-1 and TNF-α following crosslinking of cell surface-bound IgE moieties in vitro [28]. These two cytokines have been shown to play an indispensable role in the elicitation of cutaneous late-phase atopic reactions [34, 35]. IL-1 and TNF-α exert some of their biological effects via induction of E-selectin, VCAM-1, and ICAM-1 expression by endothelial cells (EC) [34, 36]. Upregulated EC adhesion molecules promote and reinforce leukocyte-EC interactions and, therefore, are a prerequisite for transmigration of inflammatory cells into inflamed tissue [37]. In delayed-type atopic reactions, the latter event is characterized by the extravasation of (Fc-IgE receptor-bearing) eosinophils and macrophages, as well as by a pronounced accumulation of T lymphocytes [3] (Fig. 4). At this particular step, IgE-amplified allergen presentation by FcεRI-expressing skin APC may decisively control the quality and quantity of allergic tissue inflammation. Even in the presence of minute allergen concentrations, this mechanism may allow effective activation and clonal expansion of skin-infiltrating allergen-specific T helper cells with a Th2-like cytokine secretion pattern [38–40] and with the capacity of mediating (IL-4-dependent) allergic tissue reactions [41]. Moreover, activated allergen-specific Th2-like cells should possess the ability to promote B cells to secrete allergen-specific IgE which again binds to FcεRI-expressing APC in skin and other tissues. If this allergen-driven, self-amplifying mechanism is operative in atopic diseases in vivo, therapeutic strategies should aim to interrupt this vicious circle by interference with: (a) FcεRI expression, (b) IgE binding to FcεRI, and/or (c) FcεRI-mediated signal transduction and antigen processing mechanisms by APC.

Acknowledgments. This work was supported, in part, by grants from the Austrian Science Foundation (S06702-MED) and from the Novartis Research Institute, Vienna, Austria.

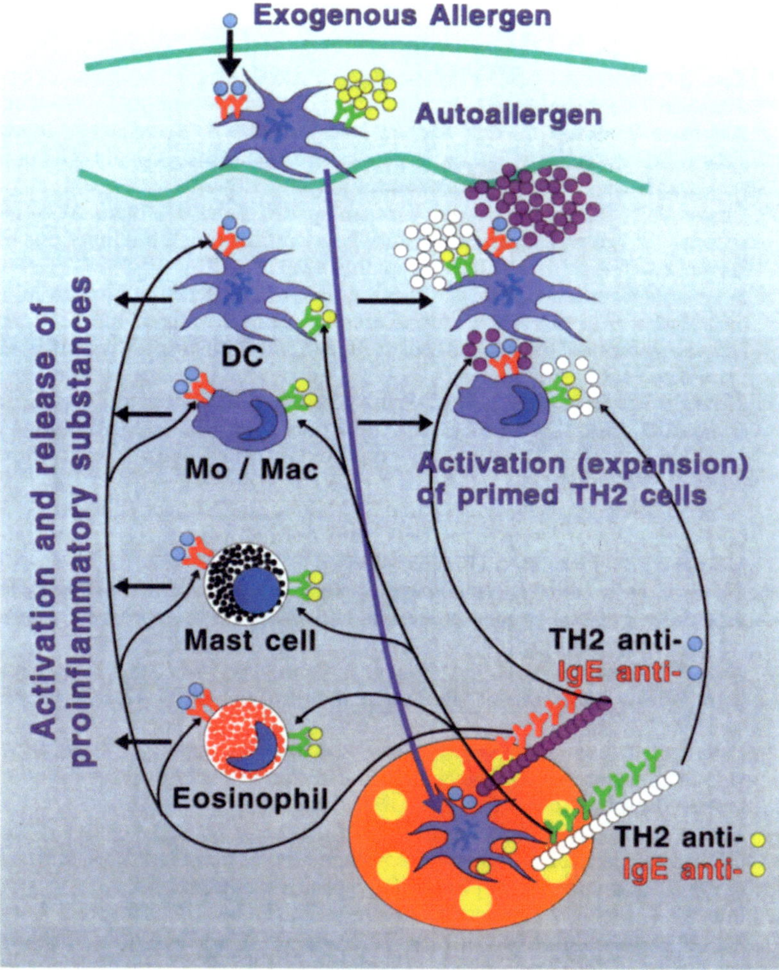

Fig. 4. The pathogenetic mechanisms operative in cutaneous delayed-type atopic inflammation. Repeated allergen exposure and genetic factors are implicated in the preferential expansion of allergen-specific Th0 cells and in their conversion into Th2-like cells. As a consequence, allergen-specific B-cells differentiate into plasma cells that produce allergen-specific immunoglobulin E (*IgE*). Upon allergen reexposure, IgE-bound skin antigen-presenting cells (Langerhans cells and dermal dendritic cells) may be directly activated by allergen-mediated crosslinking of their high affinity IgE receptors (FcεRI). This may be followed by the induction of cytokine production and secretion and, as a consequence, may result in increased expression of adhesion molecules on dermal endothelial cells and, consequently, in the influx of eosinophils and T cells. On the other hand, even in the presence of minute allergen concentrations, FcεRI-mediated amplification of allergen presentation may result in the efficient activation of allergen-specific Th2 cells which cause allergic tissue inflammation due to cytokine release. *Mo/Mac*, monocytes/macrophages; *DC*, dendritic cells

References

1. Coca RF, Cooke RA (1923) On the classification of the phenomena of hypersensitivities. J Immunol 8:163–182
2. Bruynzeel-Koomen C, van Wichen DF, Toonstra J, Berrens L, Bruynzeel PL (1986) The presence of IgE molecules on epidermal Langerhans cells in patients with atopic dermatitis. Arch Dermatol Res 278:199–204
3. Leung DYM, Schneeberger EE, Siraganian RP, Geha RS, Bhan AK (1987) The presence of IgE on monocytes/macrophages infiltrating the skin lesions of atopic dermatits. Clin Immunol Immunopathol 42:328–337
4. Bruynzeel-Koomen C, van der Donk EMM, Bruynzeel PLB, Capron M, de Gast GC, Mudde G (1988) Associated expression of CD1 antigen and Fc receptor for IgE on epidermal Langerhans cells from patients with atopic dermatitis. Clin Exp Immunol 74:137–142
5. Bieber T, Rieger A, Neuchrist C, Prinz JC, Rieber EP, Boltz-Nitulescu G, Scheiner O, Kraft D, Ring J, Stingl G (1989) Induction of FcεRII/CD23 on human epidermal Langerhans cells by human recombinant interleukin 4 and γ interferon. J Exp Med 170:309–314
6. Wang B, Rieger A, Kilgus O, Ochiai K, Maurer D, Födinger D, Kinet JP, Stingl G (1992) Epidermal Langerhans cells from normal human skin bind monomeric IgE via FcεRI. J Exp Med 175:1353–1365
7. Bieber T, de la Salle H, Wollenberg A, Hakimi J, Chizzonite R, Ring J, Hanau D, de la Salle C (1992) Human epidermal Langerhans cells express the high-affinity receptor for immunoglobulin E (FcεRI). J Exp Med 175:1285–1290
8. Haas N, Hamann K, Grabbe J, Cremer B, Czarnetzki BM (1992) Expression of the high affinity IgE-receptor on human Langerhans cells. Acta Derm Venereol (Stockh) 72:271–272
9. Osterhoff B, Rappersberger C, Wang B, Koszik F, Ochiai K, Kinet JP, Stingl G (1994) Immunomorphological characterization of FcεRI-bearing cells within the human dermis. J Invest Dermatol 102:315–320
10. Klubal R, Osterhoff B, Wang B, Kinet JP, Maurer D, Stingl G (1997) The high-affinity receptor for IgE is the predominant IgE-binding structure in lesional skin of atopic dermatitis skin. J Invest Dermatol 108:336–342
11. Maurer D, Fiebiger E, Ebner C, Reininger B, Fischer GF, Wichlas S, Jouvin MH, Schmitt-Egenolf M, Kraft D, Kinet JP, Stingl G (1996) Peripheral blood dendritic cells express FcεRI as a complex composed of FcεRIα- and FcεRIγ-chains and can use this receptor for IgE-mediated allergen presentation. J Immunol 157:607–616
12. Dessaint JP, Capron A (1990) Fcε receptor II-positive macrophages and platelets: potent effector cells in allergy and defense against helminth parasites. Semin Immunopathol 12:349–363
13. Liu FT, Frigeri LT, Gritzmacher CA, Hsu DK, Robertson MW, Zuberi RI (1993) Expression and function of an IgE-binding animal lectin (εBP) in mast cells. Immunopharmacol 26:187–195
14. Maurer D, Fiebiger E, Reininger B, Wolff-Winiski B, Jouvin M-H, Kilgus O, Kinet J-P, Stingl G (1994) Expression of functional high affinity IgE receptors (FcεRI) on monocytes of atopic individuals. J Exp Med 179:745–750
15. Maurer D, Ebner C, Reininger B, Fiebiger E, Kraft D, Kinet JP, Stingl G (1995) The high affinity IgE receptor FcεRI mediates IgE-mediated allergen presentation. J Immunol 154:6285–6290
16. Ravetch JV, Kinet J-P (1991) Fc receptors. Annu Rev Immunol 9:547–592

17. Alber G, Miller L, Jelsema C, Varin-Blank N, Metzger H (1991) Structure/function relationships of the mast cell high-affinity receptor for IgE (FcεRI). J Biol Chem 266:22613–22620
18. Mao SY, Alber G, Rivera J, Kochan J, Metzger H (1992) Interaction of aggregated native and mutant IgE receptors with the cytoskeleton. Proc Natl Acad Sci USA 89:222–226
19. Reth M (1989) Antigen receptor tail clue. Nature 338:383–384
20. Jouvin MHE, Adamczewski M, Numerof R, Letourneur O, Valle A, Kinet JP (1994) Differential control of the tyrosine kinases lyn and syk by the two signaling chains of the high affinity immunoglobulin E receptor. J Biol Chem 269: 5918–5925
21. Bieber T (1994) FcεRI on human Langerhans cells: a receptor in search of new functions. Immunol Today 15:52–53
22. Dombrowicz D, Lin S, Flamand V, Brini AT, Koller BH, Kinet JP (1998) Allergy-associated FcRβ is a molecular amplifier of IgE- and IgG-mediated in vivo responses. Immunity 8:517–529
23. Costa JJ, Weller PF, Galli SJ (1997) The cells of the allergic response: mast cells, basophils, and eosinophils. JAMA 278:1815–1822
24. Heufler C, Topar G, Koch F, Trockenbacher B, Kämpgen E, Romani N, Schuler G (1992) Cytokine gene expression in murine epidermal cell suspensions: interleukin 1β and macrophage inflammatory protein 1α are selectively expressed in Langerhans cells but are differently regulated in culture. J Exp Med 176:1221–1226
25. Matsue H, Cruz PD Jr, Bergstresser PR (1992) Langerhans cells are the major source of mRNA for IL-1β and MIP-1α among unstimulated mouse epidermal cells. J Invest Dermatol 99:537–541
26. Schreiber S, Kilgus O, Payer E, Kutil R, Elbe A, Müller C, Stingl G (1992) Cytokine pattern of Langerhans cells isolated from murine epidermal cell cultures. J Immunol 149:3524–3534
27. Nathan CF (1987) Secretory products of macrophages. J Clin Invest 79:319–326
28. Borish L, Mascali JJ, Rosenwasser LJ (1991) IgE-dependent cytokine production by human peripheral blood mononuclear phagocytes. J Immunol 146:63–67
29. Ferreri NR, Howland WC, Spiegelberg HL (1986) Release of leukotrienes C4 and B4 and prostaglandin E2 from human monocytes stimulated with aggregated IgG, IgA, and IgE. J Immunol 136:4188–4193
30. Rankin JA, Hitchcock M, Marrill WW, Bach MK, Brashler JR, Askenase PW (1982) IgE-dependent release of leukotriene C4 from alveolar macrophages. Nature 297:329–331
31. Lanzavecchia A (1996) Mechanisms of antigen uptake for presentation. Curr Opin Immunol 8:348–354
32. Maurer D, Fiebiger E, Reininger B, Ebner C, Petzelbauer P, Shi GP, Chapman HA, Stingl G (1998) FcεRI on dendritic cells delivers IgE-bound multivalent antigens into a cathepsin S-dependent pathway of MHC class II presentation. J Immunol 161:2731–2739
33. Valenta R, Maurer D, Steiner R, Seiberler S, Sperr WR, Valent P, Spitzauer S, Kapiotis S, Smolen J, Stingl G (1996) Immunoglobulin E response to human proteins in atopic patients. J Invest Dermatol 107:203–208
34. Leung DYM, Pober JS, Cotran RS (1991) Expression of endothelial leukocyte adhesion molecule-1 (ELAM-1) in elicited late phase allergic reactions. J Clin Invest 87:1805–1809
35. Mullarkey MF, Leiferman KM, Peters MS, Caro I, Roux ER, Hanna RK, Rubin AS, Jacobs CA (1994) Human cutaneous allergic late-phase response is inhibited by soluble IL-1 receptor. J Immunol 152:2033–2041

36. Petzelbauer P, Bender J, Wilson J, Pober JS (1993) Heterogeneity of dermal microvascular endothelial cell antigen expression and cytokine responsiveness in situ and in cell culture. J Immunol 151:5062–5072
37. Springer, TA (1994) Traffic signals for lymphocyte recirculation and leukocyte emigration: the multistep paradigm. Cell 76:301–314
38. Van der Heijden FC, Wierenga EA, Bos JD, Kapsenberg JL (1991) High frequency of IL-4 producing CD4$^+$ allergen-specific T lymphocytes in atopic dermatitis lesional skin. J Invest Dermatol 97:389–394
39. Kay AB, Ying S, Varney V, Gaga M, Durham SR, Moqbel R, Wardlaw AJ, Hamid Q (1991) Messenger RNA expression of the cytokine gene cluster, interleukin 3 (IL-3), IL-4, IL-5, and granulocyte/macrophage colony-stimulating factor, in allergen-induced late-phase cutaneous reactions in atopic subjects. J Exp Med 173:775–778
40. Hamid Q, Boguniewicz M, Leung DYM (1994) Differential in situ gene expression in acute versus chronic atopic dermatitis. J Clin Invest 94:870–876
41. Müller KM, Jaunin F, Masouyé J, Saurat J-H, Hauser C (1993) Th2 cells mediate IL-4-dependent local tissue inflammation. J Immunol 150:5576–5584

Anti-Inflammatory Effects of Intravenous Immunoglobulin

Y. Bar-Dayan, S. V. Kaveri, Y. Bar-Dayan, A. Pashov, Y. Shoenfeld, and M. D. Kazatchkine

Intravenous immunoglobulin (IVIg) is a therapeutic preparation of normal human polyspecific immunoglobulin (Ig) G obtained from pooled plasma of a large number of healthy donors.

Currently available IVIg preparations contain intact IgG molecules with a distribution of IgG subclasses that corresponds to that of normal serum. The half-life of infused IVIg in the immunocompetent host is 3 weeks, except for the IgG3 component that exhibits a shorter half-life of approximately 1 week. Most preparations of IVIg contain traces of IgA and trace amounts of IgM, $F(ab')_2$ fragments of IgG, soluble CD4, CD8, human leukocyte antigen (HLA) molecules (Blasczyk et al., 1993) and transforming growth factor (TGF)-β (Tekow et al., 1998).

The use of IVIg was initially restricted to the substitutive therapy of patients with primary and secondary Ig deficiencies. In the early 1980s, IVIg was first reported to increase platelet counts in children with immune thrombocytopenia associated with the Wiskott-Aldrich syndrome and in acute idiopathic thrombocytopenic purpura of childhood (Schmidt et al., 1981). In the last 10 years, IVIg has increasingly been used in the treatment of a variety of autoimmune and systemic inflammatory conditions (Dwyer, 1992). Available clinical and experimental evidence suggests that a wide spectrum of immune-mediated conditions may benefit from IVIg, including acute and chronic/relapsing diseases, autoimmune diseases mediated by pathogenic autoantibodies or by autoaggressive T-cells and systemic inflammatory disorders. The immunoregulatory and anti-inflammatory effects of IVIg are partly mediated by the ability of the Fc portion of IgG to interact with Fcγ receptors on phagocytes and lymphocytes, as well as with complement proteins in plasma. The immunomodulatory properties of IVIg are also largely dependent on the broad diversity of variable regions and antibody reactivities present in therapeutic pools as these originate from plasma of high numbers of healthy donors (Kazatchkine et al., 1994). The distinction between Fc- and variable region-dependent mechanisms of action of IVIg remains, however, somehow artificial in that immunoregulatory functions of IVIg are often amplified, or indeed made possible, by the cooperative Fc binding to Fc receptors on cells targeted by the relevant variable regions of IgG.

Symposium in Immunology VIII
Eibl/Huber/Peter/Wahn (Eds.)
© Springer Verlag Berlin Heidelberg 1999

The list of disorders reportedly responding to IVIg now includes a wide spectrum of diseases including autoimmune cytopenias (Blanchette et al., 1994; Imbach et al., 1981; Lalezari et al., 1986; McGuire et al., 1987; McIntyre et al., 1985; Oda et al., 1985), anti-Factor VIII autoimmune disease (Sultan et al., 1984), Kawasaki syndrome (Shulman, 1992), the acute Guillain-Barré syndrome (Hughes, 1997; van der Meché et al., 1992), myasthenia gravis (Gajdos et al., 1997; Gajdos et al., 1984), chronic inflammatory demyelinating polyneuropathy (Hahn et al., 1995), dermatomyositis (Dalakas et al., 1993), antineutrophil cytoplasmic antigen (ANCA)-associated systemic vasculitis (Jayne et al., 1991) and autoimmune uveitis (LeHoang et al., 1998). Preliminary data suggest that IVIg reduces the incidence of acute exacerbations in patients with chronic relapsing multiple sclerosis (Achiron et al., 1996; Fazekas et al., 1997). Recently, the use of IVIg has been suggested in chronic inflammatory conditions with the aim of reducing the need for systemic steroids (Gelfand et al., 1994).

The regimen of IVIg initially proven to be efficacious for the treatment of acute immune thrombocytopenic purpura (ITP), i.e. 0.4 g/kg body weight per day given over 5 consecutive days, has been used in most instances for the treatment of autoimmune diseases. More recently, alternative schedules of administration, e.g. 0.8–1.0 g/kg body weight per day over 2 consecutive days have been used, as suggested by the results of a controlled trial conducted in Kawasaki disease (Newburger et al., 1986).

Proposed mechanisms of action of IVIg are summarized in Table 1 (for review, see Mouthon et al., 1996). Several of these mechanisms may account

Table 1. Proposed mechanisms of action of IVIg in autoimmune and inflammatory disorders

---

Fc receptor blockade

Anti-inflammatory effects:
    Attenuation of complement-mediated tissue damage
    Alteration of the structure and solubility of immune complexes
    Induction of anti-inflammatory cytokines
    Decreased production of pro-inflammatory cytokines
    Neutralization of microbial toxins
    Modulation of expression of adhesion molecules and chemokines

Neutralization of pathogenic autoantibodies by anti-idiotypes

Neutralization of superantigens

V-region and Fc-dependent selection of immune repertoires:
    Control of emergent repertoires of bone marrow B-cells and thymocytes
    Modulation of immunoglobulin production and long-term modifications in antibody repertoires
    Modulation of cytokine production by monocytes and T-cells
    Regulation of expansion and activation of lymphocyte subsets

---

for the potent anti-inflammatory effects of IVIg that have been documented in conditions such as Kawasaki syndrome, dermatomyositis and juvenile rheumatoid arthritis. In the latter conditions, the infusion of IVIg is rapidly followed by a decrease in body temperature, sedimentation rate and in the concentration of acute phase proteins in plasma. The following chapter will summarize the current knowledge of the mechanisms by which IVIg exerts its anti-inflammatory effects. The anti-inflammatory effects of IVIg include its ability to neutralize microbial toxins, interfere with complement-mediated damage, alter the inflammatory potential of soluble immune complexes, modulate the production of pro-and anti-inflammatory cytokines and of chemokines, and the expression of adhesion molecules.

Neutralization of Microbial Toxins and Superantigens

There is evidence that IVIg exerts part of its beneficial effects in the control of the inflammatory response by neutralizing bacterial toxins (Abe et al., 1993). IVIg has been reported to be beneficial in the treatment of patients with diseases related to cytotoxin-producing pathogens, such as Kawasaki disease, the hemolytic uremic syndrome, the Guillain-Barré syndrome, chronic inflammatory demyelinating polyradiculopathy and multifocal motor neuropathy.

Inhibition by IVIg of superantigen-elicited T-cell activation was first demonstrated in the case of staphylococcal toxin superantigens that are targets for specific anti-superantigen antibodies in IVIg (Takei et al., 1993). Interleukin (IL)-2 production in response to staphylococcal enterotoxin B was also shown to be inhibited by IVIg (Takei et al., 1993). We then observed that the presence of IVIg in cultures of normal peripheral blood mononuclear cells (PBMC) stimulated with staphylococcal enterotoxin B (SEB) superantigen resulted in the rescue from apoptosis of CD3 blast cells expressing the Vβ markers of the subfamilies of T-cells which expand in the presence of SEB (Baudet et al., 1996).

Early treatment of patients with Kawasaki syndrome reduces the clinical and laboratory features of inflammation, the prevalence of coronary artery disease and protects against the formation of coronary artery aneurysms (Furusho et al., 1984; Newburger et al., 1986). One of the possible mechanisms of action of IVIg in acute Kawasaki syndrome is the neutralization of a causative microbe or toxin that results in the massive immune stimulation that characterizes the syndrome. IVIg contains high concentrations of antibodies that inhibit the T-cell response to eight different staphylococcal superantigens.

Shiga toxin (produced by Shigella disenteria 1) and SLT-1 toxin (produced by *Escherichia coli* serotype 026:H11) are considered as candidate pathogens in the primary hemolytic uremic syndrome (HUS). IVIg contains anti-toxin neutralizing antibodies, whereas the sera of healthy children do not contain such antibody activity, suggesting that IVIg may have a therapeutic role in the early stages of HUS (Ashkenazi et al., 1988). Anti-GM1 autoantibody has been claimed to be involved in some patients with the Guillain-Barré syndrome and chronic inflammatory demyelinating polyradiculopathy and is clearly associated with multifocal motor neuropathy (Yuki et al., 1995). IVIg inhibits the binding of cholera toxin to GM1 in vitro in a dose-dependent manner (Yuki et al., 1995). This effect is mediated by the $F(ab')_2$ portion of IVIg, suggesting that the binding of IVIg to GM1 or cholera toxin may neutralize the pathogenic antibodies.

Attenuation of Complement-Mediated Tissue Damage

IVIg interferes with activation and effector functions of the complement system (Table 2). Evidence for the role of IVIg in modulating the complement system was obtained in animal models of complement-mediated pathology, assays of complement uptake in vitro and studies of tissue biopsies of patients with complement-mediated diseases treated with IVIg (Basta, 1996; Basta and Dalakas, 1994).

Animal studies in vivo have demonstrated that IVIg specifically suppresses the complement-dependent hepatic clearance of IgM-sensitized guinea pig erythrocytes (Basta et al., 1989). In the model of anti-Forssman antibody-mediated shock in guinea pigs, rabbit IgG antibodies to endothelial cells induce acute complement mediated tissue damage and a lethal shock. IVIg was shown to prevent pulmonary endothelial cell lesions in 75% of treated animals, increase the median duration of survival five-fold and prevent mortality in 38% of the animals (Basta et al., 1989). In addition, the administration of IVIg in a guinea pig to rat model of cardiac xenograft-

Table 2. Inhibition of complement-mediated damage by IVIg

IVIg	binds newly generated C3b and C4b, thus reducing complement deposition and the subsequent formation of the cytolytic C5b-9 terminal complex in target tissues
IVIg	competes with serum IgG for the binding of C1q
IVIg	increases the rate of inactivation of C3b in immune complexes, thus preventing the formation of an immune complex-bound amplification of C3 convertase

ing effectively delays complement-mediated hyper-acute rejection. The latter effect is mediated by the variable regions of IVIg and correlates with complement-inhibitory activity in the IVIg preparation (Latremouille et al., 1997).

In vitro experiments demonstrated that IVIg inhibits the uptake of newly generated C3b and C4b on IgG- and IgM-coated surfaces (Basta et al., 1989). The latter observations have led to the suggestion that IVIg acts as an acceptor (chelator) for activated complement components C3b and C4b, thus preventing their binding to and accumulation in target tissues. The effects of IVIg on complement also include its capacity to competitively bind C1q, deviating C1 from binding to plasma IgG and immune complexes (Mollnes et al., 1995), and its ability to accelerate Factor I-dependent inactivation of C3b bound to immune complexes (Lutz et al., 1996). The latter mechanism may be important in preventing amplification of complement activation to occur on immune complexes, whether in the circulation or deposited in tissues.

Evidence for an effect of IVIg on complement in vivo came from the study of patients with steroid-resistant dermatomyositis (Basta and Dalakas, 1994; Dalakas et al., 1993). Patients with active dermatomyositis exhibited high baseline C3 uptake in vitro, which was decreased significantly in patients after treatment with IVIg. Serum levels of the terminal SC5b-9 complex were high at baseline and normalized after IVIg therapy. Muscle biopsies of patients treated with IVIg showed the disappearance of, or a significant decrease in, the amount of C3b and C5b-9 antigens deposited in endothelial capillaries, in association with a restoration of the capillary network (Basta and Dalakas, 1994).

The capacity of normal immunoglobulin to inhibit C3 and C4 uptake by immune complexes is not restricted to IgG. On a molar basis, monomeric serum IgA and IgM were shown to be more active than IgG in inhibiting complement activation (Miletic et al., 1996).

Changes in Structure and Solubility of Immune Complexes

By altering the amount and form of C3 and C4 bound to IgG in immune complexes, IVIg may change immune complex size and composition. IVIg further alters immune complexes by allowing free valences of complexed antigen or antibody to bind antibody molecules in IVIg (e.g. anti-idiotypic antibodies). IVIg is thus capable of modifying the structure, molecular weight, composition and phlogistic potential of immune complexes (Tomino et al., 1984). Hence, the addition of IVIg to renal biopsy material from patients with immune complex-mediated glomerulonephritis resulted in decreased amounts of IgG being deposited in glomeruli (Sato et al., 1986). Similarly, the incubation of IVIg with tissue samples obtained from patients with extra-thyroidal manifestations of Grave's disease resulted in complete disappearance of IgG and C3 deposition as a result of a change in the solubility of the immune complexes induced by IVIg (Antonelli et al., 1996).

Modulation of Production of Cytokines

An important mechanism by which IVIg exerts anti-inflammatory effects is dependent on its ability to modulate the production, release and function of pro-inflammatory cytokines (Abe et al., 1994; Andersson et al., 1994; Kazatchkine et al., 1994) (Table 3).

IVIg was shown to alter the patterns of cytokine production in vitro in cultures of PBMC stimulated with various mitogens. Thus, IVIg downregulated the production of IL-2, IL-3, IL-4, IL-5, IL-10, tumor necrosis factor (TNF)-β and granulocyte-macrophage colony-stimulating factor (GM-CSF) in mitogen-stimulated cells during the first 48 h of culture, whereas no effectof IVIg on IFN-γ production was observed (Amran et al., 1994). In cultures of purified monocytes or unfractionated PBMC, IVIg behaved as an anti-inflammatory agent. It selectively triggered the production and secretion of IL-1 receptor antagonist (IL-1ra) – the natural antagonist of IL-1 – together with IL-8, without a concomitant effect on the production of the pro-inflammatory monokines IL-1α, IL-1β, IL-6 and TNF-α by monocytes (Poutsiaka et al., 1991; Ruiz de Souza et al., 1995) (Fig. 1). The induction of IL-1ra by IVIg required both the Fc and F(ab')$_2$ moiety of IgG. It was also shown that IVIg suppresses lipopolysacharide-induced production of TNF-α and IL-1, possibly through an increase in the intracellular levels of cyclic adenosine monophosphate (cAMP) following the interaction of IVIg with Fcγ receptors on monocytes (Shimozato et al., 1990; Shimozato et al., 1991). Recent evidence suggests that the anti-cytokine effect of IVIg against TNF-α and IL-2 is mediated by the variable regions of the Igs (Menezes et al., 1997).

Table 3. Interactions between IVIg and the cytokine network

IVIg	contains natural antibodies to cytokines, cytokine antagonists and cytokine receptors
IVIg	selectively induces the production of anti-inflammatory cytokines in monocytes
IVIg	decreases the production of cytokines by activated T-cells and tends to restore the normal balance between Th1 and Th2 cells in vivo. The effect of IVIg on T-cell cytokine production requires accessory cells

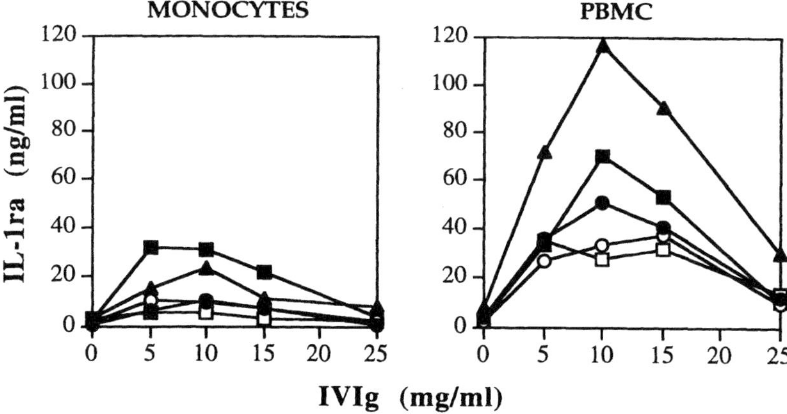

Fig. 1. Selective induction of interleukin-1 receptor antagonists (*IL-1ra*) from monocytes by intravenous immunoglobulin (*IVIg*) in vitro. Purified adherent monocytes (1×10^6 NSE$^+$ cells/ml) (*left panel*) or peripheral blood mononuclear cells (*PBMC*) (1×10^6 NSE$^+$ cells/ml) (*right panel*) from normal donors ($n = 5$) were cultured in the presence of increasing concentrations of IVIg for 24 h at 37 °C. The concentrations of IL-1ra were then determined in culture supernatants by enzyme-linked immunosorbent assay. Each donor is represented by the same symbol in both panels. (Adapted from Ruiz de Souza et al. 1995)

The effects of IVIg on proinflammatory cytokines extends to T-cells, as indicated by the study of cytokine production in vivo in animal models of Th1-mediated diseases. Animal models of rat autoimmune encephalomyelitis and adjuvant arthritis have demonstrated that IVIg treatment was capable of preventing the induction of the disease. Although some T-cell reactivity to the specific antigens was present, a significant decrease in the production of TNF-α was observed after IVIg treatment (Achiron et al., 1994; Pashov et al., 1997) (Fig. 2). In the experimental autoimmune encephalomyelitis (EAE) model, IVIg inhibits cytokine production by antigen-activated T-cells, with a stronger inhibitory effect on Th1 cytokines than on Th2-related cytokines. From data obtained in vivo in the human (Andersson et al., 1994) and the study of Th2-dependent experimental autoimmune disease (Rossi et al., 1991), it may be considered that, rather than inducing immune deviation, IVIg will affect T-cell cytokine production in a way that will tend to bring the Th1-Th2 balance of the diseased IVIg recipient close to the equilibrium state that characterizes the normal immune system. Recent evidence supports the fact that the effects of IVIg on T-cell cytokine production require the interaction of IVIg with accessory cells (Andersson, unpublished data).

The effect of IVIg on cytokine production in patients has been examined in vivo. A marked increase in the plasma levels of IL-1ra with a 1000-fold

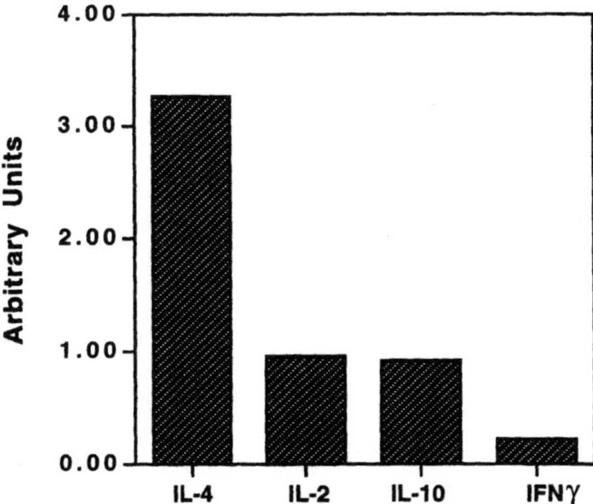

Fig. 2. Levels of interleukin (*IL*)-4, IL-10, IL-2 and interferon γ (*IFNγ*) in lymph node cells collected at day 13 after immunization from intravenous immunoglobulin-treated rats with experimental autoimmune encephalomyelitis, measured by semi-quantitative reverse transcriptase polymerase chain reaction. The intensities of bands for each protein were normalized to intensity of β-actin hand. (Adapted from Pashov et al. 1997)

molar excess of IL-1ra to IL-1β was found in patients treated with IVIg (Aukrust et al., 1994). IVIg decreased the plasma levels of TNF-α in HIV-1 infected patients, whereas the levels of soluble TNF receptors increased in HIV-infected patients following IVIg therapy (Aukrust et al., 1997).

IVIg contains natural antibodies against IL-1, TNF-α and IL-6 (Abe et al., 1994; Bendtzen et al., 1990; Svenson et al., 1990). The clinical relevance of natural anti-cytokine antibodies in IVIg is as yet unclear. It has been suggested that IVIg preparations which contain high amounts of anti-interferon (IFN)-γ inhibit lymphocyte proliferation and TNF-α secretion in the mixed lymphocyte reaction. Inhibition was reversed by the addition of recombinant human IFN-α (Toungouz et al., 1996). Thus, natural anti-cytokine antibodies may be involved in the inhibition of cytokine-mediated effects when these are produced in excess in systemic inflammatory disorders.

Modulation of Expression of Chemokines and Adhesion Molecules

During inflammation, activated endothelial cells rapidly synthesize and release chemokines and newly express, within hours, integrins involved in the adhesion, rolling and diapedesis of leukocytes (Carlos & Harlan, 1994).

Among the newly synthesized inflammatory molecules are monocyte chemoattractant protein I (MCP-1), granulocyte-colony stimulating factor (G-CSF), GM-CSF, intercellular adhesion molecule-1 (ICAM-1) and vascular cell adhesion molecule-1 (VCAM-1). IVIg plays a role in modulating endothelial cell function by inhibiting endothelial cell proliferation and downregulating the expression of key adhesion molecules and chemokines. We have recently investigated the role of IVIg in controlling endothelial cell activation in inflammatory conditions in vitro. We observed that IVIg inhibits the TNF-α- or IL-1β-induced expression of mRNA of adhesion molecules (ICAM-1 and VCAM-1) and chemokines [MCP-1, M-CSF (macrophage colony-stimulating factor) and GM-CSF] (Xu et al., 1998). These molecules have a significant role in leukocyte recruitment observed in several inflammatory diseases (Brady, 1994). IVIg was shown to decrease the plasma level of M-CSF in patients with idiopathic thrombocytopenic purpura who had high pretreatment M-CSF levels, which was suggested to cause thrombocytosis after IVIg treatment (Nomura et al., 1996).

Serum ICAM-1 levels correlate with the severity of vascular damage in acute Kawasaki disease. Increased levels of ICAM-1 correlate with high levels of TNF-α (Furukawa et al., 1992). IVIg does not block the expression of ICAM-1 by endothelial cells in vitro. Anti-TNF-α in IVIg, however, blocks the expression of ICAM-1 by vascular endothelial cells treated with supernatants of human mononuclear cells stimulated with *Lactobacillus casei* cell wall used as an in vitro model of inflammation in Kawasaki disease (Tomita et al., 1993).

Steroid-Sparing Effects of IVIg

IVIg has allowed for a reduction in the amount of steroids required in patients with allergic/inflammatory diseases including bronchial asthma, birdshot retinochoroidopathy, pemphigus and necrotizing vasculitis (Beckers et al., 1995; Gedalia et al., 1995; Gelfand et al., 1994; George et al., 1996; Taprantzi et al., 1996).

The administration of IVIg decreased the amount of systemic steroids required in patients with chronic steroid-dependent bronchial asthma (Taprantzi et al., 1996). IVIg reduced the number of CD4$^+$ T-lymphocytes and activated T-lymphocytes in bronchial biopsies from the patients. Preliminary data have also shown that IVIg causes a reduction in the free levels of the chemotactic cytokine IL-8 in serum, probably as a result of the binding of IL-8 by anti-IL-8 antibodies in IVIg.

Birdshot retinochoroidopathy is a chronic progressive bilateral posterior uveitis that occurs in individuals expressing the HLA-A29 phenotype

(George et al., 1996; LeHoang et al., 1998). IVIg has allowed a decrease in daily intakes in prednisone by at least three-fold or prevented the need for steroids for up to 5 years of follow-up in patients with the disease (Karmochkine et al., 1998).

A steroid-sparing effect of IVIg was reported in a $2\,^1/_2$-year-old child who had fever, arthritis and cutaneous necrotizing vasculitis (Gedalia et al., 1995). In patients with pemphigus, IVIg was reported as the only means of tapering off steroid therapy to acceptable, effective maintenance doses (Beckers et al., 1995).

The anti-inflammatory effects of IVIg discussed above are certainly clinically relevant in patients whose systemic inflammatory symptoms improve rapidly upon infusion of Ig. The anti-inflammatory properties of IVIg also contribute to the changes in B- and T-cell immune repertoires that underly the long term beneficial effects of Ig therapy in autoimmune and systemic inflammatory diseases.

References

Abe J, Kotzin BL, Meissner C, Melish ME, Takahshi M, Fulton D, Romagne F, Melissen B, Leung DYM (1993) Characterization of T cell repertoire changes in acute Kawasaki disease. J Exp Med 177:791–796

Abe Y, Horiuchi A, Miyake M, Kimura S (1994) Anti-cytokine nature of human immunoglobulin: one possible mechanism of the clinical effect of intravenous therapy. Immunol Rev 139:5–19

Achiron A, Barak Y, Sarova-Pinhas I, Achiron R, Gabbay U, Rotstein Z, Noy S (1996) Intravenous immunoglobulin in relapsing-remitting multiple sclerosis. In: Kazatchkine MD, Morel A (eds) Intravenous immunoglobulin research and therapy. Parthenon Publishing Group Ltd., London, pp 289–294

Achiron A, Margalit R, Hershkoviz R, Markovits D, Reshef T, Melamed E, Cohen IR, Lider O (1994) Intravenous immunoglobulin treatment of experimental T cell-mediated autoimmune disease. Upregulation of T cell proliferation and downregulation of tumor necrosis factor alpha secretion. J Clin Invest 93:600–605

Amran A, Renz H, Lack G, Bradley K, Gelfand EW (1994) Suppression of cytokine-dependent human T-cell proliferation by intravenous immunoglobulin. Clin Immunol Immunopathol 73:180–186

Andersson UG, Bjork L, Skansén-Saphir U, Andersson JP (1994) Pooled human IgG modulates cytokine production in lymphocytes and monocytes. Immunol Rev 139:21–42

Antonelli A, Palla R, Casarosa L, Fallahi P, Baschieri L (1996) IgG, IgA and C3 deposits in the extra-thyroidal manifestations of autoimmune Graves' disease: their in vitro solubilization by intravenous immunoglobulin. Clin Exp Rheumatol 14 (Suppl 15):S31–S35

Ashkenazi S, Cleary TG, Lopez E, Pickering LK (1988) Anticytotoxin-neutralizing antibodies in immune globulin preparations: potential use in hemolytic-uremic syndrome. J Pediatr 113:1008–1014

Aukrust P, Froland SS, Liabakk NB, Muller F, Nordoy I, Haug C, Espevik T (1994) Release of cytokines, soluble cytokine receptors, and interleukin-1 receptor antagonist after intravenous immunoglobulin administration in vivo. Blood 84: 2136–2143

Aukrust P, Hestdal K, Lien E, Bjerkeli V, Nordoy I, Espevik T, Muller F, Frolland SS (1997) Effects of intravenous immunoglobulin in vivo on abnormally increased tumor necrosis factor-alpha activity in human immunodeficiency virus type 1 infection. J Infect Dis 176:913–923

Basta M (1996) Modulation of complement-mediated tissue damage by intravenous immunoglobulin. In: Kazatchkine MD, Morell A (eds) Intravenous immunoglobulin and therapy. Parthenon, New York, pp 83–88

Basta M, Dalakas MC (1994) High-dose intravenous immunoglobulin exerts its beneficial effect in patients with dermatomyositis by blocking endomysial deposition of activated complements fragments. J Clin Invest 94:1729–1735

Basta M, Kirshbom P, Frank MM, Fries LF (1989) Mechanism of therapeutic effect of high-dose intravenous immunoglobulin. Attenuation of acute, complement dependent immune damage in a guinea pig model. J Clin Invest 84:1974–1981

Basta M, Langlois PF, Marques M, Frank MM, Fries LF (1989) High-dose intravenous immunoglobulin modifies complement-mediated in vivo clearance. Blood 74: 326–333

Baudet V, Hurez V, Lapeyre C, Kaveri SV, Kazatchkine MD (1996) Intravenous immunoglobulin (IVIg) enhances the selective expansion of Vb3$^+$ and Vb17$^+$ ab T cells induced by superantigen. Scand J Immunol 43:277–282

Beckers RC, Brand A, Vermeer BJ, Boom BW (1995) Adjuvant high-dose intravenous gammaglobulin in the treatment of pemphigus and bullous pemphigoid: experience in six patients. Br J Dermatol 133:289–293

Bendtzen K, Svenson M, Jonsson V, Hippe E (1990) Autoantibodies to cytokines - friends or foes? Immunol Today 11:167–169

Blanchette VS, Imbach P, Andrew M (1994) A prospective randomized trial of intravenous immunoglobulin G, oral prednisolone and intravenous anti-D in childhood acute idiopathic thrombocytopenic purpura. Lancet 344:703–707

Blasczyk R, Westhoff U, Grossewilde H (1993) Soluble CD4, CD8, and HLA molecules in commercial immunoglobulin preparations. Lancet 341:789–790

Brady HR (1994) Leukocyte adhesion molecules and kidney diseases. Kidney Int 45: 1285–1300

Carlos TM, Harlan JM (1994) Leukocyte-endothelial adhesion molecules. Blood 84: 2068–2101

Dalakas M, Illa I, Dambrosia J, Soueidan S, Stein D, Otero C, Dinsmore S, McCrosky S (1993) A controlled trial of high-dose intravenous immune globulin infusions as treatment for dermatomyositis. N Engl J Med 329:1993–2000

Dwyer JM (1992) Manipulating the immune system with immune globulin. N Engl J Med 326:107–116

Fazekas F, Deisenhammer F, Strasser-Fuchs S, Nahler G, Mamoll B (1997) Randomised placebo-controlled trial of monthly intravenous immunoglobulin therapy in relapsing remitting sclerosis. Lancet 349:589–593

Furukawa S, Imai K, Matsubara T, Yone K, Yachi A, Okumura K, Yabuta K (1992) Increased levels of circulating intercellular adhesion molecule 1 in Kawasaki disease. Arthritis Rheum 35:672–677

Furusho K, Kamiya T, Nakano H, Kiyosawa N, Shinomiya K, Hayashidera T, Tamura T, Hirose O, Manabe Y, Yokoyama T, Kawarano M, Baba K, Mori C (1984) High-dose intravenous gammaglobulin for Kawasaki disease. Lancet ii:1055–1058

182   Y. Bar-Dayan et al.

Gajdos P, Chevret S, Clair B, Tranchant C, Chastang C (1997) Clinical trial of plasma exchange and high-dose intravenous immunoglobulin in myasthenia gravis. Myasthenia gravis clinical study group. Ann Neurol 41:89–96

Gajdos P, Outin H, Elkharrat D, Brunel D, Rohan-Chabot PD, Raphael JC, Goulon M, Goulon-Goeau C, Morel E (1984) High-dose intravenous gammaglobulin for myasthenia gravis. Lancet i:406–407

Gedalia A, Correa H, Kaiser M, Sorensen R (1995) Case report: steroid sparing effect of intravenous gamma globulin in a child with necrotizing vasculitis. Am J Med Sci 309:226–228

Gelfand EW, Esterl B, Mazer BD (1994) Benefit of 12% solution of intravenous immunoglobulin in the treatment of steroid-dependent asthma. In: Kazatchkine MD, Louwagie A (eds) Immunoglobulins extending the horizons. Parthenon Publ, London, pp 49–62

George F, Goichot L, Francois A, Castiel P, Kulmann N, Cassoux N, LeHoang P, Kazatchkine MD (1996) Corticosteroid-sparing effect of intravenous immunoglobulin in birdshot retinochoroidopathy. In: Kazatchkine MD, Morell A (eds) Intravenous immunoglobulin and therapy. Parthenon, New York, pp 333–334

Hahn AF, Bolton CF, Zochodone D, Feasby TE (1995) Intravenous immunoglobulin treatment in chronic inflammatory demyelinating polyneuropathy (CIDP): a double-blind, placebo-controlled study. Brain 119:1067–1078

Hughes R, Plasma exchange/Sandoglobulin Guillain-Barré syndrome trial group (1997) Randomised trial of plasma exchange, intravenous immunoglobulin, and plasma exchange followed by intravenous immunoglobulin in Guillain-Barré syndrome. Lancet 349:225–230

Imbach P, Barandun S, d'Apuzzo V, Baumgartner C, Hirt A, Morell A, Rossi E, Schoni M, Vest M, Wagner HP (1981) High-dose intravenous gammaglobulin for idiopathic thrombocytopenic purpura in childhood. Lancet i:1228–1230

Jayne DRW, Davies M, Fox C, Lockwood CM (1991) Treatment of systemic vasculitis with pooled intravenous immunoglobulin. Lancet ii:1137–1139

Karmochkine M, Cassoux N, Goichot-Bonnat L, Lehoang P, Kazatchkine MD (1998) Steroid-sparing effect of intravenous immunoglobulin in inflammatory uveitis. (Submitted)

Kazatchkine MD, Dietrich G, Hurez V, Ronda N, Bellon B, Rossi F, Kaveri SV (1994) V region-mediated selection of autoreactive repertoires by intravenous immunoglobulin (IVIg). Immunol Rev 139:79–107

Lalezari P, Korshidi M, Petrosova M (1986) Autoimmune neutropenia of infancy. J Pediatr 109:764–769

Latremouille C, Genevaz D, Hu MC, Schussler O, Goussev N, Bruneval P, Haeffner-Cavaillon N, Carpentier A, Glotz D (1997) Normal human polyclonal immunoglobulins for intravenous use (IVIg) delay hyperacute xenograft rejection through F(ab')$_2$-mediated anti-complement activity. Clin Exp Immunol 110:122–126

LeHoang P, Jobin D, Kazatchkine MD (1998) Treatment of birdshot retinochoroidopathy with intravenous immunoglobulins. (Submitted)

Lutz HU, Stammler P, Jelezarova E, Nater M, Spath PJ (1996) High doses of immunoglobulin G attenuate immune aggregate-mediated complement activation by enhancing physiologic cleavage of C3b in C3bn-IgG complexes. Blood 88:184–193

McGuire WA, Yang HH, Bruno E, Brandt J, Briddell R, Coates TD, Hoffman R (1987) Treatment of antibody-mediated pure red-cell aplasia with high-dose intravenous gammaglobulin. N Engl J Med 317:1004–1008

McIntyre EA, Linch DC, Macey MG, Newland AC (1985) Successful response to intravenous immunoglobulin in autoimmune hemolytic anemia. Br J Haematol 60:387–388

Menezes MC, Benard G, Sato MN, Hong MA, Duarte AJ (1997) In vitro inhibitory activity of tumor necrosis factor alpha and interleukin-2 of human immunoglobulin preparations. Int Arch Allergy Immunol 114:323–328

Miletic VD, Hester CG, Frank MM (1996) Regulation of complement activity by immunoglobulin. J Immunol 156:749–757

Mollnes TE, Hogasen K, Hoas BF, Michaelsen TE, Garred P, Harboe M (1995) Inhibition of complement-mediated red cell lysis by immunoglobulins is dependent on the IG isotype and its Cl binding properties. Scand J Immunol 41:449–456

Mouthon L, Kaveri SV, Spalter SH, Lacroix-Desmazes S, Lefranc C, Desai R, Kazatchkine MD (1996) Mechanisms of action of intravenous immune globulins in immune-mediated diseases. Clin Exp Immunol 104:3–9

Newburger JW, Takahashi M, Burns JC, Beiser AS, Chung KJ, Duffy CE, Glode MP, Mason WH, Reddy V, Sanders RP, Shulman ST, Wiggins JW, Hicks RV, Fulton DR, Lewis AB, Leung DYM, Colton T, Rosen FS, Melish ME (1986) The treatment of Kawasaki syndrome with intravenous gammaglobulin. N Engl J Med 315:341–347

Nomura S, Yasunaga K, Fujimura K, Kuramoto A, Okuma M, Nomura T (1996) High-dose intravenous gamma globulin reduces macrophage colony-stimulating factor levels in idiopathic thrombocytopenic purpura. Int J Hematol 63:227–234

Oda H, Honda A, Sugita K (1985) High dose intact IgG infusion in refractory autoimmune hemolytic anemia (Evans syndrome). J Pediatr 107:744–746

Pashov A, Bellon B, Kaveri SV, Kazatchkine MD (1997) A shift in encephalogenic T cell pattern is associated with suppression of EAE by intravenous immunoglobulins (IVIg). Multiple Sclerosis 3:153–156

Poutsiaka DD, Clark BD, Vannier E, Dinarello CA (1991) Production of IL-receptor antagonist and IL-1β by peripheral blood mononuclear cells is differentially regulated. Blood 78:1275–1279

Rossi F, Bellon B, Vial MC, Druet P, Kazatchkine MD (1991) Beneficial effect of human therapeutic intravenous immunoglobulins (IVIg) in mercuric-chloride-induced autoimmune disease of Brown-Norway rats. Clin Exp Immunol 84:129–133

Ruiz de Souza V, Carreno MP, Kaveri SV, Ledur A, Sadeghi H, Cavaillon JM, Kazatchkine MD, Haeffner-Cavaillon N (1995) Selective induction of interleukin-1 receptor antagonist and interleukin-8 in human monocytes by normal polyspecific IgG (intravenous immunoglobulin). Eur J Immunol 25:1267–1273

Sato M, Kojima H, Koshikawa SJ (1986) Modification of immune complexes deposited in glomeruli in tissue sections treated with sulfonized gamma-globulin. Clin Exp Immunol 64:623–628

Schmidt RE, Budde V, Schäfer G, Stroehmann I (1981) High-dose intravenous gammaglobulin for idiopathic thrombocytopenic purpura. Lancet ii:475–476

Shimozato T, Iwata M, Kawada H, Tamura N (1990) Suppression of tumor necrosis factor alpha production by a human immunoglobulin preparation for intravenous use. Infect Immun 58:1384–1388

Shimozato T, Iwata M, Kawada H, Tamura N (1991) Human immunoglobulin preparation for intravenous use induces elevation of cellular cyclic adenosine 3′:5′-monophosphate levels, resulting in suppression of tumor necrosis factor alpha and interleukin-1 production. Immunology 72:497–501

Shulman ST (1992) Recommendations for intravenous immunoglobulin therapy of Kawasaki disease. Pediatr Infect Dis J 11:985–986

Sultan Y, Kazatchkine MD, Maisonneuve P, Nydegger UE (1984) Anti-idiotypic suppression of autoantibodies to Factor VIII (antihaemophilic factor) by high-dose intravenous gammaglobulin. Lancet ii:765–768

Svenson M, Hansen MB, Bendtzen K (1990) Distribution and characterization of autoantibodies to interleukin 1α in normal human sera. Scand J Immunol 32: 695–701

Takei S, Arora Y, Walker SM (1993) Intravenous immunoglobulin contains specific antibodies inhibitory to activation of T cells by staphylococcal toxin superantigens. J Clin Invest 91:602–607

Taprantzi P, Syrigou E, Zervaki K, Andriani E, Papdoulous N, Sinaniotis C, Saxoni-Papgeorgiou F (1996) Low-dose intravenous immunoglobulin in severe steroid-dependent childhood asthma. In: Kazatchkine MD, Morell A (eds) Intravenous immunoglobulin and therapy. Parthenon, New York, p 332

Tekow J, Reinhold D, Pap T, Ansorge S (1998) Intravenous immunoglobulins and transforming growth factor-β. Lancet 351:184–185

Tomino Y, Sakai H, Takaya M, Miura M, Suga T, Endoh M, Nomoto Y (1984) Solubilization of intraglomerular deposits of IgG immune complexes by human sera or gammaglobulin in patients with lupus nephritis. Clin Exp Immunol 58: 42–48

Tomita S, Myones BL, Shulman ST (1993) In vitro correlates of the L. casei animal model of Kawasaki disease. J Rheumatol 20:362–367

Toungouz M, Denys C, Dupont E (1996) Blockade of proliferation and tumor necrosis factor-alpha production occuring during mixed lymphocyte reaction by interferon-gamma-specific natural antibodies contained in intravenous immunoglobulins. Transplantation 62:1292–1296

van der Meché FGA, Smith PIM, Dutch Guillain-Barré Study Group (1992) A randomized trial comparing intravenous immune globulin and plasma exchange in Guillain-Barré syndrome. N Engl J Med 326:1123–1129

Xu C, Poirier B, Lavaud S, Lucchiari N, Michel O, Chevalier J, Kaveri S (1998) Modulation of endothelial cell function by normal polyspecific human immunoglobulins: a possible mechanism of action of in vascular diseases. Amer J Pathol (Submitted)

Yuki N, Ichihashi Y, Taki T (1995) Subclass of IgG antibody to GM1 epitope-bearing lipopolysaccharide of Campylobacter jejuni in patients with Guillain-Barré syndrome. J Neuroimmunol 60:161–164

Gene Therapeutic Strategies
in Inflammatory Bowel Diseases

M. F. Neurath, S. Wirtz, C. Becker, K. Barbulescu, and S. Finotto

Introduction

Inflammatory bowel diseases (IBD) comprise two major forms: ulcerative colitis (UC) and Crohn's disease (CD) [1–2]. Although the etiology of both diseases remains unknown, recent data suggest that genetic factors, environmental factors and bacterial antigens may play a key role in their pathogenesis [1–2]. However, both diseases can be discriminated in about 90% of patients by using endoscopic, radiologic and histologic criteria: Whereas UC consists of a more superficial inflammation limited to the large bowel, CD is characterized by a discontinuous, transmural granulomatous inflammation that can occur anywhere in the alimentary canal. Furthermore, there is recent evidence that both diseases are associated with changes in the intestinal immune system.

Changes in the mucosal immune system appear to play an important role in the pathogenesis of IBD [3–4], in which, in particular, an altered cytokine production by lymphocytes and macrophages has been implicated. This hypothesis is supported by the finding that mice in which the genes for certain cytokines, such as interleukin (IL)-2 or IL-10, have been inactivated by homologous recombination develop chronic enterocolitis [5–6]. In addition, overexpression of some cytokines (e.g. IL-7) results in the development of chronic intestinal inflammation. Furthermore, changes in cytokine production by macrophages and T-cells have been found in various experimental colitis models, such as adoptive transfer of normal CD45RB^{hi} T-cells from BALB/c mice to C.B.-17 SCID mice and intrarectal administration of the hapten reagent 2,4,6,-trinitrobenzene sulfonic acid (TNBS) in SJL/J mice [7–10]. Finally, recombinant cytokines (e.g. IL-10) or antibodies to cytokines (e.g. TNF-α, IL-12) have been successfully used for the treatment of established colitis in mice.

Clinical therapy of IBD with corticosteroids and immunosuppressive drugs is frequently complicated by side effects such as gastritis, hepatotoxicity, pancreatitis or osteopathy [11]. Thus, alternative treatment strategies with added specificity but reduced toxicity are highly desirable. Here, we will discuss recent progress in our understanding of gene therapeutic strategies in

Symposium in Immunology VIII
Eibl/Huber/Peter/Wahn (Eds.)
© Springer Verlag Berlin Heidelberg 1999

experimental intestinal inflammation. First, we focus on principles of the antisense approach for gene regulation. Next, we discuss the potential of such antisense techniques to downregulate various important regulatory genes in the inflamed gut. Finally, we will focus on gene delivery to the inflamed intestine by recombinant adenoviruses and discuss potential therapeutic strategies to inhibit gene activation in patients with chronic intestinal inflammation.

Antisense Strategies

The Antisense Approach

Selective inhibition of the function of regulatory proteins by antisense DNA is a fascinating approach to specifically regulate intestinal gene expression. The "antisense" approach in which the target is mRNA uses complementary DNA sequences to arrest gene transcription or mRNA translation [12–14]. These DNA sequences thus specifically overlap transcription or translation start sites of genes, thereby influencing gene expression. Since naked DNA is easily degraded by endonucleases at phosphor–oxygen bondings, antisense DNA is usually chemically modified (phosphotriesters, methylphosphonates, phosphorothioates) to increase the resistance of the DNA to endonucleases (Fig. 1) [15–16]. The most frequent modification consists of the introduction of sulfur groups in the DNA, creating so-called phosphorothioate oligonucleotides (Fig. 1). The half-life of such oligonucleotides is strikingly enhanced compared to the relatively short half-life (about 10 min in the peripheral blood) of naked DNA. It has been suggested that phosphorothioate oligonucleotides are actively taken up by cells of the immune system via receptor-mediated endocytosis (Fig. 2). In contrast, naked DNA is taken up passively via diffusion. Upon uptake, most phosphorothioate oligonucleotides are transported via endosomes and from there reach cytoplasmic and nuclear target structures (Fig. 2). Antisense DNA has been used to modify the expression of genes in vitro and in vivo [17–18]. Several ways of delivering the antisense DNA to the target tissues in vivo have been studied, including local and systemic delivery systems in mice. Interestingly, systemic administration of antisense DNA to mice via intravenous injection leads to accumulation of the DNA in the liver and kidney, whereas the blood–brain barrier prevents delivery of the antisense DNA to the brain.

Downregulation of proteins by antisense DNA has been a powerful tool to analyze their functional properties. For instance, it was shown that downregulation of various transcription factors such as c-myc, c-myb, c-fos and Pax5 by antisense DNA strongly suppresses cell proliferation [19–22]. However, various unspecific effects of some antisense DNA sequences have been

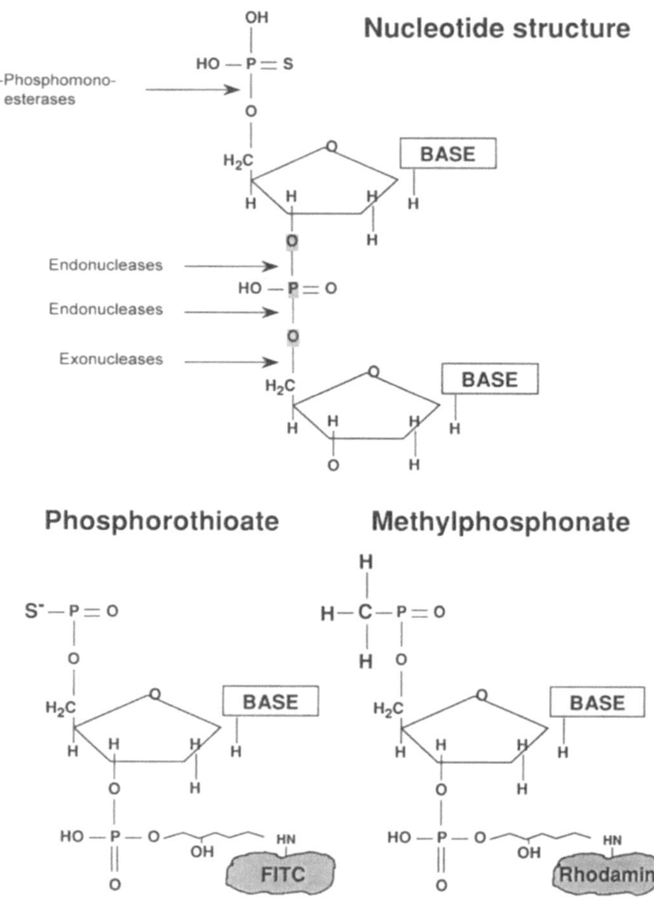

Fig. 1. Since naked DNA is easily degraded by endonucleases at phosphor–oxygen bondings, antisense DNA is usually chemically modified (phosphotriesters, methylphosphonates, phosphorothioates) to increase the resistance of the DNA to endonucleases. *FITC*, fluorescein isothiocyanate

observed, explaining the necessity for a tight control of "antisense effects" (Table 1). Various studies have shown that the composition and length of the antisense DNA is an important parameter to prevent unspecific hybridization. Therefore, one should carefully avoid repetitive sequences and design an antisense phosphorothioate oligonucleotide of appropriate length (usually 16–19 bp). Another relevant problem is the occurrence of B-cell proliferation upon antisense treatment that appears to be due to C plus G (CpG) motifs in the DNA. CpG motifs have also been recently shown to modulate cytokine production by T-cells, leading to increased production of TH1 cyto-

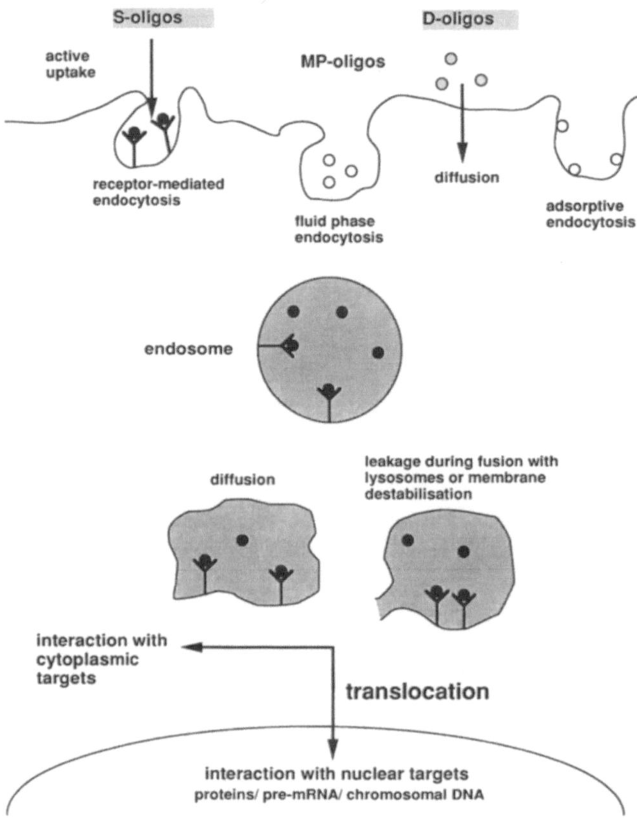

Fig. 2. Biologic fate of oligonucleotides

kines such as interferon (IFN)-γ. Other unspecific effects consist of inhibition of cell adhesion by quadruple G-containing oligonucleotides and of unspecific toxic effects of the DNA (Table 1). Thus, four key criteria should be used to demonstrate specificity of antisense DNA [23–24]:

1. Demonstration that the corresponding "sense" and control "nonsense" oligonucleotides do not have the same effect
2. Demonstration of inhibition of the target gene by definitive molecular studies and demonstration that another, non-targeted gene is normally expressed
3. Ability to reverse the antisense effect by competition with a complementary sense oligonucleotide
4. Exclusion of other explanations of the antisense effect such as the CpG effect and toxicity of the antisense DNA.

Table 1. Unspecific effects of antisense-DNA

1. Unspecific hybridization
2. C-plus G effect
3. Quadruple G effect
1. Activation or inactivation of other genes
2. B-cell proliferation
3. Inhibition of adhesion
AS: AGAGT T: ACTCT
AS: CACTTTCGCACGTA
AS: CACGGGGTATAGC

Antisense in Inflammatory Bowel Disease

In our laboratory, we have recently tried to apply the antisense strategy to the treatment of chronic intestinal inflammation in mice and humans [25–28]. We reasoned that the transcription factor nuclear factor (NF)-κB might be a suitable target for antisense DNA. This regulatory factor was described a decade ago as a nuclear protein that bound a site in the immunoglobulin κ enhancer. It is now well established that NF-κB comprises a family of transcription factors with major physiological relevance in a variety of biological processes, most notably immune responses and inflammation [29–35]. Family members include so far NF-κB1 (p50 and its precursor p105), NF-κB2 (p52 and its precursor p100), p65 (RelA), c-Rel (Rel), and RelB. The functional importance of NF-κB in acute and chronic inflammation is based on its ability to regulate the promoters of a variety of genes whose products, such as cytokines, adhesion molecules and acute phase proteins, are critical for inflammatory processes.

Here, we describe a method to treat established intestinal inflammation by local or systemic application of antisense phosphorothioate oligonucleotides, targeting the translation start site of murine NF-κB p65 [25]. In an initial series of studies, we determined NF-κB levels in lamina propria macrophages from mice with trinitrobenzene sulfonic acid (TNBS)-induced colitis or IL-10$^{-/-}$ colitis. A striking increase of NF-κB DNA binding activity in nuclear extracts from lamina propria cells was observed and subsequent shift-Western blotting experiments identified the p65 subunit of NF-κB as a major component of the retarded NF-κB complex. We then designed a specific antisense phosphorothioate oligonucleotide (murine p65 antisense: 5′-GAAACAGATCGTCCATGGT-3′) targeting the translation initiation site of murine p65 to reduce expression levels of p65 (Fig. 3). The p65 antisense oligonucleotide strikingly reduced the expression of p65 at the protein level.

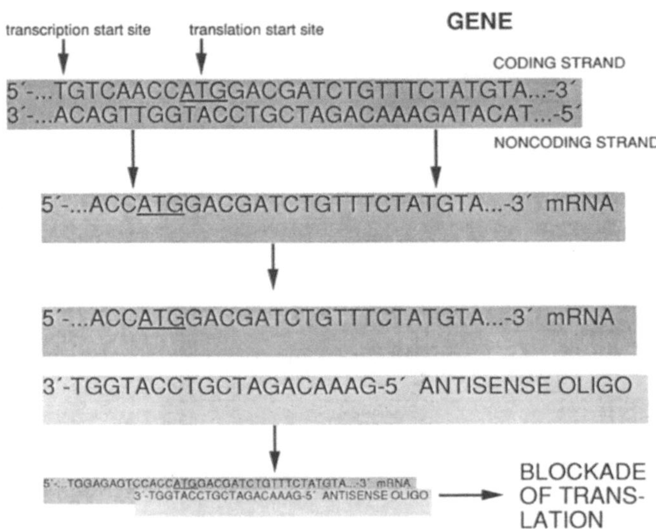

Fig. 3. Murine p65 gene sequence

Next, phosphorothioate oligonucleotides were administered to mice with chronic TNBS-induced colitis or IL-10$^{-/-}$ colitis either as a single intravenous injection or applied locally into the colon by injection via a catheter. We found that a single intravenous injection of 800 μg p65 antisense oligonucleotides abrogated clinical signs of established intestinal inflammation. Antisense-treated mice no longer had diarrhea and started to gain weigth. In contrast, no significant clinical changes were observed in mice treated with control phosphorothiate oligonucleotides. Furthermore, systemic administration of p65 antisense oligonucleotides was more effective in treating established colitis than daily systemic administration of glucocorticoids. However, we found that high doses (> 1500 μg) of p65 antisense oligonucleotides led to toxic side effects, including hepatitis, suggesting that a local approach might be safer for the treatment of mice.

Accordingly, we performed studies using local application techniques and found that TNBS-induced colitis could be successfully treated by a single local administration of the p65 antisense oligonucleotide. There was no apparent sign of toxicity of the p65 antisense oligonucleotide at the concentration used as evaluated by hematocrit and thrombocyte levels of the antisense-treated mice. Moreover, macrophages obtained from the lamina propria of p65 antisense-treated mice produced significantly lower amounts of IL-1, IL-6 and TNF-α mRNA in cell culture.

Based on these data that suggested a predominant role for NF-κB p65 in two murine models of chronic intestinal inflammation, we focussed in further studies on the question of whether there is a deregulated activity of p65 in CD in humans. Accordingly, we purified lamina propria macrophages from bowel specimens in patients with CD using negative selection techniques and analyzed the expression of NF-κB p65 in stimulated and unstimulated cells by Western blot analysis. As assessed by densitometry, we found a significant upregulation of p65 levels in patients with CD ($p < 0.01$). There was on average a 14.2-fold increase of p65 expression in unstimulated and a 36.5-fold increase in lipopolysaccharide-stimulated lamina propria macrophages in patients with CD compared to macrophages obtained from control specimens. This finding was consistent with an increased production of proinflammatory cytokines by lamina propria macrophages in patients with CD. When lamina propria macrophages from CD patients were co-cultured with p65 antisense oligonucleotides, a strongly reduced production of IL-1, IL-6 and TNF-α was found, supporting the idea that p65 is a key factor in deregulating these cytokines in CD. The data provide direct evidence for the central importance of p65 in experimental intestinal inflammation and suggest the potential therapeutic utility of p65 antisense oligonucleotides for the treatment of patients with chronic intestinal inflammation.

Taken together, we had explored the molecular mechanisms that regulate experimental TNBS-induced colitis and colitis in IL-10$^{-/-}$ mice. First, we found a striking overexpression of the transcription factor NF-κB p65 in both models of colitis; second, we showed that local or systemic administration of an antisense oligonucleotide that specifically downregulates p65 expression led to an abrogation of established colitis; and third, we showed that antisense-induced p65 suppression was accompanied by reduced production of various important proinflammatory cytokines by lamina propria cells. These data suggest a continuous activation of NF-κB in intestinal inflammation (possibly due to products of the bacterial flora) as an important mechanism for pathogenesis of chronic colitis. Furthermore, the results implicate the potential utility of p65 antisense treatment in patients with chronic intestinal inflammation.

Lamina propria macrophages in both the TNBS- and IL-10-colitis models produced high levels of the proinflammatory cytokines IL-1, IL-6 and TNF-α, consistent with the cytokine profiles found in patients with CD. Based on this observation, we then focussed, in further molecular studies, on the expression of NF-κB, a key transcription factor of mononuclear cells that had been previously implicated in the transcriptional control of the promoter activity of these genes [29–35]. We found a striking overexpression of NF-κB by macrophages in TNBS-induced colitis and demonstrated that p65 was a major component of the NF-κB complex. This finding prompted us to design a strategy to inhibit NF-κB function.

In initial studies, we found that lamina propria macrophages that were co-cultured with a specific p65 antisense oligonucleotide failed to secrete high levels of IL-1, IL-6 and TNF-α. Having shown the ability of the antisense oligonucleotide to specifically downregulate the expression of several important proinflammatory cytokines, we then analyzed the effects of the p65 antisense oligonucleotide on established chronic colitis in vivo. It was found that TNBS-induced colitis and IL-10$^{-/-}$ colitis can be successfully treated by systemic administration of p65 antisense oligonucleotides, even after the lesion is established. Perhaps even more strikingly, we found that TNBS-induced colitis could be successfully treated by a single local administration of the p65 antisense oligonucleotide. This finding suggests that the presence of p65 is essential to maintain TNBS-induced colitis and a persistent local activation of macrophages with concomitant cytokine response.

The above data suggested the existence of pathologic cytokine gene transcription in patients with CD. Although some NF-κB family members are apparently important in preventing inflammatory responses (e.g. RelB), it was found that nuclear NF-κB levels are strikingly increased in CD patients. In particular, the p65 subunit was highly activated in epithelial cells and lamina propria macrophages from patients with active CD and UC. These data are consistent with immunohistochemical data indicating an increased expression of NF-κB p65 in active IBD. In addition, it was recently demonstrated that a specific p65 antisense oligonucleotide can block p65 expression and proinflammatory cytokine production by lamina propria macrophages in patients with active CD and UC. Furthermore, in a murine model of colitis, p65 antisense treatment led to an abrogation of chronic intestinal inflammation. In spite of these data on the role of NF-κB p65 in inflammatory bowel disease, many additional questions have to be solved. In particular, there are only few data concerning the role of other inhibitors of NF-κB (IκB) family members in epithelial cells and T-cells in the gut. In addition, the expression of IκB family members and their degradation mechanisms in IBD have only been partially characterized. Interestingly, recent data showed an altered regulation of IκB degradation in native colonic epithelial cells [36–37]. In addition, adenoviral-mediated delivery of a mutant NF-κB-repressing IκB protein resulted in inhibition of IL-8 production by intestinal epithelial cells. Furthermore, pharmacological inhibition of IκB degradation strongly reduced IL-8 secretion by intestinal epithelial cells. Finally, recent evidence suggests that NF-κB is important in regulating ICAM-1 expression in the intestine [38]. Interestingly, an ICAM-1 antisense DNA approach is currently being clinically tested in patients with CD (Table 2) and it will be

Table 2. Current clinical ICAM-1 antisense trial (ISIS) in CD

1. Target: ICAM-1; placebo-controlled, randomized, double-masked study in CD
2. Patient with steroid-resistant CD and moderate activity
3. Result: remission > 40% and response rate > 50%

interesting to determine the efficacy and safety of this drug compared to anti-NF-κB p65 strategies.

Inhibition of NF-κB activity has been recently suggested as a major component of the anti-inflammatory activity of glucocorticoids that are frequently used for the treatment of chronic intestinal inflammation in humans [1–2, 39–40]. Our data provide a molecular explanation for the effect of local or systemic treatment with glucocorticoids in chronic colitis in humans (Fig. 4) [25]. Furthermore, they provide direct evidence for a predominant role of the p65 subunit of NF-κB in two murine models of chronic intestinal inflammation and our data strongly suggest that activation of p65 is essential to maintain chronic experimental colitis. Interestingly, further studies in humans showed an upregulation of p65 expression by lamina propria macrophages in patients with CD and specific downregulation of p65 in these cells strongly reduced production of IL-1, IL-6 and TNF-α. Therefore, one may speculate that local antisense therapy directed at mucosal p65 in CD could offer a novel and promising way to safely treat these patients with added specificity compared to standard immunosuppressive drugs.

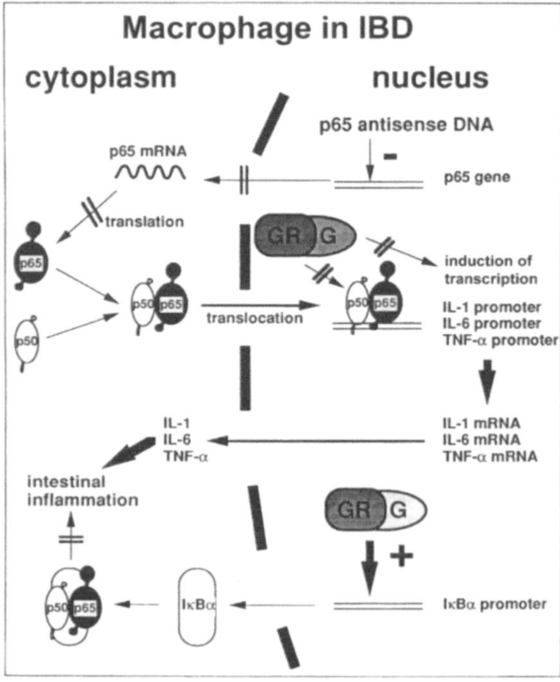

Fig. 4. Macrophage in inflammatory bowl diseases (*IBD*). *IL*, interleukin; *TNF-α*, tumor necrosis factor α; *G*, glucocorticoids, *GR*, glucocorticoid receptor, *IκBa*, inhibitor of NF-κBα

Adenoviral Expression Systems

Adenoviral Vectors

Adenoviral vectors have been widely used as vehicles for gene therapy in mice [41–42]. They are stable vectors that infect a broad range of cell types and are not cell-cycle limited. The length of the insert is usually limited to 8 kb of foreign DNA. One disadvantage of adenoviral systems is that most adenovirally-transduced genes are silenced after only 1–2 weeks in vivo. Furthermore, a failure of systemically administered vectors to be expressed in most extravascular tissues has been described. Interestingly, recent studies have shown prolonged expression of adenovirally-transduced genes in the gut of immunocompromised mice. This method may thus allow long-term expression of adenovirally-transduced genes in the gut [43].

Adenoviruses in Inflammatory Bowel Disease

The use of adenoviruses to express genes in the inflamed intestine has recently been explored. These studies have shown that IL-4 expression by adenoviral vectors strongly suppresses experimental colitis in rats. With regard to NF-κB, recent studies have analyzed the potential of a NF-κB-repressing IκB protein to specifically prevent NF-κB activation in the gut. For instance, Jobin and coworkers [36–37] showed activation of NF-κB in epithelial cells in response to IL-1 and an altered regulation of IκBα degradation in native colonic epithelial cells. Such enhanced resistance of epithelial cells to IκBα proteolysis suggested a potentially increased responsiveness to therapeutic blockade. Indeed, adenovirally-mediated delivery of a mutant NF-κB-repressing IκBα protein resulted in inhibition of IL-8 production by intestinal epithelial cells. These data suggest the potential of adenovirally-expressed IκB protein to inhibit intestinal inflammation and further studies are necessary to confirm this hypothesis.

Acknowledgements. The research of M. F. N. was supported by grants from the Innovationsstiftung Rheinland-Pfalz and the Gerhard Hess program of the DFG (Ne490/3-1).

References

1. Podolsky DK (1991) Inflammatory bowel disease. New Engl J Med 325:928–938
2. Strober W, Neurath MF (1995) Immunological diseases of the gastrointestinal tract. In: Rich RR (ed) Clinical Immunology, Chapter 94. Mosby, St. Louis, pp 1401–1428
3. Strober W, Kelsall BL, Fuss I, Marth T, Ludviksson B, Ehrhardt R, Neurath MF (1997) Reciprocal IFN-γ and TGF-β responses regulate the occurrence of mucosal inflammation. Immunol Today 18:61–64
4. Strober W, Fuss I, Kelsall B, Marth T, Ehrhardt R, Ludviksson B, Neurath MF (1996) Mucosal immune regulation and dysregulation: The pathogenesis of inflammatory bowel disease. In: Sleisenger (ed) Gastrointestinal Disease. Update 4. Saunders Corp, pp 1–10
5. Sadlack B, Merz H, Schorle H, Schimpl A, Feller AC, Horvak I (1993) Ulcerative colitis-like disease in mice with a disrupted interleukin-2 gene. Cell 75:253–261
6. Kühn R, Löhler J, Rennick D, Rajewsky K, Müller W (1993) Interleukin-10-deficient mice develop chronic enterocolitis. Cell 75:263–274
7. Powrie F, Leach MW, Mauze S, Menon S, Caddle LB, Coffman RL (1994) Inhibition of Th1 responses prevents inflammatory bowel disease in scid mice reconstituted with CD45RB[hi] CD4[+] T cells. Immunity 1:553–562
8. Morrissey PJ, Charricr K, Braddy S, Liggitt D, Watson JD (1993) CD4[+] T cells that express high levels of CD45RB induce wasting disease when transferred into congenic severe combined immunodeficient mice. Disease development is prevented by cotransfer of purified CD4[+] T cells. J Exp Med 178:237–246
9. Neurath MF, Fuss I, Kelsall BL, Stüber E, Strober W (1995) Antibodies to IL-12 abrogate established experimental colitis in mice. J Exp Med 182:1281–1290
10. Neurath MF, Fuss I, Kelsall B, Presky DH, Waegell W, Strober W (1996) Experimental granulomatous colitis in mice is abrogated by induction of TGF-β-mediated oral tolerance. J Exp Med 183:2605–2616
11. Kornbluth A, Salomon P, Sachar D (1995) Crohn's disease. In: Fordtran, Sleisinger (eds) Gastrointestinal disease. Pathophysiology, diagnosis, management. W. Saunders Corp, Philadelphia, pp 1270–1304
12. Helene C, Toulme JJ (1990) Specific regulation of gene expression by antisense, sense and antigene nucleic acids. Biochim Biophys Acta 1049:99–125
13. Stein CA, Cheng Y-C (1993) Antisense oligonucleotides as therapeutic agents – is the bullet really magical? Science 261:1004–1012
14. Wagner RW, Matteucci MD, Lewis JG (1993) Antisense gene inhibition by oligonucleotides containing C-5 propyne pyrimidines. Science 260:1510–1515
15. Loke SL, Stein C, Zhang X (1988) Delivery of c-myc antisense phosphorothioate oligodeoxynucleotides to hematapoietic cells in culture by liposome fusion: specific reduction in c-myc protein expression correlates with inhibition of cell growth and DNA synthesis. Curr Top Microbiol Immunol 141:282–288
16. Venturelli D, Travali S, Calabretta B (1990) Inhibition of T-cell proliferation of a myb antisense oligomer is accompanied by selective down-regulation of DNA polymerase alpha expression. Proc Natl Acad Sci USA 87:5963–5967
17. Krieg AM (1995) CpG motifs in bacterial DNA trigger direct B cell activation. Nature 374:546–549
18. Holt JT (1995) A "senseless" immune response to DNA. Nature Med 1:407–408
19. Voltieri M, Venturelli D, Care A (1991) Antisense myb inhibition of purified erythroid progenitors in development and differentiation is linked to cyclin activity and expression of DNA polymerase alpha. Blood 77:1181–1190

20. Nishikura K, Murray JM (1987) Antisense RNA of proto-oncogene c-fos blocks renewed growth of quiescent 3T3 cells. Mol Cell Biol 7:639–648.
21. Heikkila R, Schwab G, Wickstrom E (1987) A c-myc antisense oligodeoxynucleotide inhibits entry into S phase but not progress from G0 to G1. Nature 328: 445–449
22. Wakatsuki Y, Neurath MF, Max EE, Strober W (1994) The B cell-specific transcription factor BSAP regulates B cell proliferation. J Exp Med 179:1099–1108
23. Helene C (1991) Rational design of sequence-specific oncogene inhibitors based on antisense and antigene oligonucleotides. Eur J Cancer 27:1466–1471
24. Wagner RW (1994) Gene inhibition using antisense oligodeoxynucleotides. Nature 372:333–335
25. Neurath MF, Pettersson S, Meyer zum Büschenfelde KH, Strober W (1996) Local administration of antisense phosphorothioate oligonucleotides to the p65 subunit of NF-κB abrogates experimental colitis in mice. Nature Med 2:998–1004
26. Neurath MF, Pettersson S (1997) Predominant role of NF-κB p65 in the pathogenesis of chronic intestinal inflammation. Immunobiol 198:91–98
27. Neurath (1997) Antisense strategies for treatment of chronic intestinal inflammation. Med Forsch 10:39–48
28. Neurath MF, Fuss I, Schürmann G, Pettersson S, Arnold K, Müller-Lobeck H, Strober W, Herfarth C, Meyer zum Büschenfelde KH (1998) Deregulation of NF-κB family members in patients with inflammatory bowel disease. Ann New York Acad Sci USA, in press.
29. Grilli M, Chiu JJ, Lenardo MJ (1993) NF-κB and Rel: participants in a multiform transcriptional regulatory system. Int Rev Cytol 143:1–11
30. Baeuerle P, Henkel T (1994) Function and activation of NF-κB in the immune system. Annu Rev Immunol 12:141–153
31. Baldwin AS (1996) The NF-κB and IκB proteins: new discoveries and insights. Annu Rev Immunol 14:649–662
32. Ryseck RP, Bull P, Takamiya M, Bours V, Siebenlist U, Dobrzanski P, Bravo R (1992) RelB, a new Rel family transcription activator that can interact with p50-NF-κB. Mol Cell Biol 12:674–683
33. Mercurio F, Didonato J, Rosette C, Karin M (1992) Molecular cloning and characterization of a novel Rel/NF-κB family member displaying structural and functional homology to NF-κB p50/p105. DNA Cell Biol 11:523–537
34. Rice NR, Ernst MK (1993) In vivo control of NF-κB activation by IκBα. EMBO J 12:4685–4695
35. Beg AA, Baldwin AS (1993) The IκB proteins: multifunctional regulators of Rel/NF-κB transcription factors. Genes Dev 7:2064–2072
36. Jobin C, Haskill S, Mayer L, Panja A, Sartor BR (1997) Evidence for altered regulation of IκBα degradation in human colonic epithelial cells. J Immunol 158: 226–234
37. Jobin C, Panja A, Iimuro Y, Brenner DA, Sartor RB (1997) Potential novel therapy for the intestine: adenoviral-mediated gene delivery of an NFκB super-repressor blocked proinflammatory gene expression in human intestinal epithelial cells. Gastroenterology 1997:A874
38. Morise Z, Brand S, Komatsu S, Russell JM, Granger DN, Grisham MB (1997) Inhibition of ICAM-1 expression and mucosal injury by a selective proteasome inhibitor in a model of NSAID-induced gastropathy: role of NFκB. Gastroenterology 1997:A775
39. Scheinman RI, Cogswell PC, Lofquist AK, Baldwin AS (1995) Role of transcriptional activation of IκBα in mediation of immunosuppression by glucocorticoids. Science 270:283–286

40. Auphan N, DiDonato JA, Rosette C, Helmberg A, Karin M (1995) Immuno suppression by glucocorticoids: inhibition of NF-κB activity through induction of IκBα synthesis. Science 270:286–290
41. Smith T, Mehaffey D, Kayda D, Saunders J, Yei S, Trapnell B, McClelland A, Kaleko M (1993) Adenovirus mediated expression of therapeutic plasma levels of human factor IX in mice. Nat Genetics 5:397–402
42. Raper SE, Wilson JM (1998) Making space for intestinal gene therapy. Gastroenterology 112:1753–1765
43. Brown GR, Thiele DL, Silva M, Beutler B (1998) Adenoviral vectors given intravenously to immunocompromised mice yield stable transduction of the colonic epithelium. Gastroenterology 112:1586–1594

Pathology of Rheumatoid Arthritis: Molecular and Inflammatory Aspects

S. Gay and R. E. Gay

Rheumatoid arthritis (RA) is a chronic systemic disorder with a progressive destruction of joints. The hallmarks of the disease include: (a) inflammation, (b) abnormal humoral and cellular immune responses, and (c) synovial hyperplasia.

Inflammation is the basis of joint pain and several systemic manifestations mediated by inflammatory cytokines such as interleukin (IL)-1 and tumor necrosis factor (TNF)α (Keyszer et al. 1994). A large number of additional inflammatory mediators, including arachidonic acid metabolites, vaso-active amines, and neuropeptides contribute further to the systemic effects of the disease. Past and current therapies have resulted in the development of "anti-rheumatic" drugs which are anti-inflammatory to relieve pain and discomfort. However, these drugs have shown only very limited success in inhibiting the progression of joint destruction. Furthermore, these agents have major adverse effects involving largely the gastrointestinal system. To explore the effect of cyclooxygenase (COX) inhibition by novel COX-2 inhibitors, as well as drugs with a dual inhibitory effect on COX and 5-lipoxygenase (5-LOX), we developed assays for the detection of COX-1 and -2 mRNA in synovial cells and tissues (Franz et al. 1997a) to study the molecular interplay between these molecules.

Abnormal cellular and humoral immune responses represent another hallmark of RA. Autoantibodies, particular rheumatoid factors (RFs), and autoantibodies against cartilage-derived matrix molecules are often present. Accumulation of T-cells, particularly those expressing $CD4^+$, $CD45Ro^+$, is detected in the synovium. Expansion of $CD4^+$ $CD28^-$ T-cells has been correlated with the clinical phenotype of RA, in particular in patients with extra-articular complications (Weyand and Goronzy, 1997). The strong association between major histocompatibility genes with RA point to an important role of T-cells. Detailed studies on the contribution of human leukocyte antigen (HLA) polymorphism elucidated the disease process by modulating the disease course, determining disease progression, and influencing the clinical pattern of the disease (Weyand and Goronzy, 1997). Recent studies in T-cell-receptor (TCR) signaling have shown a defective phosphorylation in the TCR in association with decreased intracellular concentrations of antioxidants in synovial T-cells, which may explain their inactive state (Maurice

Symposium in Immunology VIII
Eibl/Huber/Peter/Wahn (Eds.)
© Springer Verlag Berlin Heidelberg 1999

et al. 1997). The activation of B-cells is another characteristic feature of the RA synovium. For example, increased frequencies of IgG$^+$ and IgA$^+$ B-cells specific for cartilage collagen type II have been detected in synovial fluid and tissue (Rudolphi et al. 1997).

Synovial hyperplasia is characterized by large numbers of infiltrating macrophages (Burmester et al. 1997) and a proliferation of resident synovial fibroblasts with a "transformed appearance" (Fassbender 1983). However, it needs to be stressed at this point that "transformed appearance" does not imply uncontrolled proliferation. These cells appear in a state of cellular activation and represent an aggressive phenotype (Firestein 1996). They are characterized by the elevated production of proto-oncogenes, various cellular transcription factors, and adhesion molecules (Müller-Ladner et al. 1996a), but do not reveal an increased rate of proliferation (Aicher et al. 1994). The upregulation of proto-oncogenes is associated with the production of both matrixmetallo- and cysteine-proteinases (Müller-Ladner et al. 1996a). The most recent data reveal that both somatic mutations in the p53 tumor suppressor gene (Firestein et al. 1997) and the novel apoptosis-inhibiting molecule, sentrin (Franz et al. 1997b), are expressed in rheumatoid synovium. These data indicate that the expression of both molecules contributes to the transformed-appearance phenotype, as well as the prevention of Fas- and TNF receptor-mediated apoptosis, and might thereby extend the lifespan of these invasively-growing cells.

However, little is known about the etiology and initiation of the disease. The conundrum of RA has puzzled researchers for decades. What is the initial step in pathogenesis? The association of certain major histocompatibility complex (MHC) class II molecules, in particular defined HLA DR B1 alleles sharing a common epitope, has been repeatedly demonstrated (Weyand and Goronzy, 1997). Since MHC class II molecules are known to function in the restricted presentation of peptides to CD4$^+$ T-cells, in the shaping of the CD4$^+$ TCR- repertoire, as well as the presentation of superantigens to CD4$^+$ T-cells, T-cells play an important role in the pathogenesis of RA. On the other hand, Firestein and Zvaifler (1990) have challenged the importance of T-cells in RA based on the observation that only negligible amounts of T-cell-specific cytokines, such as IL-2, IL-3, IL–4, interferon (INF)γ and TNFβ, can be detected in RA joints. However, it is well established that both T- and B-cell responses against autoantigens, such as collagen type II, take place (Rudolphi et al. 1997). Since new studies related to the evaluation of early synovitis are just emerging, the future may hold the answer to the question: What comes first? One major impediment to uncovering the early features and sequence of events in the etiopathogenesis of RA has been the lack of an appropriate animal model. Earlier studies in animals developing spontaneously joint destruction (O'Sullivan et al. 1995), in particular the MRL-lpr/lpr mouse, have guided studies on the molecular and cellular pathways of rheumatoid joint destruction and resulted in the concept that two cellular mechanisms may explain joint destruction (Gay et al. 1993). There is now clear evidence that both *T-cell-independent* as well as *T-cell-dependent* pathways lead to joint destruction.

The recent finding that synovial fibroblasts derived from patients with RA maintain their aggressive behavior in the absence of human T-cells and macrophages in the severe combined immunodeficiency (SCID) mouse model (Müller-Ladner et al. 1996b), strongly support the role of T-cell-independent pathways. However, these data do not discount the contribution of macrophages and T-cells to joint destruction. The production of cytokines and matrix-degrading enzymes by macrophages (Burmester et al. 1997) undoubtedly contributes significantly to the destruction of cartilage and bone. Taken together, these data set important targets for new therapeutic strategies in the development of inhibitors of synovial hyperplasia by inducing apoptosis, inhibitors of synovial attachment to cartilage, and matrix-degrading enzymes delivered by novel approaches, including gene transfer (Hummel et al. 1997).

The SCID mouse model did not only serve us as a useful model to study the molecular and cellular mechanisms of rheumatoid joint destruction, but also to explore the feasibility of new approaches to therapy.

We follow three strategies:
1. *The transfer of protective genes regulating the effect of cytokines.* These studies were performed in collaboration with C. Evans and P. Robbins from the University of Pittsburgh, Pennsylvania. To investigate the effect of gene transfer using a gene encoding the naturally occurring inhibitor of IL-1, IL-1 receptor antagonist (IL-1Ra)-transduced synovial fibroblasts from patients with RA were co-implanted with normal human cartilage in SCID mice (Müller-Ladner et al. 1997). The transduced fibroblasts continued to secrete IL-1Ra for 60 days. Cartilage that had been co-implanted with the *Lac*-Z marker gene exhibited progressive chondrocyte-and fibroblast-mediated invasive cartilage destruction. Most remarkably, no pericullar chondrocyte-mediated degradation was observed in cartilage that had been co-implanted with RA synovial fibroblasts transduced with IL-1Ra. However, neither the delivery of IL-1Ra nor the subsequent transfer of TNFα Rp55 resulted in a significant inhibition of the fibroblast-mediated cartilage invasion. In contrast, more than 50% of the MFG-human-IL-10 retrovirus-transfected RA fibroblasts incorporated the retrovirus-delivered gene sequences and resulted in a significant reduction of synovial invasion (Müller-Ladner et al. 1996c). Since IL-10 is thought to inhibit several proinflammatory and proliferative pathways (Geng et al. 1994), our results support the concept that overexpression of IL-10 in the joint might be a successful approach to inhibit cartilage destruction in RA. The results

of the first human clinical trial to assess the safety, feasibility, and efficacy of transferring a potentially anti-arthritic cytokine gene to human joints with RA are forthcoming (Evans et al. 1996) and the tissues examined in our laboratory.

2. *The transfer of ribozymes cleaving the mRNA of matrix-degrading enzymes* collagenase (MMP-1) and cathepsins B and L, is explored with W. Zacharias from the University of Alabama, Birmingham.

3. *The transfer of genes inhibiting signaling mechanisms of the Ras-Raf-MAPK (mitogen-activated protein kinase) cascade* in the activation of synovial fibroblasts. These studies are carried out in cooperation with M. Nawrath in K. Mölling's Institute for Virology at the University of Hospital of Zürich (Hummel et al. 1997). First results from these studies show that a distinct in vitro expression of a c-Raf mutant protein could be achieved by retroviral gene transfer of a c-Raf-negative mutant into RA synovial fibroblasts. However, this transfer did not sufficiently inhibit synovial fibroblasts in patients with RA from invading normal human cartilage in the SCID mouse model. These data suggest that Raf-independent pathways, e.g., the Src-Myc pathway, are participating in the activation of synovial fibroblasts in RA.

Future studies on both the T-cell-dependent, as well as the T-cell-independent pathways operating in the pathogenesis of RA are designed to determine the sequence of events to better target the molecular and cellular events taking place in the destruction of joints in RA.

References

Aicher WK, Heer AH, Trabandt A, Bridges SL Jr, Schroeder HW Jr, Stransky G, Gay RE, Eibel H, Peter HH, Siebenlist U, Koopman WJ, Gay S (1994) Overexpression of zinc-finger transcription factor Z-225/Egr-1 in synoviocytes from rheumatoid arthritis patients. J Immunol 152:5940–5948

Burmester GR, Stuhlmüller B, Keyszer GM, Kinne RW (1997) Mononuclear phagocytes and rheumatoid synovitis: Mastermind or workhorse in arthritis? Arthritis Rheum 40:5–18

Evans CH, Robbins PD, Ghivizzani SC, Herndon JH, Kang R, Bahnson AB, Barranger JA, Elders EM, Gay S, Tomaino MM, Wasco MC, Watkins SC, Whiteside TL (1996) Clinical Protocol: Clinical trial to assess the safety, feasibility and efficacy of transferring a potentially anti-arthritic cytokine gene to human joints with rheumatoid arthritis. Human Gene Therapy 7:1261–1280

Fassbender HG (1983) Histomorphologic basis of articular cartilage destruction in rheumatoid arthritis. Coll Rel Res 3:141–156

Firestein GS (1996) Invasive fibroblast-like synoviocytes in rheumatoid arthritis. Passive responders or transformed aggressors? Arthritis Rheum 39:1781–1790

Firestein GS, Echeverri F, Yeo M, Zvaifler NJ, Green DR (1997) Somatic mutations in the p53 tumor suppressor gene in rheumatoid arthritis synovium. Proc Natl Acad Sci USA 94:10895–10900

Firstein GS, Zvaifler NJ (1990) How important are T cells in chronic rheumatic synovitis? Arthritis Rheum 33:768–773

Franz JK, Hummel KM, Aicher WK, Müller-Ladner U, Gay RE, Gay S (1997a) Sentrin – a novel anti-apoptosis molecule is strongly expressed in synovium of patients with rheumatoid arthritis (RA). Arthritis Rheum 40:S116

Franz JK, Hummel KM, Aicher WK, Petrow PK, Müller-Ladner U, Gay RE, Gay S (1997b) In situ detection and quantification of cyclooxygenase (COX)1 and 2 mRNA in rheumatoid arthritis (RA) and osteoarthritis (OA) synovium. Arthritis Rheum 40:S249

Gay S, Gay RE, Koopman WJ (1993) Molecular and cellular mechanisms of joint destruction in rheumatoid arthritis: two cellular mechanisms explain joint destruction? Ann Rheum Dis 52:S37–39

Geng Y, Gulbins E, Altman A, Lotz M (1994) Monocyte deactivation by interleukin 10 via inhibition of tyrosine kinase activity and the Ras signaling pathway. Proc Natl Acad Sci USA 91:8602–8606

Hummel KM, Gay RE, Gay S (1996) Novel strategies for the therapy of rheumatoid arthritis. Brit J Rheum 36:265–267

Hummel KM, Petrow PK, Nawrath M, Müller-Ladner U, Neidhart M, Pavlovic J, Gay RE, Mölling K, Gay S (1997) Retroviral gene transfer of a c-raf dominant negative mutant does not inhibit synovial fibroblasts (SF) from patients with rheumatoid arthritis (RA) to invade normal human cartilage in the SCID mouse model. Arthritis Rheum 40:S120

Keyszer GM, Heer AH, Gay S (1994) Cytokines and oncogenes in cellular interactions of rheumatoid arthritis. Stem Cells 12:75–86

Maurice MM, Nakamura H, von der Voort EAM, van Vliet AI, Staal FJT, Tak PP, Breedveld FC, Verwij CL (1997) Evidence of the role of an altered redox state in hyporesponsiveness of synovial T cells in rheumatoid arthritis. J Immunol 158:1458–1465

Müller-Ladner U, Gay RE, Gay S (1996a) Structure and function of synoviocytes. In: Koopman WJ (ed) Arthritis and Allied Conditions. A Textbook of Rheumatology. Williams and Wilkins, pp 243–253

Müller-Ladner U, Kriegsmann J, Franklin BN, Matsumoto S, Geiler T, Gay RE, Gay S (1996b) Synovial fibroblasts of patients with rheumatoid arthritis attach to and invade normal human cartilage when engrafted into SCID mice. Am J Path 49:1607–1615

Müller-Ladner U, Franklin BN, Roberts CR, Robbins PD, Gay RE, Evans CH, Gay S (1996c) Gene transfer of interleukin 10 into human synovial fibroblasts and implantation into SCID mouse. Arthritis Rheum 39:S160

Müller-Ladner U, Roberts CR, Franklin BN, Gay RE, Robbins PD, Evans CH, Gay S (1997) Human IL-1RA gene transfer into human synovial fibroblasts is chondroprotective. J Immun 158:3492–3498

O'Sullivan FX, Gay RE, Gay S (1995) Spontaneous arthritis models. In: Henderson B, Edwards JCW, Pettipher ER (eds) Mechanisms and Models in Rheumatoid Arthritis. Academic Press, London, pp 471–483

Rudolphi U, Rezepka R, Kaufmann SH, von der Mark K, Peter HH, Melchers I (1997) The B cell repertoire of patients with rheumatoid arthritis. II. Increased frequencies of IgG[+] and IgA[+] B cells specific for mycobacterial heat-shock protein 60 or human type II collagen in synovial fluid and tissue. Arthritis Rheum 40:1408–1419

Weyand CM, Goronzy JJ (1997) Pathogenesis of rheumatoid arthritis. Med Clin North Am 81:29–55

Subject Index

actin   83
adenoviral vectors   194
adjuvant arthritis   177
ADP-ribosylation   79
AGM (aorta, genital ridge, mesonephros)   141
allergens   163
alternative splicing   137
aminoethyl-ITU   71
aminoguanidine   70
ANCA   172
annexin II   50
antagonistic analogue   105
antagonistic effect   107
antibiotics   94
anti-GM1 autoantibody   174
anti-idiotypic antibodies   175
antisense DNA   186
arachidonic acid   15, 23, 100
atopy   159
autoallergenic immune response   166
autoantibodies   171
autoimmune
- cytopenias   172
- encephalomyelitis   177
autoimmunitiy   3 pp.

baboons   69
bacterial
- cell wall   90
- pathogens   129
- protein toxins   123
- sepsis   89
bactericidal/permeability increasing protein (BPI)   100
birdshot retinochoriodopathy   179
bone resorption   50
bronchial asthma   179

546C88   69
C3 convertase   51
cardiac index   74
cardiotrophin-1 (CT-1)   135

cathepsin S   164
cathepsin K   50
CD4   171
CD4$^+$ TCR-repertoire   200
CD8   171
CD14   101
CD23   161
cell activation   101, 103
cellular responsiveness   149
chemokines   178
ciliary neurotrophic factor (CNTF)   135
circulatory failure   71, 72
collagenous capsule   49
complement   3 pp., 174
- activation   128
- C5   54
- depletion   55
- factor B   55
- factor H   54
- system   51
concomitant immunity   45
cord blood cell   142
CpG motifs   187
cPLA$_2$ 22
Crohn's disease   185
cross reactivity   108
cross-talk   22
CT-1   135
cyclooxygenase (COX)   199
cyst   44
cytokines   31, 47, 80, 90, 100, 176, 185
cytoskeleton   127
cytosolic PLA$_2$ 15, 22

dendritic cells (DC)   159
3-deoxy-D-manno-oct-2-ulosonic acid   94
dermatomyositis   172
designer cytokine   145
differentiation-inhibiting activity   150
diffusion chamber   45
diseases (see syndromes)
down regulatory control proteins   53
Echinococcus granulosus   43

Symposium in Immunology VIII
Eibl/Huber/Peter/Wahn (Eds.)
© Springer Verlag Berlin Heidelberg 1999

elastase 126
endothelial cells 179
endotoxic conformation 98
endotoxins 89, 128
eNOS 64
eosinophil 54
epitheloid cells 49
extramedullary hematopoiesis 141

F(ab')$_2$ 171
factor H 53
FADD 32
Fas antigen 32
Fcγ receptors 171
fetal liver hematopoiesis 147
Flt-3-ligand 142

gene transfer 201
germinal layer 47
giant multinucleated cells 49
glucocorticoids 193
GM-CSF 176
gp130 137
– stimulation during development 148
gp130-deficient mice 149
gram-negative bacteria 90, 94, 96
– sepsis 91, 104
granulocytes 99, 126
granulomatous-type response 49
Guillain-Barré syndrome 172

hematopoiesis 146
hematopoietic progenitor cells
– in vitro expansion of 151
– primitive 144
hemolytic uremic syndrome (HUS) 174
hepatic genes 139
hepatocellular injury 73
high affinity IgE receptor FcεRI 160
high-density lipoprotein (HDL) 102
HLA 171
HLA-A29 179
humans with septic shock 74
hydatid cyst
– fluid 48
– wall 47, 55
hydatid disease 43
1-hydroxy-2-guanidine 70
hyper-IL-6 146
hypotension 65

IκB 31
ICAM-1 179
IFN-γ 176

IgA 171
IgG subclasses 171
IgM 171
IKK-α 35
IKK-β 35
immune complexes 175
immunoglobulins 107
immunoreceptor tyrosine-based activation
    motif 161
immunotherapy 110
in vitro expansion of hematopoietic
    progenitor cells 151
inducible NOS 64
inflammation 3 pp., 15 pp., 49
inflammatory
– bowel disease 185
– lipid mediators 17
– reactions 125
– response 47
innate immunity 43
iNOS 64
– activity, selective inhibitor of 68
integrins 178
interleukin 1 20, 34
– receptor antagonist (IL-1Ra) 201
interleukin-1α 176
interleukin-1β 176
interleukin-2 176
interleukin-3 142, 176
interleukin-4 176
interleukin-5 176
interleukin-6 135, 176
– structure function analysis of 136
interleukin-10 176, 190
interleukin-11 135
intestinal
– immune system 185
– inflammation 194
intravenous immunoglobulin (IVIg) 171
invariant chains 164
IRAK 34
isothioureas (ITUs) 71
ITP 172

JNK 34

Kawasaki syndrome 173
Kdo 94
kidney 20

laminated layer 44, 47
Langerhans cells (LC) 159
L-arginine 64
leukemia inhibitory factor (LIF) 135

leukotriens   15
lipid A   92
lipopolysaccharide (see LPS)
liver injury   71
LPS (lipopolysaccharide)   24, 79, 89
– binding protein (LBP)   102
LPS-uptake   84
lung vascular injury   129
lymphocytes   185
lysophospholipids   23

macrophage mannose receptor   23
macrophages   99, 185
MAP kinase kinase kinase (MAPKKK)   35
MAPK (mitogen-activated protein kinase)
   15, 22
matrixmetallo and cysteine-proteinases
   200
MCP-1   179
M-CSF   179
membrane damage   123
mesangial cells   20
metalloproteases   137
MHC class II   164
mitogen-activated protein kinase (MAPK)
   15, 22
monocytes   99
monoclonal antibodies   107
MRL-lpr/lpr mouse   200
multicentre study   74
multiple organ dysfunction syndrome
   (MODS)   63
myasthenia gravis   172

L-N^G-(L-iminoethyl)lysine (L-NIL)   72
N^G-methyl-L-arginine (L-NMMA)   65
N^G-nitro-L-arginine methylester
   (L-NAME)   69
necrotizing vasculitis   179
neuronal differentiation   143
neutralizing agents of endotoxin   110
NF-κB   189
NIK   35
nitrate   68
nitric oxide (NO)   64, 126
– synthase (see NOS)   64
nitrite   68
NOS inhibitors   66
nuclear factor (NF)-κB   24, 31

O-antigens   92
oncosphere   43
oncostatin M (OSM)   135
organ failure   128

osteoclast differentiation   144
outer membrane   90
oxygen extraction   74

paracrine   143
parasite evasion mechanisms   46
pemphigus   179
peroxynitrite   66
Phospholipase A$_2$ (PLA$_2$)   15
– receptor mutant mice   23
phosphorothioate oligonucleotides   186
phosphorylation   22, 81
PKC (protein kinase C)   22
PLA$_2$ receptor mutant mice   23
platelet activating factor   15
polysaccharides   48
pore-forming toxins   123
prednisone   180
primitive hematopoietic progenitor cells
   144
prostaglandins   15
protease   136
protective immunitiy   46
protein tyrosine kinase   162
protein kinase C (PKC)   15, 22
proto-oncogenes   200
protoscoleces   43, 54
pseudo-chemokine effects   127
pulmonary
– edema   126
– hypertension   66

Ras-Raf-MAPK (mitogen-activated protein
   kinase) cascade   202
rBet v I   163
renal dysfunction   72
repair of membrane lesions   125
respiratory burst   127
retrovirus-transfected RA fibroblasts   201
rheumatoid
– arthritis   173, 199
– factors (RFs)   199
ribozymes   202
RIP   32
rPhl p II   163

SCID mouse model   201
secretory PLA$_2$ 16
– receptors   23
selective inhibitor of iNOS activity   68
sentrin   200
septic
– cascade   104
– shock   104

shedding   137
– metalloproteinases   127
Shiga toxin   174
signal transduction   103
SLT-1 toxin   174
soluble receptors   135
sPLA$_2$ receptors   23
stem cell factor (SCF)   142
steroids   179
streptolysin-O   124
superantigens   173
syndromes / diseases (names only)
– Crohn's disease   185
– Guillain-Barré syndrome   172
– Kawasaki syndrome   173
synergisms   128
synovial hyperplasia   199
systemic inflammatory response syndrome
    (SIRS)   63

targeted deletion   3 pp.
T-cell clones (TCCs)   164
T-cell-dependent joint destruction   201
T-cell-independent joint destruction   201
T-cell-receptor (TCR) signaling   199
T-cells   173
TGF-β   171, 176
Th1   177

Th2   177
therapeutic interventions   63
TNBS-induced colitis   190
TNF (tumor necrosis factor)   31, 32, 136
– receptors   32
TNF-α   20, 90, 101, 191
– Rp55   201
TNF-R1   32
TNF-R2   32
toxins   123
– α-toxin   124
TRADD   32
TRAF   33
TRAF2   34
TRAF6   34
transcription factor   24, 189
transforming growth factor (TGF)-β$_2$ 21
transgenic   138
transsignaling   138
tumor necrosis factor   (see TNF)

ulcerative colitis   185

vascular hyporeactivity   65
VCAM-1   179

1400 W   72

xenografting   174

Springer
and the
environment

At Springer we firmly believe that an
international science publisher has a
special obligation to the environment,
and our corporate policies consistently
reflect this conviction.
We also expect our business partners –
paper mills, printers, packaging
manufacturers, etc. – to commit
themselves to using materials and
production processes that do not harm
the environment.

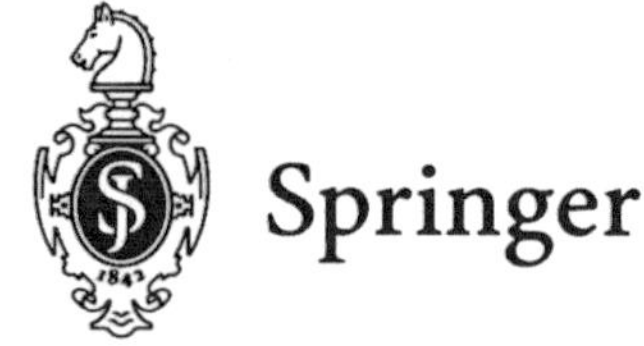

Made in the USA
Monee, IL
07 July 2026

56546129R00133